Advanced Osteopathic Technique
PPT Manipulation and Synergetic Bio-Mechanics

True science begins from a starting point that is pure and uncontaminated from others misconceptions and prejudices. Bad science sets out from a mid-point and builds on the misconceptions and prejudices that have gone before, and that which has so far failed to be demonstrated.

The science behind this book starts from the very beginning and provides a step by step set of new and practical theories on bio-mechanics and manipulation that can be demonstrated.

A

Advanced Osteopathic Technique
PPT Manipulation and Synergetic Bio-mechanics
By J.R.Bayliss

Other publications by J.R.Bayliss:

DVD: Spinal Mechanics and Bony Locking *For Health Professionals*
by John Bayliss DO and Peter O'Toole
ISBN 0-9550936-0-0

Book: The Theory of Synergetic Spinal Mechanics and PPT Manipulation
by John Bayliss
Out of print

**Book: The Theory of Synergetic Spinal Mechanics and PPT Manipulation
Edition 2**

by J.R. Bayliss
ISBN 0-9550936-2-7

Published by: John Bayliss
3, Moor Lane
Chessington
Surrey KT9 1BJ
England UK
www.spinalmechanics.com

ISBN 978-0-9550936-3-5

B

Data collected from thousands of patient record findings over a 25 year period, plus literally thousands of experiments and numerous mini research projects went into formulating the original theories and their practical application that are described and demonstrated in this book.

Osteopath John Bayliss is the originator and developer of all the 'Synergetic Bio-Mechanic' theories and 'PPT' manipulation.

Acknowledgments

I would like to thank all the people who both encouraged me and took an active role in helping me write this book:

Behind the camera:
Lindsey Gleeson
Daniel Bayliss
James Bayliss

Front Cover design: Daniel Bayliss

The models:
Lisa Hood: *L3-right-right*
Matthew Swan: *L3-left-right*
Sam Lipop: *Walking backwards*
Daniel Bayliss: *Hands*
Paul Middlecott: *PPT manipulations*
Rafaela Arce Dantas: *PPT manipulations*
Lindsey Gleeson: *Rib ergonomics/neck*
Dan Hood: *Rib cage/Shoulder joints*
Mark Gleeson: *Feet*

Sub-editing:
John Day
Daniel Bayliss

_____

About the Author

J.R.Bayliss DO is a UK Osteopath who trained with the 'College of Osteopaths Educational Trust.'
He has a background in psychology and engineering drawing and drew all of the illustrations.

C

Introduction

When I studied Osteopathy back in the eighties no one could tell us in bony terms what an Osteopathic lesion was in any meaningful way. We were given fancy quotes from famous Osteopaths about the soft tissue changes they thought took place but very little about how the joints themselves physically locked. We were taught that a lesion can be side-bent left and rotated right or rotated and side-bent right in flexion or extension etc... but that was how H Fryette described spinal articulation? None of this made any sense to me, there was clearly a vacuum of knowledge within the profession that was being glossed over and this vacuum prevailed at the time of writing this book and for many, it still does.

With the aid of a dissected plastic spine, I set out to discover for myself the answer to these questions:

- How do spinal joints articulate singularly and in liaison with other joints?

- How do the sacroiliac joints articulate in harmony with their surrounding joints?

- Why are the sacroiliac facets shaped the way they are?

- What forces create spinal articulation?

- What are the bony mechanics behind an osteopathic lesion. The actual mechanics that cause a joint to tighten to the point where it degrades the integrity of the local tissue chemistry?

- How can I make the benefits of my manipulations last longer?

- How can I make my manipulations more patient friendly?

- How do I genuinely manipulate with greater efficiency?

- How do I manipulate the neck safely?

- How do I manipulate and balance the pelvic joints for longer lasting results?

This book takes the reader through a series of simple step by step home experiments which they can do for themselves to prove the validity of my theories. It contains a myriad of photographs and illustrations to accompany the detailed explanations and reveals the mechanics behind PPT manipulation.

D

Contents

Page Index

F

G

H

Warning:
Be very, very careful if you try out the movements that cause bony subluxations, they can lock your back in an instant. (I found that out the hard way). The responsibility is yours.

K

Chapter One

An Introduction to Sacroiliac and Spinal Articulation

Introduction

Synergetic bio-mechanics is a vast subject and when reading this book the order of the topics may at first seem haphazard but this is because there are so many different aspects and parts that come together to form the whole. Be patient and you will see it all come together and work as one flowing mechanism. This level of detail and completeness has never been attempted before. Bio-mechanics tends to be a complicated and dry subject, so to make visualization and learning easier I have put in an array of coloured illustrations and photographs. It really helps to have individual bones and joints in your hands as you read through the chapters.

PPT manipulation

Originally I called my new and exciting manipulative techniques 'Passive Prone Technique'. This was because the patients would relax passively in a prone position while the techniques took place. Since then the techniques have evolved and now cover the whole body and not just the sacroiliac and spinal joints. For this reason I have changed their description to 'Passive Patient Technique'.

What is the difference between PPT's and classical manipulative techniques?

What sets PPT's apart is that these techniques remove the corrupt forces that create Osteopathic lesions (not just the underlying bony locking). When the forces that create an osteopathic lesion are reversed the local bony locking just falls away. PPT's are not gapping techniques so there is usually no audible click. Because the lesion is removed, the manipulation becomes much more of a permanent fix when the spine becomes weight bearing again.

Classical techniques are based on placing the patient in awkward uncomfortable positions to counter all the local forces and fully lock the errant joint. This is followed by wrenching the joint apart by a technique known as 'gapping'. Gapping techniques, however refined produce an audible click and run a high risk of temporally traumatizing the joint. Because the forces that created the osteopathic lesion are not fully countered there is a fairly good chance that the local bony locking will reappear very shortly after the body becomes weight bearing again.

Research on the Sacroiliac Articulation

Recent Research

Recent research using advanced Roentgen Stereophotogrammetric Analysis (RSA) imaging techniques has revealed some of the intricate movements that take place during sacroiliac facet articulation. But this complex and detailed information has not practically advanced our understanding of human movement, rather, it has added confusion. Osteopaths and Chiropractors scratch their heads when the sacroiliac articulation is mentioned and revert to old semi-dislocation theories like the 'Nutation' and 'Three pole' theories especially as an explanation for their sacroiliac manipulations.

Research results have been further complicated by other recently published research using the same RSA technology claiming that nobody has so far successfully managed to manipulate and change the position of a lesioned sacroiliac joint from its pre-manipulative position. This leaves the question open as to whether the original sacroiliac joint articulation research was imaged on lesioned joints?

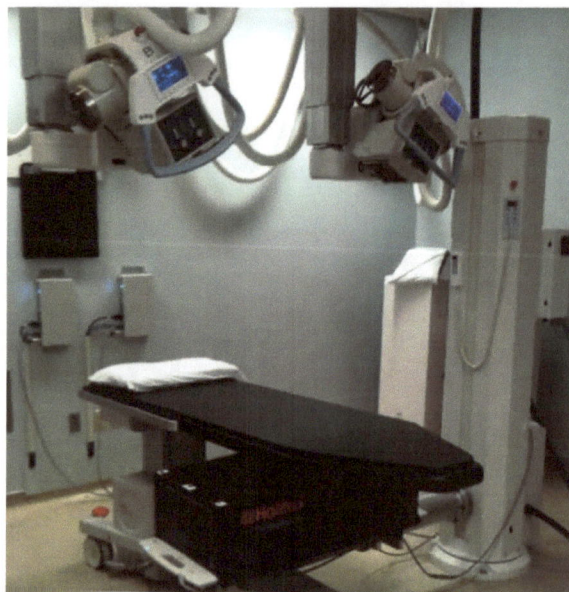

Figure 0001
RSA Imaging equipment

Being unable to correct misaligned sacroiliac joints is very bad news for manipulators who thought they were doing this routinely. I have put forward what I think could be a working solution using PPT's. Future research will tell.

Function Governs Structure

Osteopaths have a phrase '**Structure Governs Function**' and the above research was based on this philosophy, seldom is the phrase '**Function Governs Structure**' used. However, this was how I approached the subject, logically working backwards from the function we expect a joint or set of joints to be capable of achieving, to accommodate the every day movements humans take for granted.

I was able to work out an entirely new set of theories that throw new light on the published sacroiliac research. This includes how all the individual joints of the human skeleton articulate with each other harmoniously and synergetically to produce walking, rotation, side-bending and breathing.

After identifying the forces that create spinal movement I was able to work out what would happen if these same forces became corrupted. From this I was able to establish how joint subluxations occur and how they tighten to the point where local pathological tissue changes take place within the joint, originally theorized as an 'osteopathic lesion'. With this information I was able to develop a set of gentle osteopathic manipulative techniques that simply unravel the conflicting forces.

On the following page I have shown the formulae for sacroiliac and spinal movement. Bony subluxations are caused when one of these forces is misapplied. Osteopathic lesions are caused when pelvic side-shift and weight bearing are misapplied and compounded by rotation during forward or backward bending.

Formulae for Sacroiliac and Spinal Articulation

Previous thinking assumed that muscles were the sole governing force in the creation of spinal movement. However, with the new synergetic understanding of the forces that create sacroiliac and spinal articulation, we now know that this is incorrect.

The following formulae account for the way the sacroiliac joints articulate and their governing influence on lumbar and thoracic vertebral articulation.

Normal mechanism for sacroiliac articulation during walking:
- KF + LWbss + PSSss = acetabulum: anterior, superior, medial. (Leading leg forward)
- KF - LWBos + PSSos = acetabulum: posterior, inferior, lateral. (Weight bearing leg backward)

Normal sacroiliac articulation during pelvic rotation:
- KF - LWBos + PSSos = Pelvic rotation to opposite side

Normal sacroiliac articulation during pelvic side-bending:
- KF + LWbss + PSSss = Pelvic side-bending to same side

Normal mechanism for lumbar *(lumbar extension)* articulation during rotation > side-bending:
- Pelvic KF - LWBos + PSSos = Lumbar Rotation os > Lumbar Side-bending os

Normal mechanism for lumbar *(lumbar flexion)* articulation during side-bending > rotation:
- Pelvic KF + LWBss + PSSss = Lumbar Side-bending ss > Lumbar Rotation ss

Normal mechanism for thoracic *(thoracic flexion)* articulation during side-bending > rotation:
- Pelvic KF + LWBss + PSSss = Lumbar Side-bending ss > Lumbar Rotation ss

IMPORTANT:
The thoracic spine cannot physiologically rotate and side-bend in thoracic extension
Cervical articulation is driven by muscles

KEY:
- ss = same side
- LWB = leg weight bearing
- KF = knee flexion
- PSS = pelvic side-shift
- os = opposite side
- > secondary movement

3

An Introduction into the Design of the Sacroiliac Facets - Part One

Mechanics behind the design of the sacroiliac joints

The most accurate description of the sacroiliac (S/I) facets would be to describe them as a complex set of facets along an elongated contoured axes. The sacral facets do not physically slide up and down or slide round the iliac facets. Rather their multi facets make contact due to the combination of pelvic side-shift and weight distribution.

Do this self test: Pelvis

Stand up on your right leg and lift your left leg and move it forward in the same way you would when you walk (do not let your foot touch the floor just yet).

Note that your pelvis on the right side has side-shifted to the right and now takes your full body weight.

Now lean forward until your weight is taken fully on your left leg and then lift your right leg forward. Note that your pelvis has now side-shifted to the left.

The two arcs

The pelvic movement you have just confirmed is shown in **figure 0002** (Feet are shown in blue and pelvis in faded red). You can see two distinct tracking radii on either side. The 'X' and 'Y' arcs. Arc 'Y' has a tighter radius than arc 'X'. This tells us that the sacroiliac facets would need two different articulatory contoured surfaces in order to account for this difference.

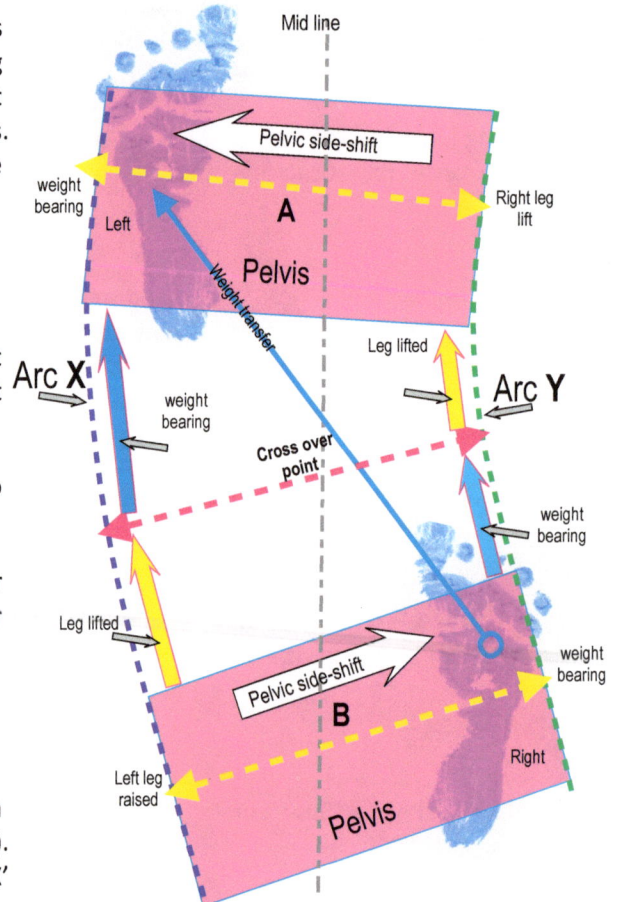

Figure 0002 Showing a theoretical S/I facet tracking arc during walking. Arcs are created by movement forward and pelvic side-shift.

Notice that there are three crossover points shown in **figure 0002.** These points illustrate where weight and side-shift cross over from each other. One point is within each pelvis (shown by yellow dotted arrows) and one midway between(shown as a red dotted arrow). If we remove one pelvis to simplify, there are two crossover points:

1) One within the pelvis. (Full weight bearing with side-shift on one side)

2) One midway between a leg stride. (Equal weight distribution in the mid-line. See next page)

The sacroiliac facets have to account for these two factors. It is logical to assume that the cross over point for the facets at the pelvic crossover point would be big and sturdy because they have to take the full weight of the body on one side. In **figure 0002** this would be on the the right side of pelvis 'B'. Whereas the facets at the midway crossover point would only need be of medium size because there is an equilibrium of weight distributed through both legs at this point.

4

An Introduction into the Design of the Sacroiliac Facet - Part Two

We can deduce that the left S/I facets from the midway crossover point would become gradually bigger and more robust as weight and side-shift transfer to that side.

So we can speculate that the facets would look something like a pear on its side, see **figure 0003**.

For completeness we will do another self test to prove the existence of the mid-way facet crossover point.

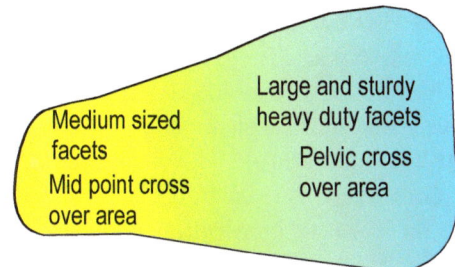

Medium sized facets

Mid point cross over area

Large and sturdy heavy duty facets

Pelvic cross over area

Figure 0003

Illustrates the theoretical shape of a sacral facet and the logical areas where cross might take place

Do this self test: Cross over point

Stand up on your right leg and lift your left leg and move it forward in the same way you would when you walk. When your left foot touches the floor you will find a point where your weight is divided equally through both legs. Note, at this point the pelvic side-shift is in the midline.

With all this information we are able to conclude that the medium sized facets somehow account for the midway crossover points. (Remember S/I facets are located on either side).

The pear shape shown in **figure 003** vaguely resembles a typical S/I facet and confirms the design of a weight bearing end and a medium weight bearing end.

Next we need to look at how the S/I joints account for the differences in the radial arcs.

Figure 0004 is a photograph of the left sacral facet

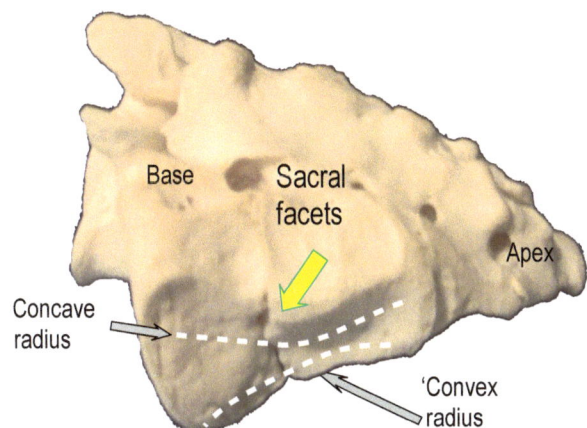

Base   Sacral facets

Apex

Concave radius

'Convex radius

Figure 0004

is a a side-view photograph of the left sacral facet surfaces to illustrate the existence of the convex 'Y' radius the concave 'X' radius

surfaces. Two radial arcs can be found running parallel along the facet surfaces. One is convex and the other concave. We need to look at why this is.

Do this self test

Place your right foot on the floor and side-shift your pelvis to the right. Now put your left leg fully forward as if you were going to walk forward and bring it to the ground. Notice that in completing this action your foot has been guided to align itself straight ahead. To achieve this what you should have felt , contrary to **figure 0002**, was the left leg moving forward in a concave arc rather than a convex one. You are at the crossover point. Now begin to transfer your weight to your left foot and move forward until you are taking all of your weight on your right leg with pelvic side-shift to the left. Notice that in completing the second half of this stride your left leg had to move in a convex arc. Again notice that your foot has been guided to align straight ahead.

An Introduction into the Design of the Sacroiliac Facet - Part Three

Figure 0005 shows how the tracking would look in the last self test. If you refer to **figure 0004,** you can see that the facets on the inferio-anterior side of the sacrum are concave. Their most likely function therefore is of a non-weight-bearing nature. These facets guide the hip and legs. Conversely the function of the superio-posterior convex facets would be weight bearing as well as hip and leg guiders.

Recap

1) The superio-posterior S/I facets are weight-bearing and guide the hips and legs in a convex arc.

2) The inferio-anterior S/I facets are non-weight-bearing and guide the hips and legs in a concave arc.

3) At either end of the S/I facets there is a crossover point where weight bearing changes to non weight bearing.

4) The anterior area of the S/I facets have a larger more robust surface to take the full weight of the body on one leg.

5) The posterior area of the S/I facets have a medium sized surface and are designed to take the full weight of the body equally on both legs.

6) Contact between the sacral and iliac facets are made in the direction of non-weight bearing to weight bearing. This equates to an oblong rotation.

Figure 0006 shows a photograph of a sacral facet with the S/I joint factors we have deduced added. For completeness, the dividing ridge that runs horizontally along the middle of the S/I facets has also been added.

Not all S/I facets are shaped exactly the same, some have more or less convexity than others and some have more or less concavity or a mixture of both. Every human has an individual gait.

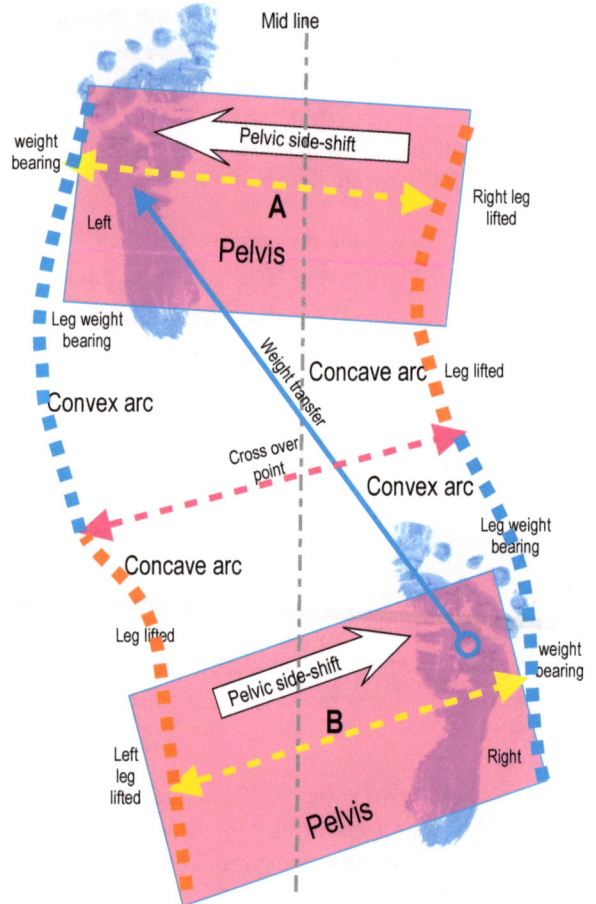

Figure 0005

Showing the true tracking arc the shape of the sacroiliac facets create during walking.

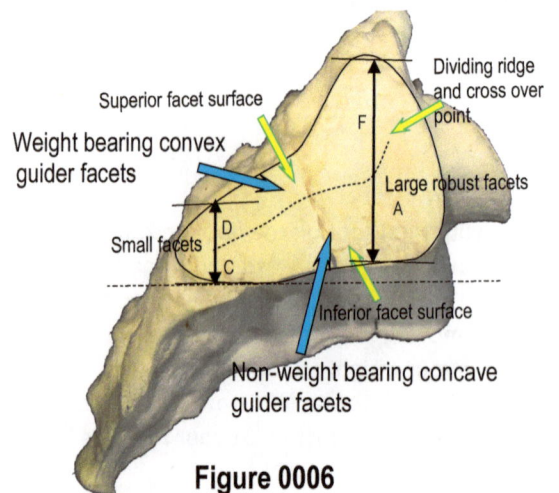

Figure 0006

Side-view of a sacral facet

The Mechanism that Drives the Sacroiliac Joints

The driving force that causes the sacroiliac joints to articulate is rarely spoken about, if ever.

The first thing you notice about the sacroiliac joint facets is that they do not fit together properly. The S/I joints are incorrectly presumed to be sliding joints, when a more apt description would be rocking contact joints.

The sacral facets are held tightly against the iliac facets by a web of very strong ligaments. The ligaments have to be strong because the sacral facets have to articulate with the iliac facets whilst keeping the weight bearing Sacrum stabilized, see **figure 0019a**.

With spinal weight bearing down and through the sacroiliac facets it would require an enormous amount energy to create enough direct force to drive any form of sacroiliac articulation.

If the sacroiliac articulations were muscle driven we would expect to see some seriously strong small muscles. **Figures 0007** and **0008** show all the sacral muscle attachments but none of these muscles would be capable of providing the direction and power needed to articulate any form of sacroiliac articulation. It can therefore be concluded that the energy needed to drive the S/I joints is coming from another source.

So we need to look for an energy source that is more powerful than the sum of the weight bearing down on the base of the sacrum and through the sacroiliac facets.

The answer to this riddle is simple. It is weight itself, or rather the distribution of weight. When body weight bears down it encounters an equal upward ground resistance known as the 'reactive force' travelling back up the legs. This meeting of opposing forces occurs at every cell in the body.

If a person stands on two legs body weight is divided by the pelvis and equally transferred through each leg. If the person transfers their body weight to one side of their pelvis the single leg on that side bears the full weight of the body.

However, it is physiologically impossible to transfer weight to one leg without side-shifting the pelvis towards the weight bearing leg. Without the side-shift the person would fall over.

If we take the pelvis as one point where body weight and ground resistance collide and equal each other out, it would take very little energy to lever the pelvis laterally under weight bearing conditions. This makes pelvic side-shift a very powerful and efficient driving force.

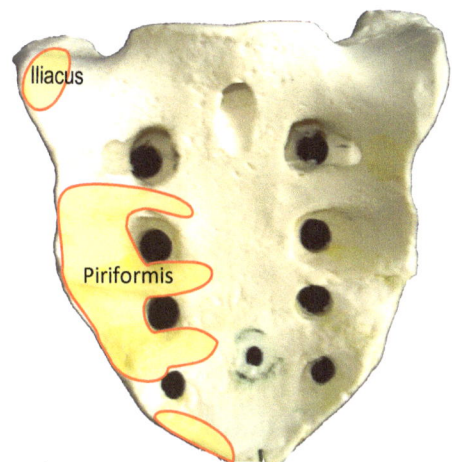

Figure 0007
Anterior view of sacral muscle attachments

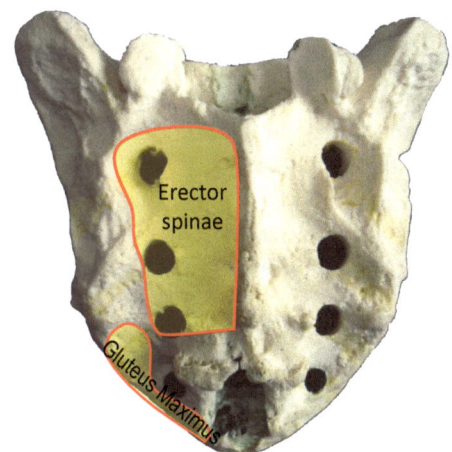

Figure 0008
Posterior view of sacral muscle attachments

Pelvic Side-Shift Blocking

The dilemma facing pelvic side-shift is not so much about the mechanism needed to push it laterally, because the energy needed would be minimal, it is about the mechanism needed to block the side-shift from going too far. It is also about returning the pelvis to the mid line.

Figure 009 is a stick view of the spine, pelvis and legs. The muscles etc are represented in blue and the gravity forces in red-yellow arrows. The muscle and gravitational forces are all equal. This keeps the body in the midline.

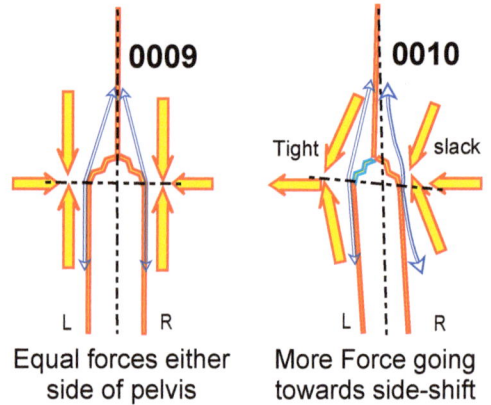

0009

Equal forces either side of pelvis

0010

Tight   slack

L   R

More Force going towards side-shift

If the pelvic muscles on the right in **figure 0010** relax and those on the left remain tight, this would generate enough muscle energy to side-shift the pelvis to the left.

See **figure 0011**. The strong quadrates lumborum muscles reside above the pelvis on either side. They originate along the iliac crests and insert along the inferior posterior border of the twelfth ribs and the posterior lateral surfaces of the transverse processes of the upper four vertebrae. The angles of the tendons would allow this powerful muscle to graduate pelvic side-shift.

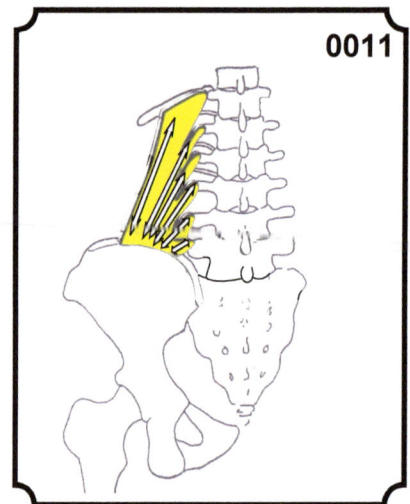

0011

Posterior view of Quadratus Lumborum Muscle

See **figure 0012**. Below the pelvis, the forces created by pelvic side-shift are greater than in the lumbar because of body-weight factors. Therefore, resistance to the pelvic side-shift requires more blocking power. This comes mainly in the form of the strong elastic Iliotibial Tract and its tension governing muscle the Tensor Fasciae Latae. The Gluteal and Piriformis muscles may also have a part to play in this process. The Iliotibial Tract is a strong fibrous sheath that acts as a strap that runs down the side of each thigh and graduates the side-shift to avoid jolts, and with the Tenser Fasciae Latae muscle, limits the amount of side-shift. The iliotibial tract originates from the Ilium and terminates at the lateral knee. It is generally considered a knee stabilizer. During side-shift it becomes stretched. This elastic stretch helps to spring the pelvis towards the midline.

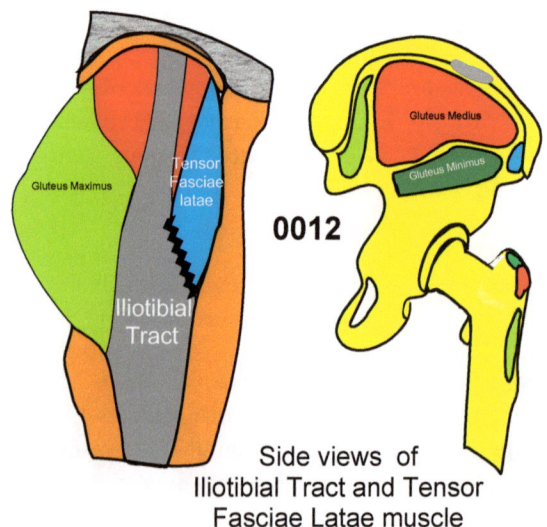

Gluteus Maximus

Tensor Fasciae latae

Iliotibial Tract

Gluteus Medius

Gluteus Minimus

0012

Side views of Iliotibial Tract and Tensor Fasciae Latae muscle

Sacroiliac Imaging Research

On the previous pages we deduced the type of axes the sacroiliac facets would need to function efficiently and the source of the huge amount of energy that would be required to generate movement. It is therefore time to take a back step and look at some of the introspective research that has been undertaken in recent years using highly accurate imaging technology and see how their results might fit in.

Wang and Dumas determined that the sacrum articulated about an orthogonal Axes. These axes are illustrated in **figure 0013**. Orthogonal in mathematical terms means two lines at right angles to each other. However, as you can see this does not apply to the **Y**, y axes.

In illustration, **figure 0013** using axes 'X' as an example, the primary axis of movement is shown by the larger red arrow X' and = superio-inferior; and the minor axis of movement by the smaller red arrow 'x' and = lateral-lateral. In summary, the forces at work cause the sacrum to move in a superio-inferior direction whilst moving marginally to the left and right.

With the use of tantalum metal markers *Sturesson et al* used highly accurate Roentgen Stereophotogrammetric Analysis (RSA) to assess sacroiliac facet articulation. Their findings suggested that 1.3 degrees of rotation took place around a 3D helical screwing axis. Of this, 90% of the movement was recorded around the **X** axis, vaguely described as 'nutation' (nodding). The 'nutation' theory was originally recorded by *Weisl*. The other 10% axes were responsible for the magnitude of rotation and their translation and were represented by the addition of the x, **Y**, Y and **Z**, z axes.

However, it was found that no two sacroiliac joints followed the exact same axes and varied from side to side. Other contemporary studies have found between 1- 2 degrees of articulation along the **X** axis, with a greater evolvement of the **Z** axis. See page 2.

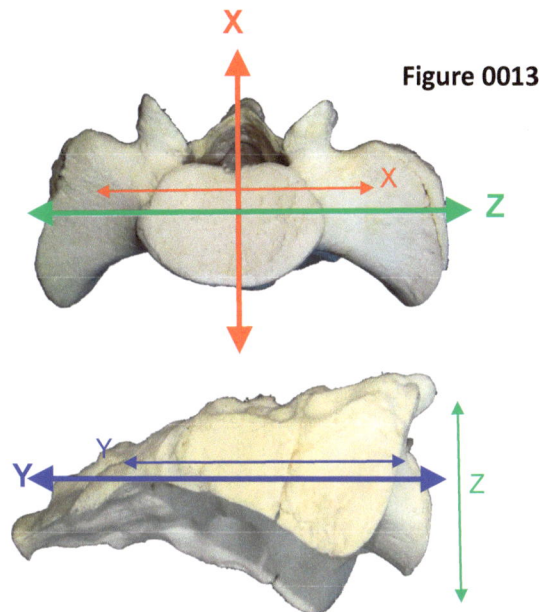

Figure 0013

Anterior and side-views of Sacrum
Wang M, Dumas GA determined the presence of XYZ Orthogonal Axes. Prime axes are shown in bolder lines and their minor axes are shown in thinner lines.

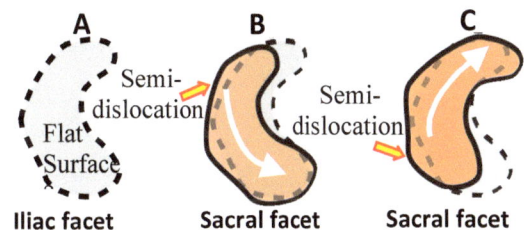

Figure 0014
Nutation theory

This research however, does not explain human pelvic movement, though for some it confirmed the validity of the semi-dislocation 'nutation' theory see **figure 0014**. The question is, how does this imaged information fit in with the type of axes we deduced on the previous pages? Also, how would the driving force created by pelvic side-shift translate into these small recorded movements?

Figure 0014 on the next page provides a summary of these movements.

The Sacroiliac Dividing Ridge

No two sacroiliac facets are identical, in some the surfaces are clearly defined and in others they are almost flat. However, they all share the consistent characteristic ridge running like a rail along the middle that divides the facet into two halves. In the iliac facet shown in **figure 0015** the ridge is well defined.

Axes **X**, x and **Z**, z in **figure 0013** are identical, though each places a different emphasis on their major and minor movements. This would indicate that there are two distinct axes in play.

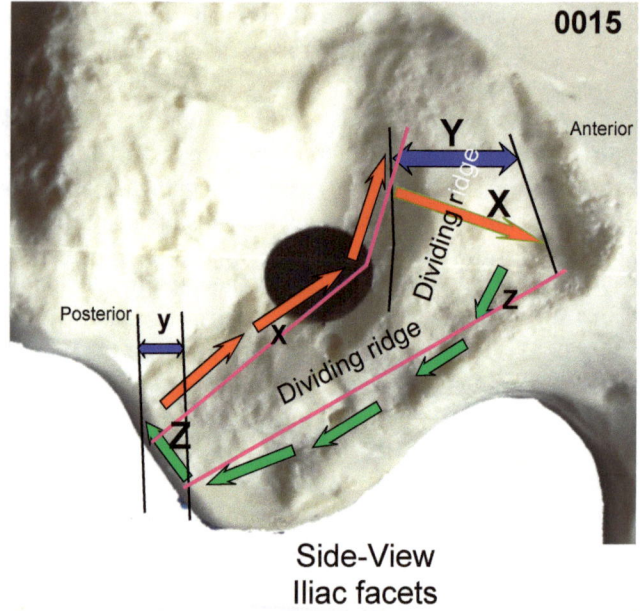

Side-View
Iliac facets

We know from **figure 004** page 5, that movement takes place along horizontal axes during ambulation. The elongated axes that the facets follow require a method of returning to their starting position without incurring a head-on collision with the facets returning the other way. The most efficient way to do this would be to divide the two facet surfaces with a middle ridge/island so that the two way traffic is separated and able to flow in opposite directions.

At the anterior and posterior ends of the sacroiliac facets the dividing ridge would have to be crossed. The most obvious way to do this without dislocating the joint would be to rock the facets over the ridge in a kind of see-saw action, see **figure 18**. If the sacrum were to slide over the perimeter edge it would semi-dislocate the joint. See **figure 0014** on the previous page.

The angle and distance at the cross over is very different at either end of the facets and accounts for several of the different axes. In **figures 0015 and 0016** the superio-inferior 'X, x' axes are illustrated by the red arrows. The minor superio-inferior 'Z, z' axes by the green arrows. The major and minor anterio-posterior 'Y, y' axes by the purple arrows. The lateral axes needs to be viewed from different angles.

Sacral Axis	Major Movement	Minor Movement
X, x	**Supero-inferior**	Lateral left-right
Y, y	Antero-posterior	Antero-posterior
Z, z	**Lateral left-right**	Supero-inferior

Figure 0016
Chart showing summary of researched sacroiliac articulation.

How Translation Occurs

Figure 0017 illustrates three different boxed views of the sacrum. **A** shows the sacrum in neutral, **B** with rotation to the left and **C** with rotation to the right. Remember, with an actual sacroiliac joint the side-view is concealed.

In illustrations **B** and **C** notice how that the sacrum moves laterally during rotation when the axis runs along the middle.

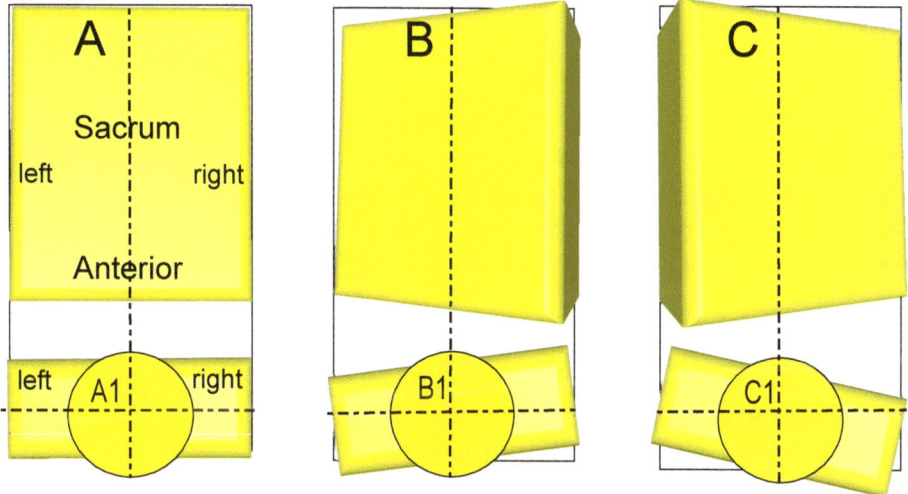

Figure 0017

Views of sacrum from above and anterior showing the sacral side-shift that would take place during rotation with middle axis

If we were able to observe the sacrum performing these axes of rotation in cross section it would be seen that the sacrum moves marginally from side to side. This would account for the **Z** and x axes. Viewed from the side this same action would account for the the superio-inferior **X** and z axes. Greater discrepancies would be seen lesioned joints.

The anterior view illustrations in **figure 0017** B1 and C1 show how the sides of the sacrum tilt along this mid-line axis. With reference to the red and green arrows illustrated in **figure 0015** on the previous page, it is not hard to envisage how these crossover points would fit in. The more angled dividing ridge is more pronounced at the anterior end than at the posterior end. This would explain the difference in the minor x lateral right-left and the **Z** major lateral right-left axes. When all these axes are added together a number of translation movements occur simultaneously and or in series depending on which part of the cycle the joint is at, at the time.

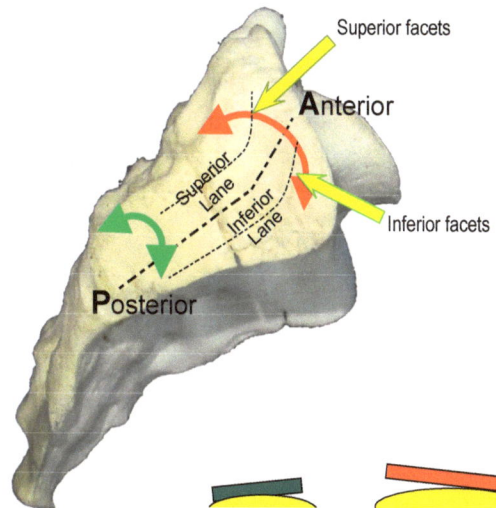

Figure 0018

Side-view of sacral facets illustrating how sacral articulation occurs in a healthy joint.

Figure 0018 illustrates the rocking mechanism that makes it possible for the facet cross over to take place. The two cross over points differ in both angle and size of movement. Together with the concave and convex facet surfaces on both sides working in opposite lanes, the working joint under microscope would appear to be constantly fluctuating with no apparent axes, especially if the facets on both sides were in lesion.

The Purpose of the Long Sacroiliac Ligaments

When the pelvic ligaments are observed it can be seen that there are two long posterior ligaments on either side of the pelvis:

The sacrotuberous ligament, see **figure 0019**, attaches and anchors to the ischial tuberosity of the Ischial bone and stretches to the lateral sides of the sacrum and coccyx and lap over the sacrum as far as the spines. There is also a part that goes from the ischial tuberosity to the PSIS.

Figure 0019a for completeness shows the short and strong posterior S/I ligaments.

The second long ligament is the sacrospinous ligament, see **figure 0020** and attaches and anchors to the ischial spine and stretches under the sacrotuberous ligament to attach to the sides of the sacrum and coccyx.

From a mechanical point of view a longer ligament would have more stretch than a shorter one.

Logically the placement of a longer ligament would indicate that there is some kind of shock-absorbing mechanism taking place in this area of the sacrum. So why at the apex of the sacrum?

To absorb the weight of the side-shifted body would require some considerable strength and rigidly. A short thick ligament would be better suited to this task. Hence the thick sacro-dorsal ligaments that lace the joint.

Cross over points

There are two cross over points, one at the anterior end and one at the posterior end of the S/I joint. These are shown as 'A and 'P' in **figure 18** on the previous page.

A) Where one leg is posterior and fully weight bearing whilst the other is lifted in the air with the foot anterior.

P) The point where the leading leg is anterior and touches the ground and then becomes load bearing with the trailing leg taking equal weight. At this cross over point without damping the leading leg contact with the ground would be jerky or even jolt.

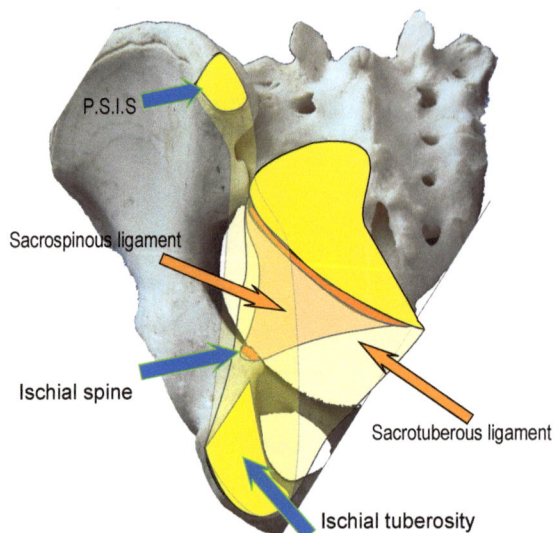

P.S.I.S

Sacrospinous ligament

Ischial spine

Sacrotuberous ligament

Ischial tuberosity

Figure 0019
Posterior view of the long sacral ligaments

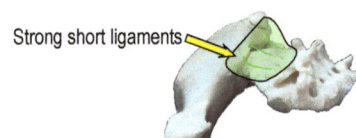

Strong short ligaments

Figure 0019a
Posterior view of the S/I posterior ligaments

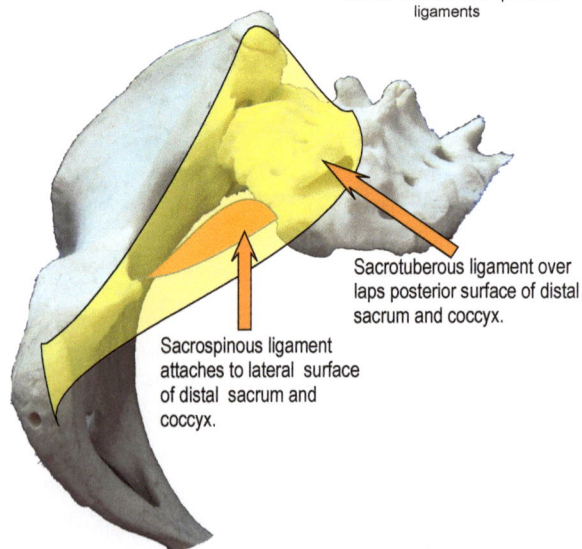

Sacrotuberous ligament over laps posterior surface of distal sacrum and coccyx.

Sacrospinous ligament attaches to lateral surface of distal sacrum and coccyx.

Figure 0020
Position of ligaments seen from underneath pelvis

12

The Mechanics Behind the Long Sacroiliac Ligaments

Recap

To arrive at **figure 0006** on page 6, it was deduced with some accuracy that the superio-posterior facets of the S/I joints are load bearing and that the inferio-anterior facets are non weight bearing.

To arrive at **figure 0015** on page 10, the role of the dividing ridge that runs horizontally along the S/I joint facet surfaces was defined. This ridge has two cross over points, one at either end where the sacral facets can rock over the iliac facets.

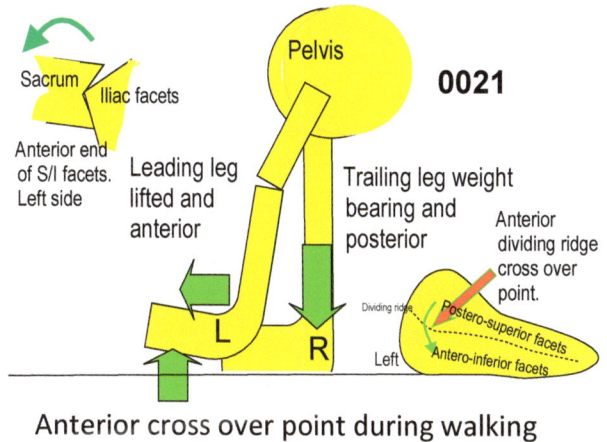

0021

Anterior cross over point during walking

Mechanics of the long sacroiliac ligaments

When the left leading leg is put forward as per **figure 0021** left S/I facet contact will have just crossed over the anterior dividing ridge to the lower anterio-inferior guider facets. At this point the side of the sacrum on the left will be angled so that contact is made with the anterio-inferior facets. The direction of facet contact in this example will be anti-clockwise.

See **figure 0022**. When the leading left foot touches the ground, the posterior cross over point will have been reached. Once the cross over point has been crossed body weight begins its transfer to the left leg. At this point the body weight is equally balanced between the leading left leg and the posterior right leg.

See **figure 0023**. To make this transition from non-weight bearing to weight-bearing as smooth as possible the long ligaments absorb the impact of the cross over and guide the anterio-inferior sacral facets onto the posterio-superior facets.

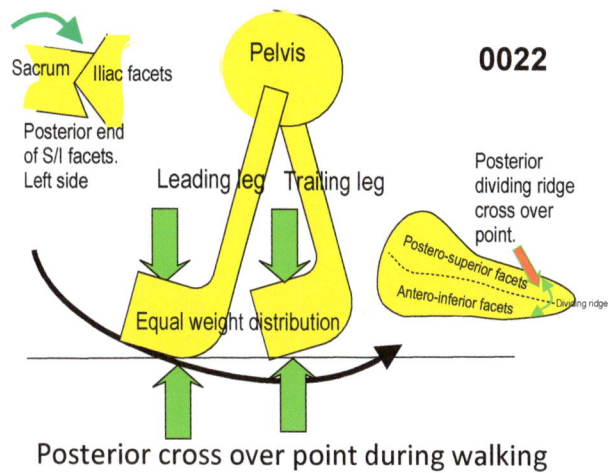

0022

Posterior cross over point during walking

Long Ligaments dampen

In more detail, attached to the left sacral apex area, the long ligaments pull and dampen the transitional rotation by pulling the left side of the sacrum towards the ischial ramus and ischial spine. See **figures 0019** and **0020**. These ligaments also help to keep a firm contact with the posterio-superior facets in this vulnerable area.

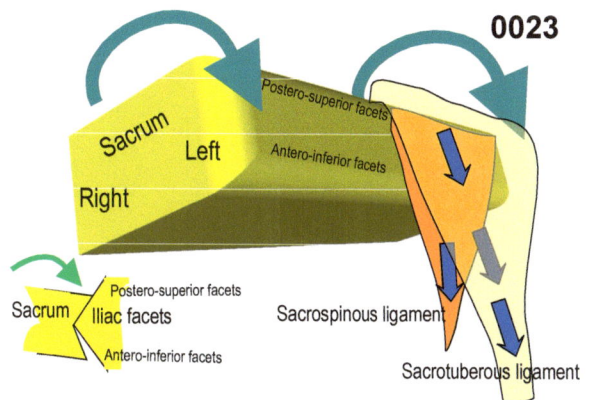

0023

The Sacroiliac superio-posterior facets are brought together by long ligaments.

13

Theoretical Load Bearing Stresses Placed on the Innominate Bones

The pelvis is a complicated bony structure and clearly it is not entirely feasible to represent the forces therein by analogy to simple structures such as beams or frames. However, if the pelvis is seen as a beam, with the acting downward force (bodyweight) vertical at mid span and reactions vertically upwards at each end (femurs acting as struts), connections being 'ball joints' let into the beam, then the forces would be as shown in **figure 0024**.

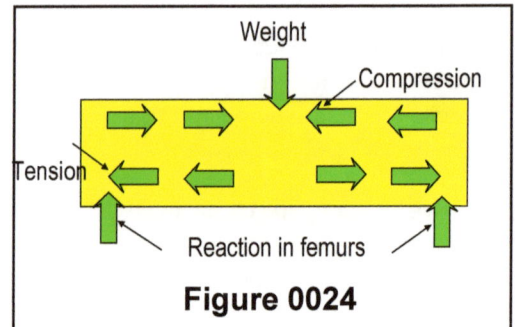
Figure 0024

There would be local forces in the ends of the beam in the form of a stress bubble as shown in **figure 0025**.

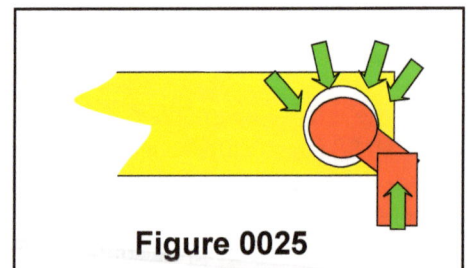
Figure 0025

If the pelvis was to be seen as a simple frame, with the same actions and reactions, there would be both tension and compression in different parts of the structure, as shown in **figure 0026**.

For a joint to remain static, all forces must balance. If, for example, mainly downward force is not vertical but can only be supported vertically (a femur in an upright position), then there must be a balancing force somewhere, a triangle of forces applies as shown in **figure 0027**.

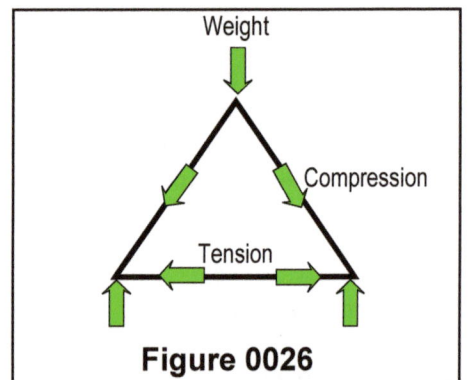
Figure 0026

And if this was to be applied to one side of the pelvis there would be tension, as shown in **figure 0028**.

It is suggested that, as the pelvis is not a simple structure, the forces would look something like those shown in **figure 0029**.

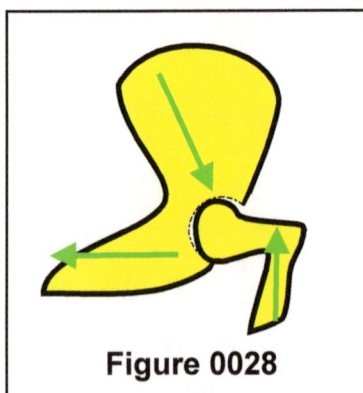
Figure 0028

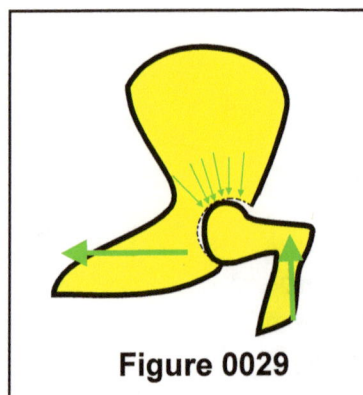
Figure 0029

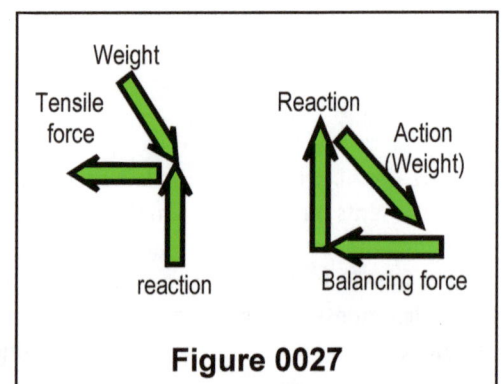
Figure 0027

Load Bearing Stresses Placed on the Sacroiliac Joints

Weight bearing forces travelling down the lumbar spine arrive at an angle when they link with the base of the sacrum. See **figure 0030**.

From **figure 0030a** it can be seen that the flexed shape of the lumbar spine acts much like a spring. It flexes when weight is bounced through it, typically when a person is walking. This softens the impact on the S/I joints.

Figure 0031 is a photograph of the underside of a sacrum. Note that the tapered sides of the sacral facets are wedge shaped and lodge against the reciprocally shaped iliac facets.

Figure 0032 illustrates the point of pivot. This very important area is where the sacral facets pivot on the iliac facets. It is the hub of the sacroiliac/iliosacral joints and the axes that allows the sacral facets to move about the iliac facets and vice-versa.

When a person is stationary and standing upright the point of pivot is where body weight passes through the iliosacral/sacroiliac joints. Such a point also allows for readiness of motion in any direction.

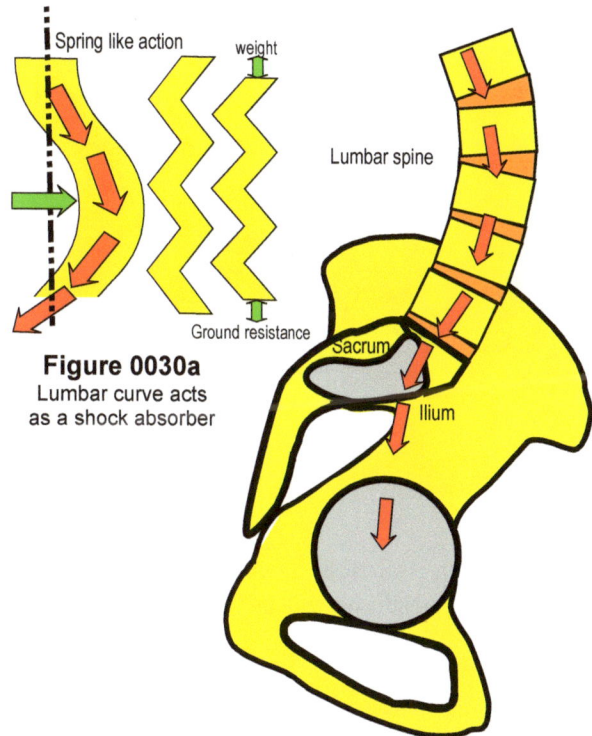

Figure 0030a
Lumbar curve acts as a shock absorber

Figure 0030
Illustrating how weight is absorbed and distributed

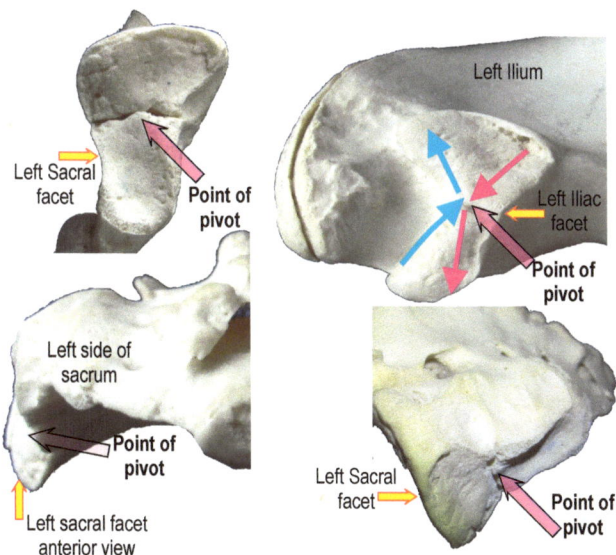

Figure 0032
Illustrates the pivot point from which all sacroiliac and iliosacral movement is able to take place

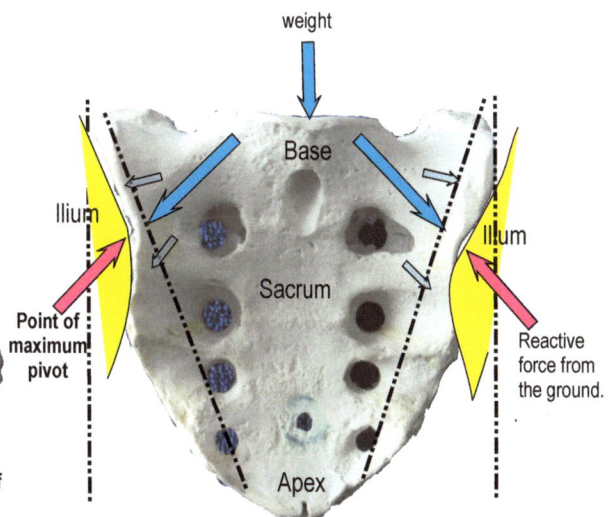

Figure 0031
Illustrates the blocking wedge shape of the sacral facets

15

Pelvic and Vertebral Side-Shift

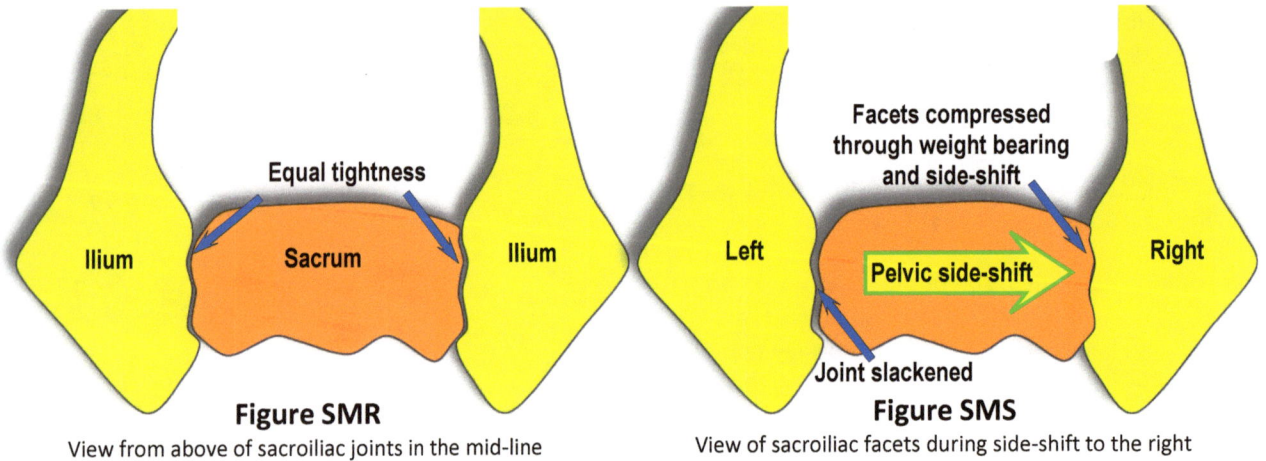

Figure SMR
View from above of sacroiliac joints in the mid-line

Figure SMS
View of sacroiliac facets during side-shift to the right

Figure SMR illustrates the sacroiliac joints from above in neutral. In this position the joints encounter an equal distribution of weight bearing and compression through both sides.

Figure SMS illustrates the sacroiliac joints when pelvic side-shift takes the weight and compression to the right. The right side of the joint becomes compressed whilst conversely, the left side of the sacroiliac joint, muscles and ligaments becomes slackened.

Vertebral side-shift

There is a distinct difference between side-bending and side-shift. Whilst this is a very obvious point, it has been illustrated in **figures SMT** and **SMU** as this is not a distinction that should be missed.

Another feature of side-shift is that the muscles to the opposite side to the side-shift which is to the left in **figure SMU**, become slackened. This can be useful to bear in mind when massaging or releasing tight and inflamed muscle groups.

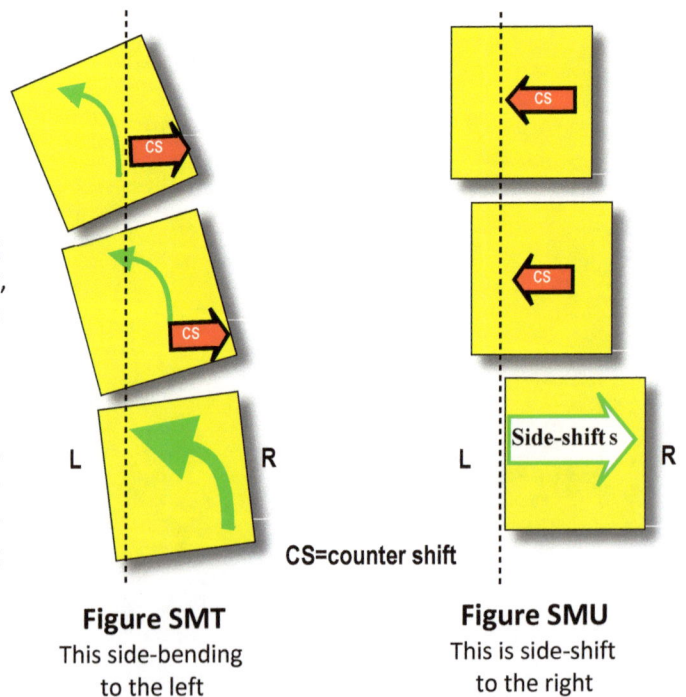

CS=counter shift

Figure SMT
This side-bending
to the left

Figure SMU
This is side-shift
to the right

Side-Shift
General Observations Continued

Figure SMV illustrates the musculo-skeletal frame positioned in the mid-line. In the mid-line the spine and pelvis are at their strongest and most resilient. Equal forces emanate from left and right and from below and above.

Figure SMW illustrates the effect on the musculo-skeleton frame when pelvic side-shift is taken to the left. In our example there is tightness on the left side of the spine and sacroiliac joints and relaxation on the right. This creates strength to the joints and tissue on the left and pliability to the joints and tissue on the right.

Figure SMWa is an illustration of a bow, (as in a bow and arrow). 'A' is the bow under normal tension. 'B' shows the bow flexed to the left. This flexion causes the top and bottom of the bow to lose height and the string to become loose. This is basic physics and applies to the musculo-skeletal frame.

Whilst caution should be exercised when treating the looser and therefore more vulnerable right side of the body, this is an asset that can be turned to huge advantage in clinical practice.

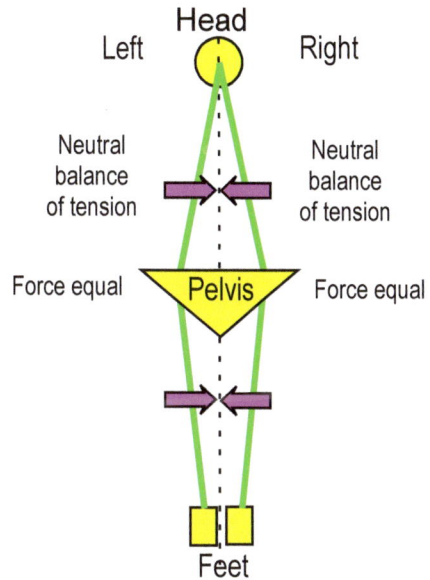

Figure SMV

This is a non weight bearing body frame with the pelvis in the mid line

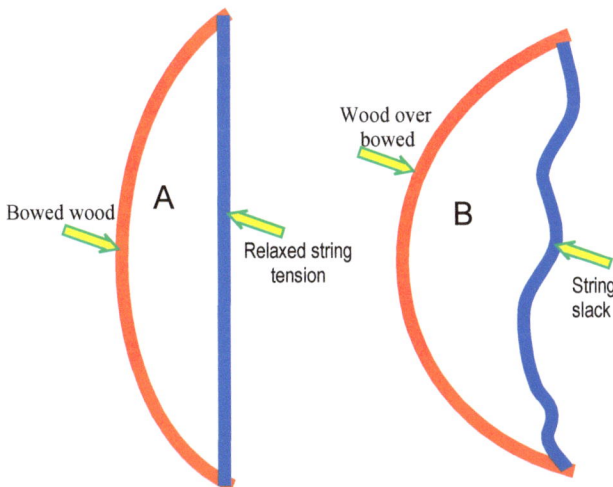

Figure SMWa

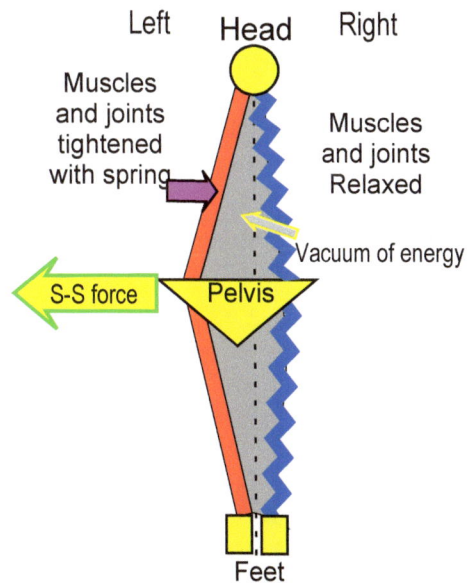

Figure SMW

This is a non weight bearing body frame with pelvic side-shift to the left

Mechanics of Spinal Articulation

Overview

The workings of the spine can be likened in many ways to the workings of a grandfather clock. As the pendulum swings from side to side, so the cog wheels above turn clockwise and anti-clockwise. And from this long lever the precise time can be produced. The beauty of a pendulum action is that it takes very little energy to create a lot of power.

The synergetic principle theorizes that human spinal articulation is driven by the pelvic pendulum action and counter balanced by muscle. When working perfectly the sacroiliac and vertebral joints articulate synchronously, with precision and with minimal energy.

Where to start

It is impossible to look at a single joint or series of joints in a certain area such as the sacroiliac, lumbar, thoracic or cervical in isolation because the body does not work like that. The body works as a complete interacting mobile unit.

I originally started by examining one of the most basic of all human movements; walking.
Walking involves many different forces, the main ones being:

- Weight bearing and weight leaning
- Leg lifting and leg direction
- The changing angles of the ilia and hip joint
- The changing angles of the knees and ankle/feet joints
- The reciprocal action of the sacroiliac joints
- The lumbar vertebrae accommodation for this action
- The thoracic vertebrae accommodation for this action
- The rib cage accommodation to ensure continued breathing and
- The action of pelvic side-shift

With so many forces to contend with, walking becomes a very complicated three dimensional movement that requires all the forces to work in harmony with each other.

Previous theories

Previous theories tended to focus on particular joints with no regard to how that joint interacted with the surrounding joints. Research is carried out this way and becomes its Achilles heel. Theories must start from a sound, demonstrable basis. I have read many books on spinal mechanics and there is not one of them where I have not had to re-read a certain paragraph repeatedly to make sense of what the author was saying. This was due to several factors, but the main one was that they were starting the explanation for their bit-part theories from a mid point. It was like coming into their version of a theory that they had surmised from a part of someone else's theory which had also been surmised from a mid point. This led to many varying theories from different factions and no one theory could be said to be better than another. What was needed was to establish a solid foundation on which future working theories could be accurately predicted and that is what I set out to discover.

Terminology

Flexion and Extension

Modern day generalizations have crept into osteopathic terminology. The two that hold back scientific progress when looking at detailed vertebral movement, are the terms applied to the individual and overall movement of forward and backward bending, flexion and extension.

To flex is to bring two ends closer together. If I arc the lumbar or cervical spines (bring the two ends together) they become in a state of flexion (backward bending). If I arc the two ends of the thoracic spine together the vertebrae become in a state of flexion (forward bending), the opposite. When looking at vertebra on a segmental level, which is what this book does, the generalization for all forward bending articulation as flexion and and all backward as extension is imprecise and unscientific and becomes a real problem when making an accurate description.

What I am saying is that if I am to describe the relative positions of L1 in relation to T12 I cannot accurately say that they are both are in a state of flexion when clearly one will be in extension.

The term subluxation

I have used the term 'subluxation' because part of the subject of this book is about simple bony locking and semi-dislocation. The 'Taber's Cyclopedic Medical Dictionary' definition of a subluxation is 'a partial or incomplete dislocation' and this is the sense it is being used in. An '**Osteopathic Lesion**' or '**Chiropractic Subluxation**' are broader terms that account for the additional forces that are brought to bear on a subluxation that tighten and lock the subluxation in place. These forces are theoretically thought to create changes to the local pathology of the surrounding nerves, blood supplies, lymph, soft tissue and muscles etc. In practice this would seem to be the case.

L3/L4 as a starting point

When describing the movement of the spine, the L4/L3 vertebral joint is probably the most illustrated articulation. In most pictures L3 is shown in lumbar extension (neutral and forward bending) in a state of rotation and side-bending. L3 is a good starting point as it is the midpoint of the five lumbar vertebrae. The law of physics determines that the design of the lumbar facets allow for four possible major movements, shown below. The major movements for L3 are:

1) **Rotation**

2) **Side-bending**

3) **Extension**

4) **Flexion**

Local side-shift is a minor movement of accommodation.

Basics of the
'G' and 'M' Forces

The mechanism behind the L3 articulation

During a typical L3 articulation two distinct forces come into play, abbreviated by: '**G**' and '**M**'

• **G:** *The overall spinal movement created by the angle and weight exerted on the pelvis followed by pelvic side-shift*

• **M:** *The local counter-force within each joint exerted by opposing muscle forces directed by balance.*

We know that the most probable force driving the sacroiliac articulation is pelvic side-shift. Nature never lets an asset as powerful as this sit idle and so logic dictates that pelvic side-shift has a dual purpose. That purpose becomes apparent when linked to balance.

To survive, humans must be able to stand upright to be at their most efficient. To accomplish this they have been provided with a sense of balance and spatial awareness. These senses emanate from the middle ears and to a lesser extent the eyes. One of the prime functions of these senses is to keep the head and body upright and vertical. It does this by directing the muscles below the head to counter the pelvic side-shift.

Do this self test

Stand upright and look in a mirror and then push your pelvis to one side. Note that your head stays in the midline to keep you balanced. What you are witnessing are the '**G** and **M**' forces at work.

When the pelvis side-shifts left as shown in **figure 0032**, the inner ears demand a powerful muscular counter force in the opposite direction to maintain an upright position and balance of the body.

The magenta box labelled '**B**' represents a typical vertebra closest to the pelvis. The force of the pelvic side-shift to the left drives the vertebra to the left. Conversely, the orange box labelled '**A**' represents a typical vertebra above and therefore closer to the cranial counter-force of balance. As can be seen, this counter-force resists and drives the vertebra to the right.

It is this meeting of two opposite forces that create a local shearing force within each vertebral joint and this is what drives vertebral articulation.

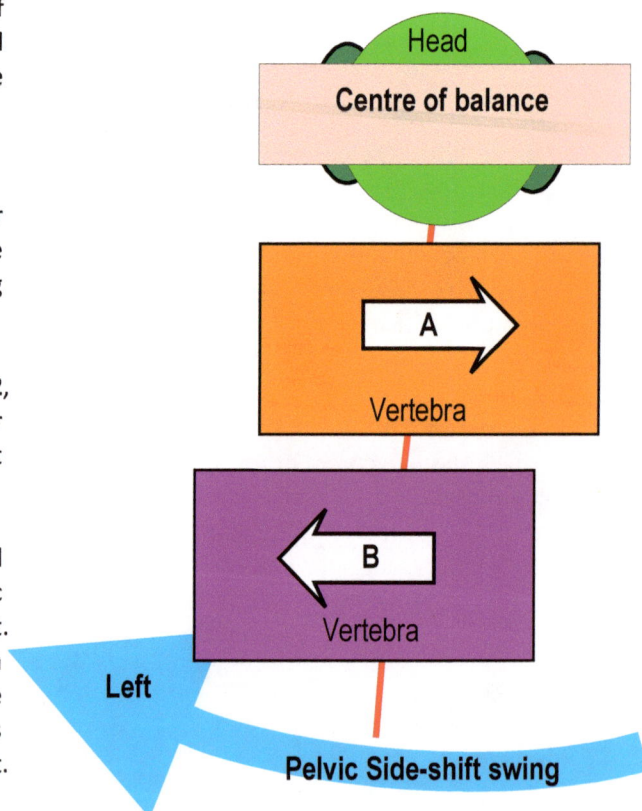

Figure 0032
is an Illustration of the gravitational pelvic 'G' force and muscle 'M' force.

Experiment to Illustrate the 'G' and 'M' Force Interaction.
Side-bending and Rotation to Opposite

Do these self experiments

In this experiment you use your clasped hands as two mock vertebra and your forearms and elbows as mock pelvis and legs. The test explains the mechanism for how the lumbar joints side-bend and rotate to opposite sides in true lumbar flexion.

Starting position to produce **side-bending and rotation to opposite sides**. (Example is side-bending left with rotation right).

Your right hand represents L4 and your left, L3.

See **figures 0033 and 0034.** Sit in front of a desk and place a book about 2 inches (5 cm) thick in front of you and to your right. Clasp your right and left hands together with your fingers tightly interlaced. Rest your right elbow on the book to give it height and your left elbow on the desk. Push your left elbow away from you a couple of inches (5 cm) to simulate left knee flexion. (You would lose height on the left side with left knee flexion; hence the book)

Look at your linked hands and notice that due to the thickness of the book, the raised right elbow has caused both hands to side-bend to the left and due to the forward placement of the elbow both hands are aligned to the right.

See **figures 0035** and **0036**. Place your weight on your left elbow and draw your right elbow side-ways towards the left to simulate pelvic side-shift to the left and observe that your hands rotate to the right and move towards your body and simulate backward leaning. This is the generalized **'G' force** that affects the spine as a whole.

Loosen your hands a little and repeat the test. This time notice how the <u>thenar</u> eminence of your right hand (L3) slides and side-bends right over the <u>thenar</u> eminence of your left hand (L4) as you side shift your right elbow toward the left. This is the **'M' force** and the local movement that takes place within the joint.

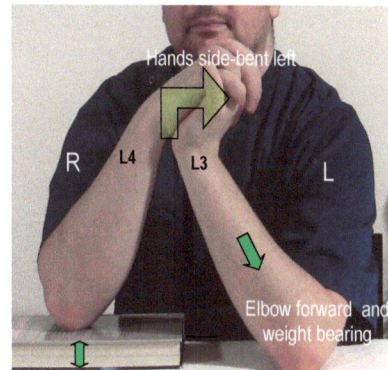

Figure 0033
Front view of stage one for lumbar flexion. Side-bending

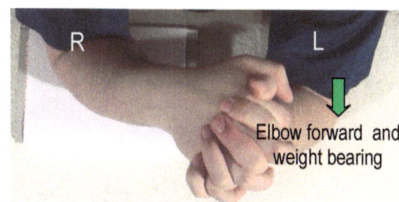

Figure 0034
View from above of stage one
for in lumbar flexion. Side-bending.

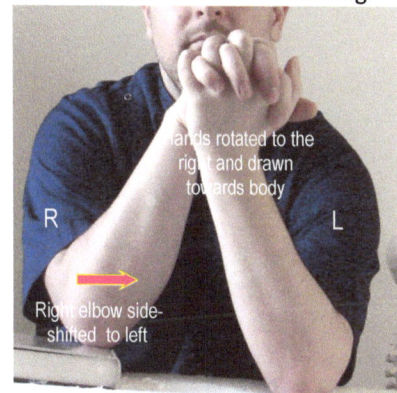

Figure 0035
Front view of stage two in lumbar flexion.

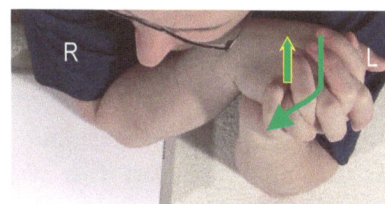

Figure 0036
View from above of stage two in lumbar flexion.

Experiment to Illustrate 'G' and 'M' Force Interaction. Rotation and Side-bending to the Same Side

This next experiment is to test **rotation and side-bending to the same side**. (Example is with rotation and side-bending to the right). Again in this experiment you use your clasped hands as two mock vertebra and your forearms and elbows as mock pelvis and legs. The test explains the mechanism for how the lumbar joints rotate and side-bend to the same side in true lumbar extension.

Your right hand represents L4 and your left, L3.

See **figures 0037** and **0038.** Sit in front of a desk and place a book about 2 inches (5 cm) thick in front of you and to your right. Clasp your right and left hands together with your fingers interlaced. Rest your right elbow on the book and place your weight on it. Push your left elbow away from you a couple of inches to simulate the left knee flexion.

With weight on your right elbow you have to lift your left elbow.

Look at your linked hands and notice that due to the thickness of the book and the forward position of your raised right elbow, both hands now rotate to the right.

See **figures 0039** and **0040**. Keep your weight on your right elbow and draw your left elbow sideways towards the right to simulate pelvic side-shift to the right. Observe that your left elbow/hand rises higher than the right to maintain balance and that both of your hands side-bend to the right. Note also that your hands have moved away from your body and simulate forward leaning. This is the generalized **'G' force** that affects the spine as a whole.

Loosen your hands and repeat the test. This time notice that the hyperthenar eminence of your left hand (L3) side-bends right over the hyperthenar eminence of your right hand (L4)as you side shift your left elbow toward the right. This is the **'M' force** and the local movement that takes place within the joint.

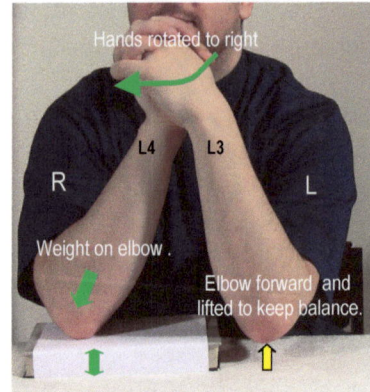

Figure 0037

Front view of stage one for lumbar extension. Rotation

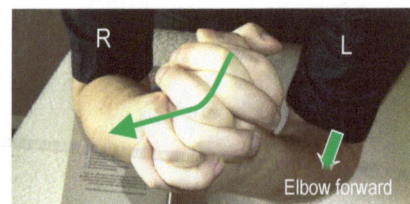

Figure 0038

View from above of stage one for lumbar extension.

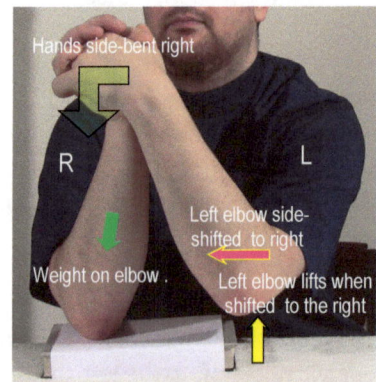

Figure 0039

Front view of stage one for lumbar extension. Side-bending

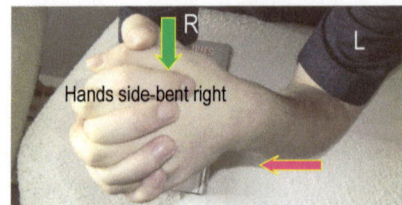

Figure 0040

View from above of stage one for in lumbar extension. Side-bending

Chapter Two

Physiology of the Sacroiliac Joints

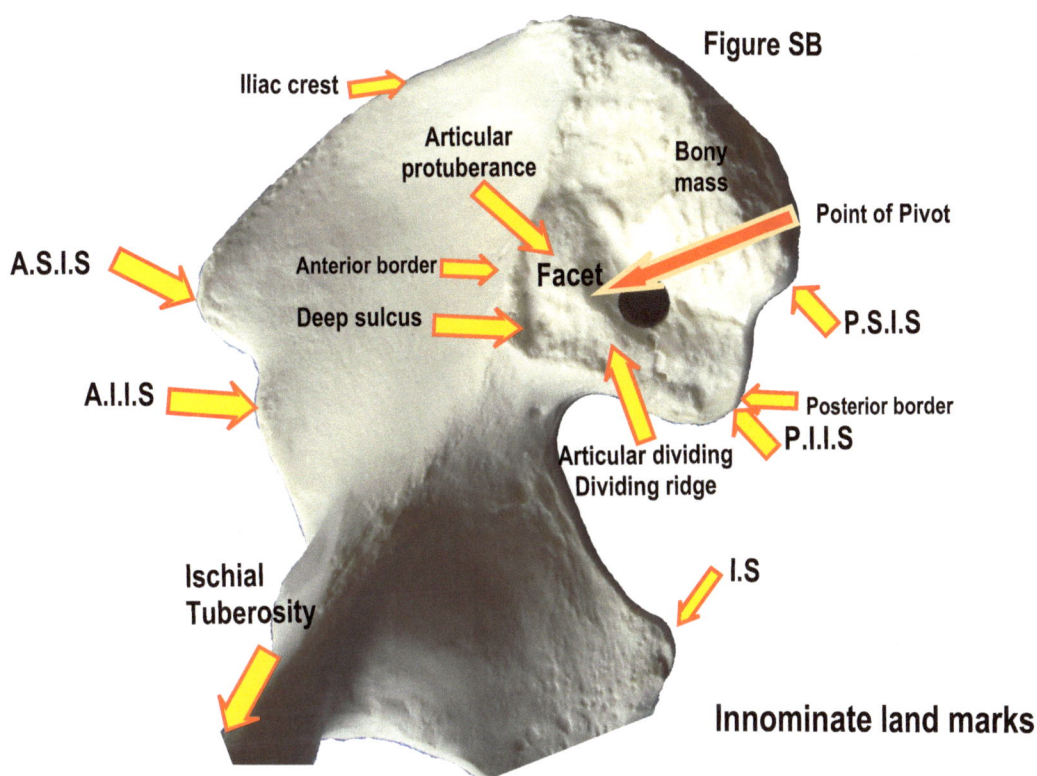

Figure SB

Iliac crest
Articular protuberance
Bony mass
Point of Pivot
A.S.I.S
Anterior border
Facet
Deep sulcus
P.S.I.S
A.I.I.S
Posterior border
P.I.I.S
Articular dividing
Dividing ridge
Ischial Tuberosity
I.S

Innominate land marks

The sacroiliac joint

There are many variations in the shapes and sizes of the sacroiliac articular facets and it is this that seems to have confounded many theorists seeking to discover their secrets in the past. However, all sacroiliac facet shapes share certain common similarities and these are explained further in this chapter. **Figure SB** shows a plastic mould of a right Ilium and details the bony architecture of its articular facet.

At the superior border of the Iliac facet there is a bony mass that would buffer excessive posterior shift of the sacrum. Dividing the Iliac facets in half is a bony ridge that runs from the anterior facets to the posterior facets. There is a deep sulcus at the anterio-inferior border on some types of facet that prohibit inferior sacral facet shift. In other types of facets the anterior ridge of the sulcus is less pronounced. A more pronounced ridge will produce a more efficient walking and running gait, whereas a flatter ridge would produce a type of mincing gait more suited to swimming and cycling.

Bayliss Sacroiliac Theory

Working sacroiliac theory overview

For a theory on the sacroiliac joints to work, it has to fill certain criteria. It has to make due allowance for the action of walking and other methods of motion, together with spinal rotation and side-bending, in both forward and backward bending.

Joints are not designed to semi-dislocate as part of their normal articulation process and the sacroiliac joint is no exception to this rule. We learned from the last chapter that the sacroiliac joints, via pelvic side-shift and side-bending act as a precursor for spinal rotation to take place. This means that the sacroiliac facets must have been designed to take these movements into account.

The theory that follows, fulfils all the above criteria.

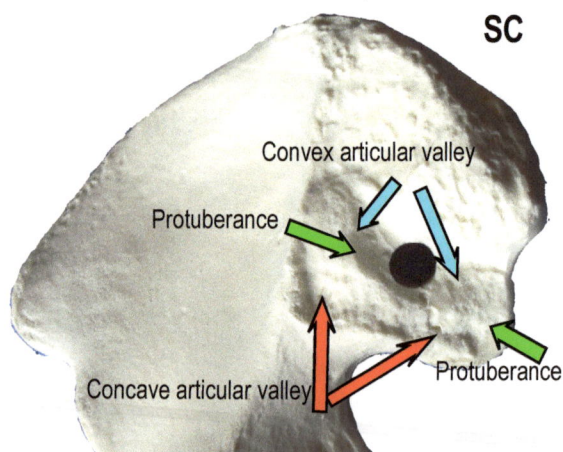

SC

Convex articular valley

Protuberance

Concave articular valley

Protuberance

The theory

Refer to **figure SC**. The iliac facets are divided by a bony ridge running along the vertico-horizontal length. This ridge divides the articular facets in half as illustrated in **figure SD**.

We established in the last chapter that the superior facet group, illustrated in **figure SD** and shown in blue can be categorized as 'load bearing' and the inferior facet group shown in magenta as 'guider facets'.

The weight bearing superior facets have a general convex shape and therefore purpose.

The guider inferior facets have a general concave shape and therefore purpose.

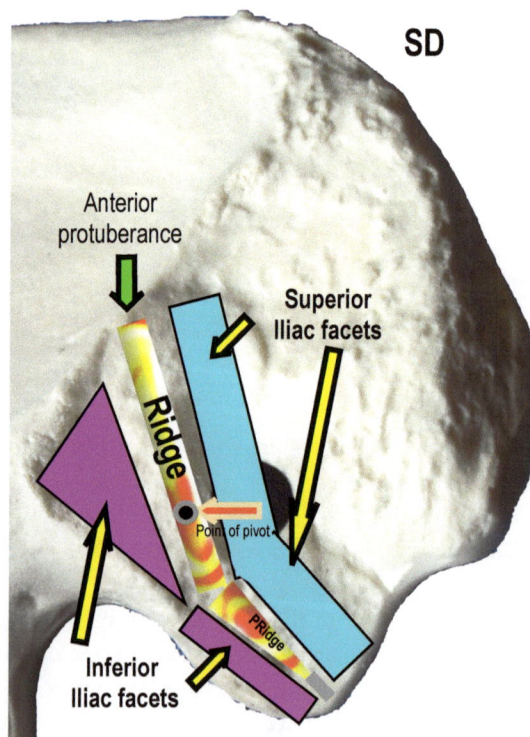

SD

Anterior protuberance

Ridge

Superior Iliac facets

Point of pivot

PRidge

Inferior Iliac facets

Summary

Superior facets are load bearing and generally convex.

Inferior facets are generally concave and guide the non- weight-bearing leg.

The point of pivot is shown for completeness.

Iliac Facet Shape

The four pictures below are exaggerated illustrations of the iliac facet surface contours

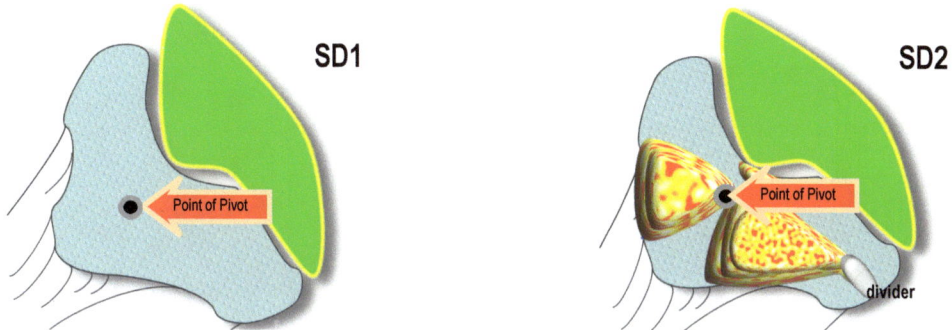

SD1

Point of Pivot

SD2

Point of Pivot

divider

Figure SD1 provides a closer look at an Iliac facet without any contours or articular surfaces added. The green colouring represents the bony mass. The bony mass acts as a buffer, should too much weight be placed on the posterior facets.

In **figure SD2** the irregular bony ridge running along the middle is shown in mottled yellow. At first sight the articular contours look like a design by committee, but nothing could be further from the truth. These contours are designed as part of a complex elongated swivel joint. The light grey contour to the far right in the illustration is a divider.

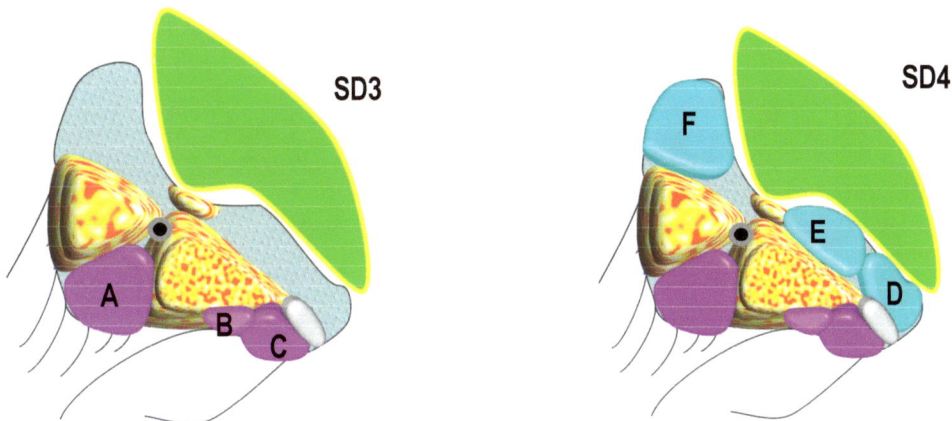

SD3

A

B

C

SD4

F

E

D

In **figure SD3** the inferior guider facets have been added. Note that they are not continuous. *Facet A* is the true anterior articular surface and is there to guide the thigh/leg forward, medially and upward in a non-weight-bearing capacity. *Facet B* has a transitory function and is there to guide the thigh/leg towards the ground. Once the foot touches the ground, *facet* C acts as a transitory weight bearing cross-over point to the transitory load bearing *facet D*, shown in **figure SD4.** At this point the weight of the body is taken equally on both feet.

As more weight is transferred to the supporting leg, the upward ground-resistance causes the transitory weight bearing *facet E* to engage. Finally when the full weight of the body is taken on the supporting vertical leg, the meeting of the ground-resistance returning up the leg causes the main load bearing *facet F* to engage. It is probable that some S/I joint facets have more articulator surfaces but the above six are the main ones.

Anatomy of the Sacral Facets

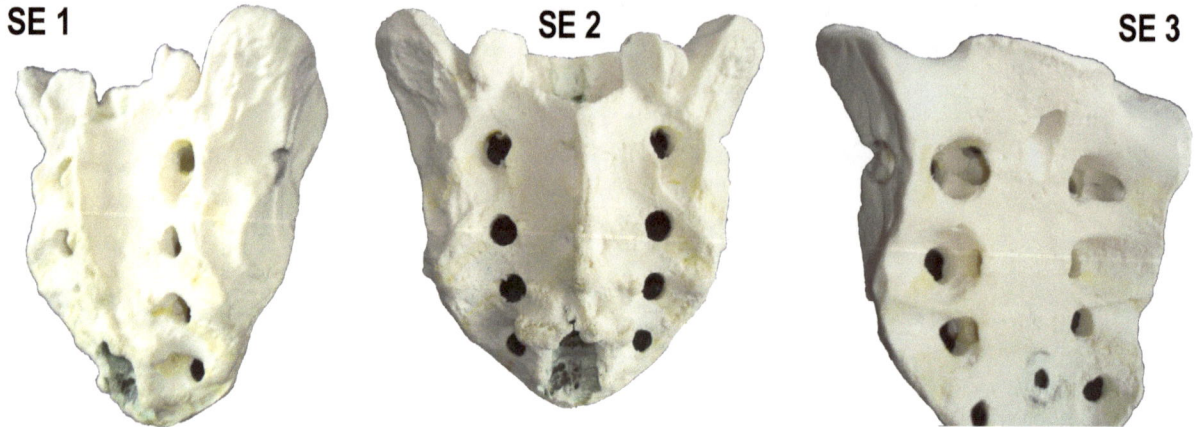

SE 1

SE 2

SE 3

Like the innominate bones, when you first look at the shape of the sacrum it looks like design by committee. But it is so cleverly designed that even huge variations in the basic shape still work relatively efficiently.

The shape of the Sacral facets are predominantly concave, in contrast to the Iliac facets which are predominantly convex. When the articular surfaces of the Sacrum and Ilium are placed together their complimentary contours form a snug but slightly loose fit.

The function of the sacrum is to act as a lever and counter lever between the two innominate bones and form a solid mobile base for the spine.

The complex shape of the sacral facets may not be immediately obvious. For simplicity **figure SE6** illustrates how the facets can be divided into two groups; inferior (magenta) and superior (blue).

These two groups can be further divided into six individual facets. These individual facets are illustrated in **figure SE7**.

(1) represents the convex shape of the posterior splitter protuberance and *(2)* the concave shape of the anterior splitter protuberance.

If you compare these contours with **figures SE1**, **SE2**, **SE3** and **SE5** it can be seen that they match.

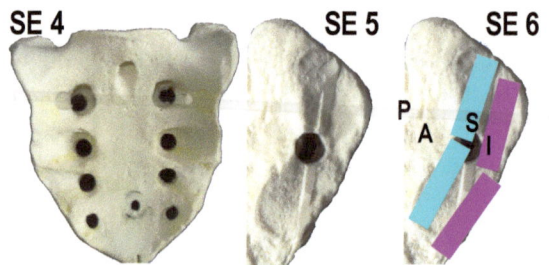

SE 4   **SE 5**   **SE 6**

Sacral views angled vertically
for illustration

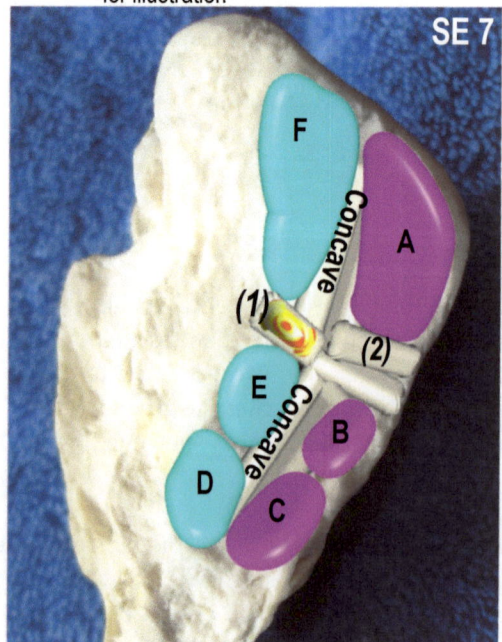

SE 7

Sacroiliac Facet Engagement

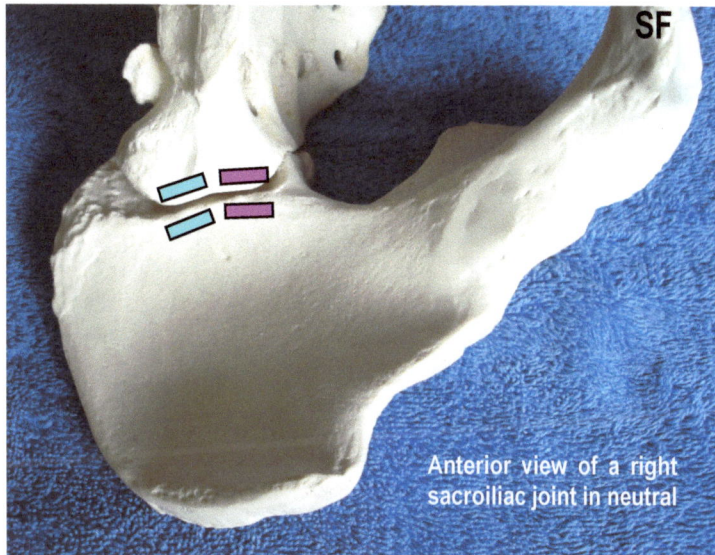

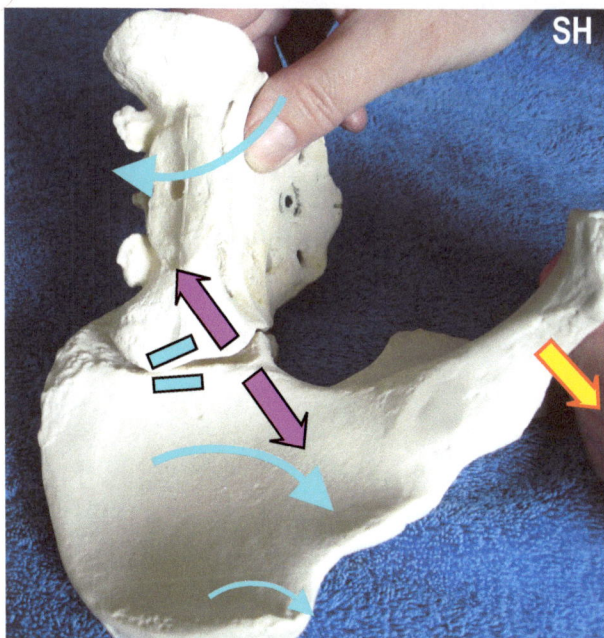

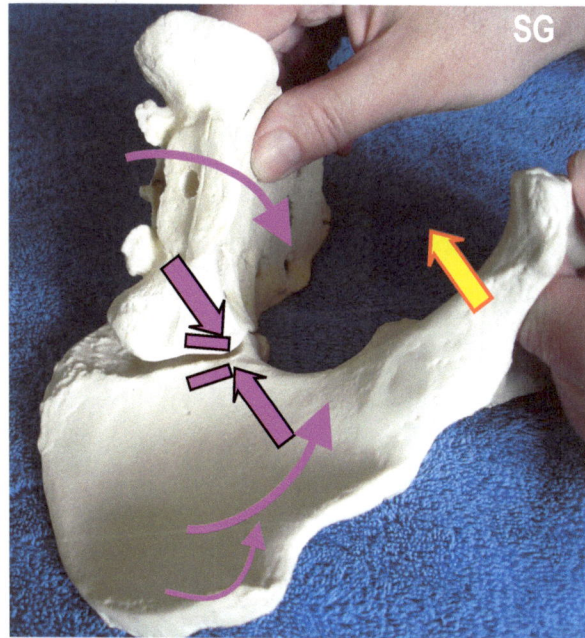

Anterior view of a right
sacroiliac joint in neutral

Figure SF is an anterior view of the right sacroiliac joint. The coloured oblong lines have been drawn in to highlight the shape of the joint.

Figure SH illustrates the superior facets of the Sacrum and the Ilium engaged and are shown in blue. Note that the pubic crest and anterior superior iliac spine have moved laterally.

Figure SG illustrates the inferior facets of the Sacrum and Ilium engaged and are shown in magenta. Note that the pubic crest and anterior superior iliac spine have moved medially.

Innominate Movements

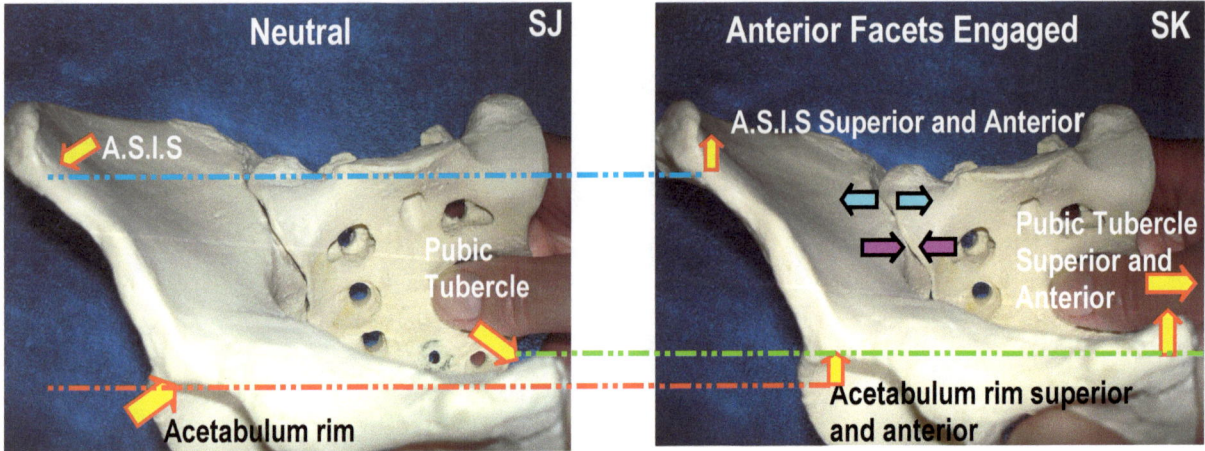

Figure SJ shows the sacroiliac joint in neutral and **figure SK,** with the superior facets engaged. Lines of reference have been added to highlight the differences between the bony landmarks.

Figure SK shows the positions the right Ilium and hip joint take to raise the right leg anteriorly, medially and superiorly.

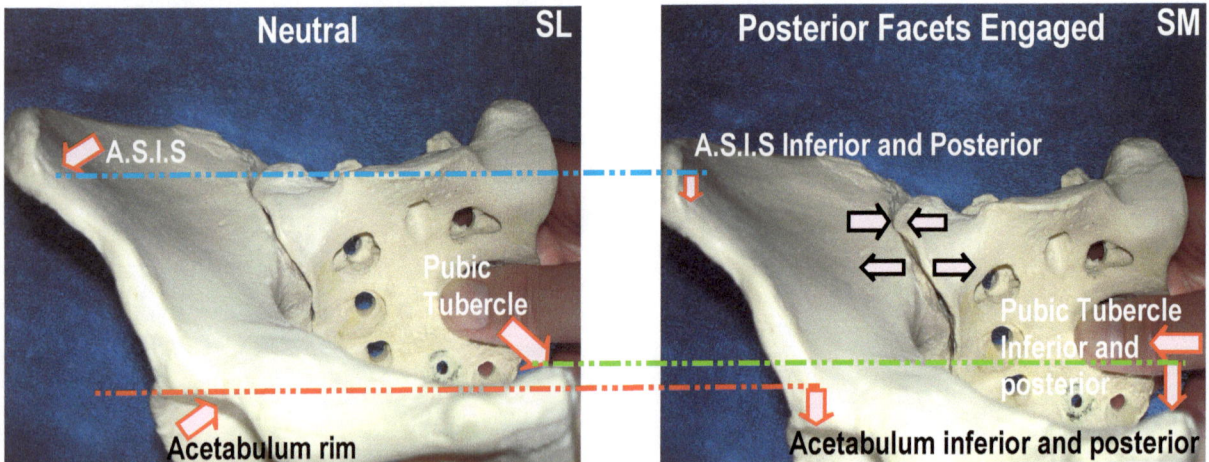

Figure SL shows the sacroiliac joint in neutral and **figure SM,** with the superior facets engaged. Lines of reference have been added to highlight the differences between the bony landmarks.

Figure SM shows the positions the right Ilium and hip joint take to lower the weight bearing right leg posteriorly, laterally and inferiorly.

Sacroiliac Principal of Reciprocation

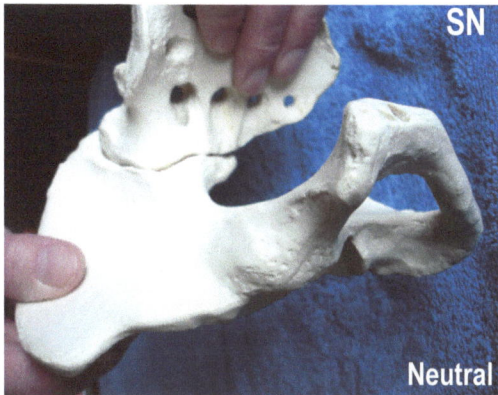

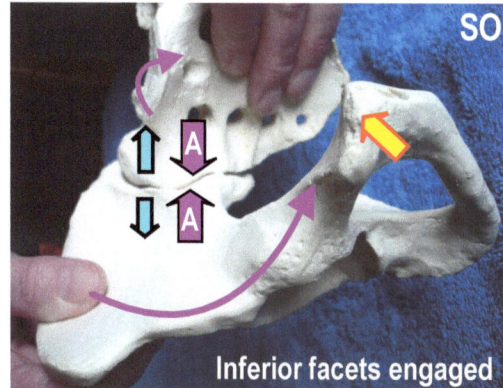

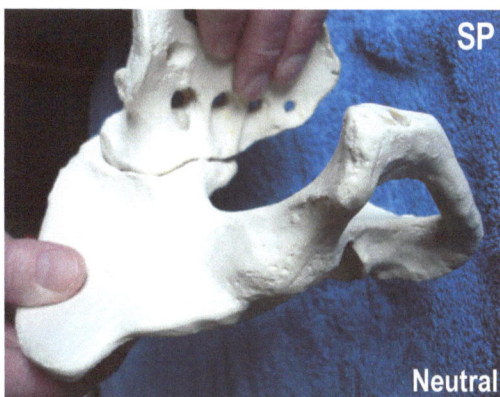

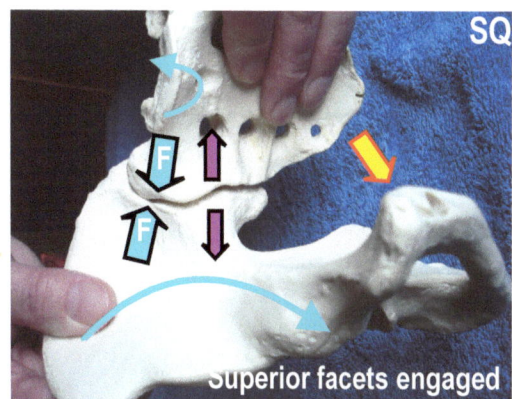

Above are more comparison photographs. **Figure SO** shows the position of the Ilium when the 'A' facets engage. **Figure SQ** shows the position of the Ilium when the 'F' facets are engaged.

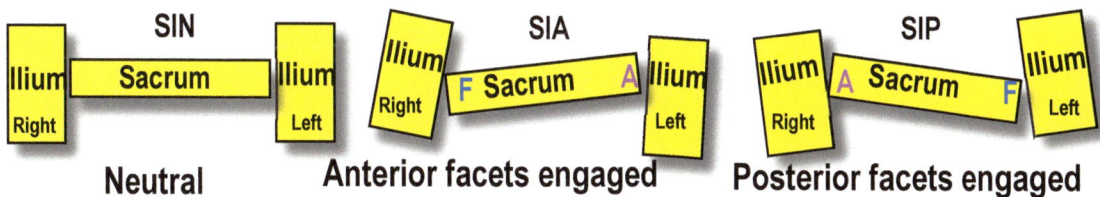

The illustrations above show the reciprocal action of the sacroiliac articulation. **Figure SIN** shows the neutral position.

When the 'A' facets engage on the left, shown in **figure SIA**, the 'F' facets are levered to engage on the right. When the 'F' facets engage on the right, shown in **figure SIP**, the 'A' facets are levered to engage on the left.

Pelvic Alignment and Motion

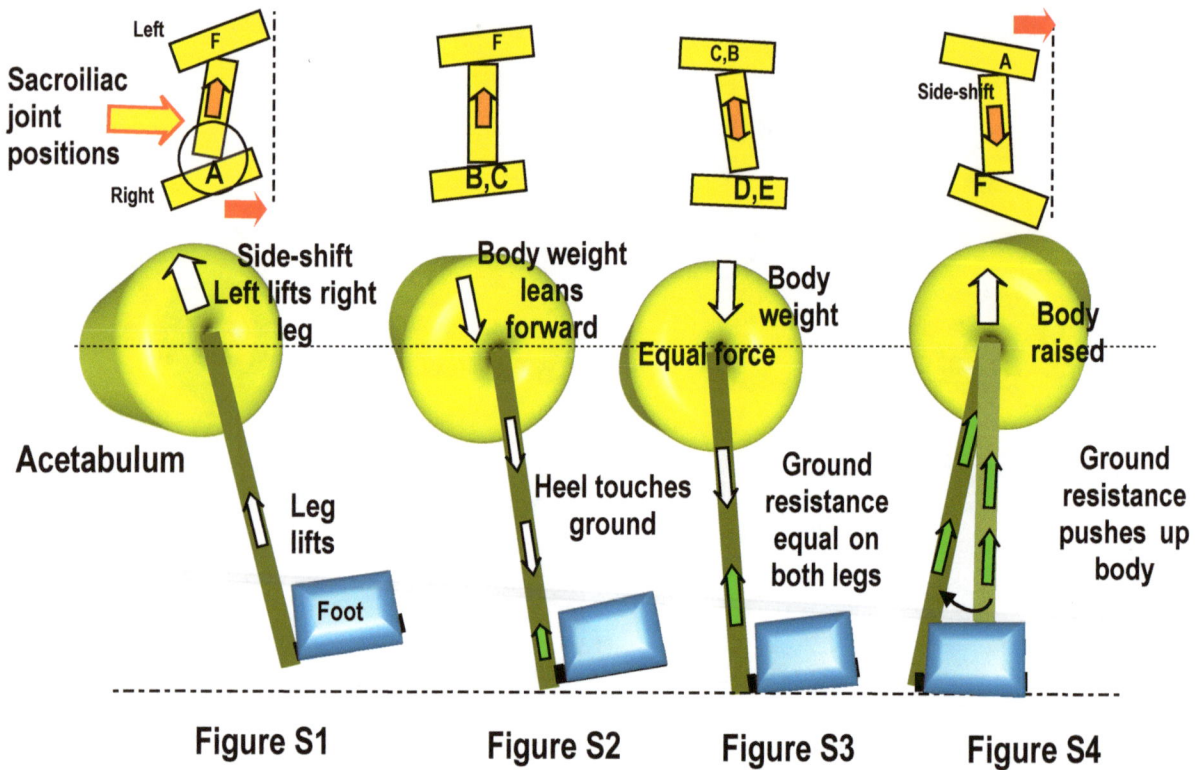

Figure S1 **Figure S2** **Figure S3** **Figure S4**

Basic walking mechanism

The illustration above represents the positions the right leg and foot take during the action of walking. **Figure S1** shows the position of the right leg when the weight bearing and pelvic side-shifts is to the left. This action levers and engages the right 'A' sacroiliac facets. With the aid of the limb muscles, the right leg moves anteriorly, medially and superiorly.

Figure S2 shows the transitory position of the leg as the upper body weight inclines forward into the direction of motion. *Weight and side-shift are still on the left*. This action causes the right leg to contact the ground and lever the ilium to engage the facets 'B' and 'C'.

Figure S3 shows the position of the leg as equal weight is placed on both legs. The position of the leading right leg is anterior and the left, posterior. This causes the Ilium to lever and engage the 'D' facet through to 'E' on the right, and the facets 'C' through to 'B' on the left.

Figure S4 shows the position of the leg in the final stage. Upward ground resistance travels up the right leg and lifts the pelvis on the same side. When weight bearing and side-shift transfer to the right, the right 'F' sacroiliac facets engage. In turn the articular surface on the left side of the sacrum is levered to engage the 'A' sacroiliac facets.

Rotation Right in Lumbar Extension

Rotation right in lumbar extension

When the left knee is flexed and body weight is directed and balanced through the right leg, as shown in **figure SR**, the 'F' sacroiliac joint facets engage. To achieve this action the pelvis as a whole is lifted on the left and rotated to the right and mildly side-bent right. This introduces general rotation and side-bending to the right in the lumbar spine.

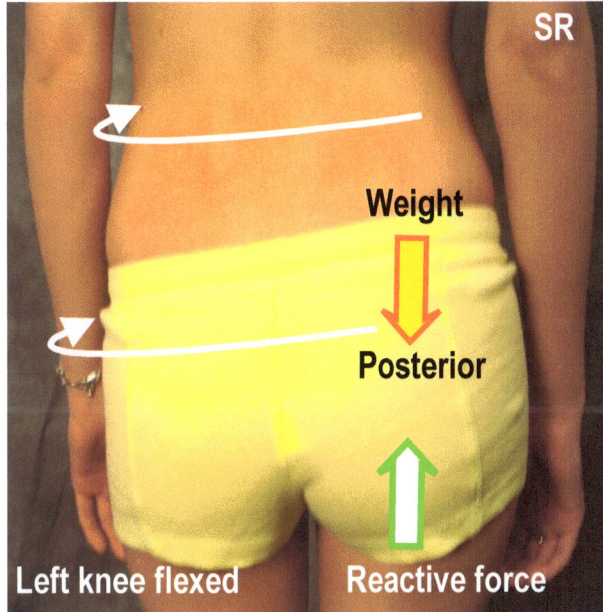

Reciprocal facet action   **Weight**

Left sacroiliac facets   **Right sacroiliac facets**

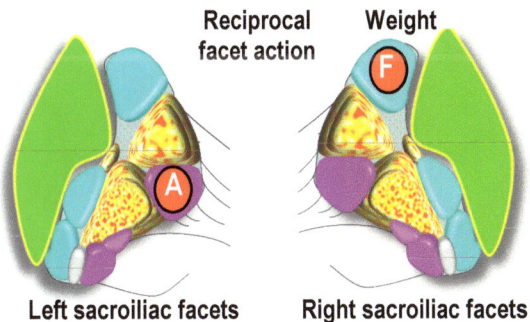

SR

Weight

Posterior

Left knee flexed   Reactive force

Pelvic side-shift

When the pelvis side-shifts to the right, as shown in **figure SS,** the pelvis levels and the local lumbar vertebrae are given the necessary 'G' force side-shift they need to individually rotate and side-bend to the right.

Key:

TP's   = Transverse processes

   = Upward ground resistance

   = Transverse processes side-bent

Reactive force = Ground resistance returning up the legs.

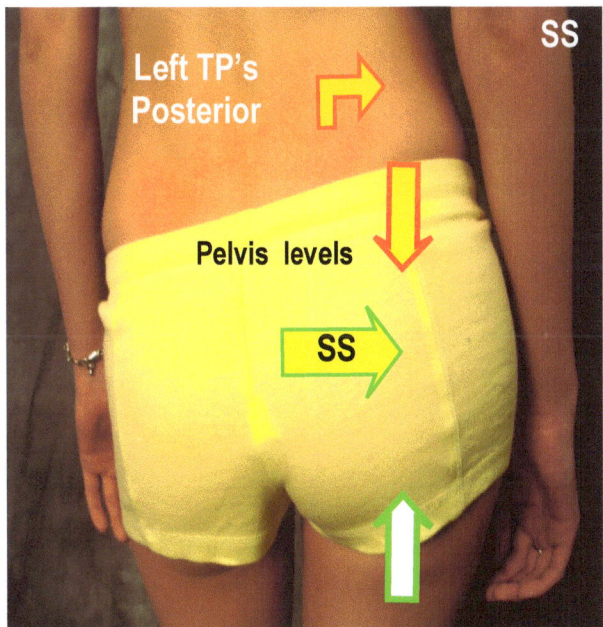

SS

Left TP's Posterior

Pelvis levels

SS

Rotation Right in Lumbar Flexion

Rotation right in lumbar flexion

When the left knee is flexed and body weight is directed through the left leg, as shown in **figure ST,** the 'A' sacroiliac facets engage. This 'G' force causes the pelvis as a whole to side-bend to the left and rotate to the right. This causes the lumbar spine to generally side-bend left and rotate right.

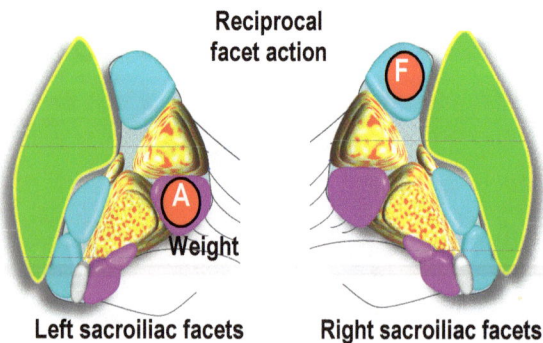

Reciprocal facet action

Left sacroiliac facets   Right sacroiliac facets

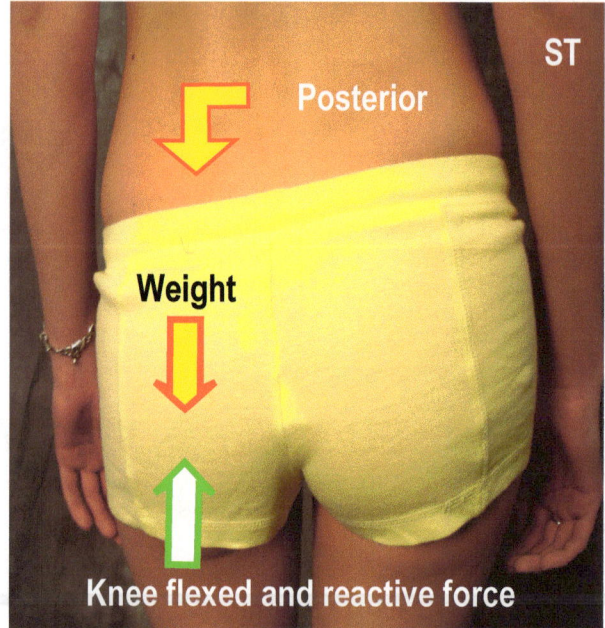

ST

Posterior

Weight

Knee flexed and reactive force

When the pelvis side-shifts to the left as shown in **figure SU**, the pelvis further side-bends left and rotates right and the local lumbar vertebrae are given the necessary 'G' force side-shift they need to individually side-bend left and rotate to the right.

Try these movements yourself

Throughout this book the pelvic movements described in these opening chapters are constantly being referenced.

The G force rule

It is fundamentally important that you understand how weight direction plus knee flexion produce the essential general 'G' force.

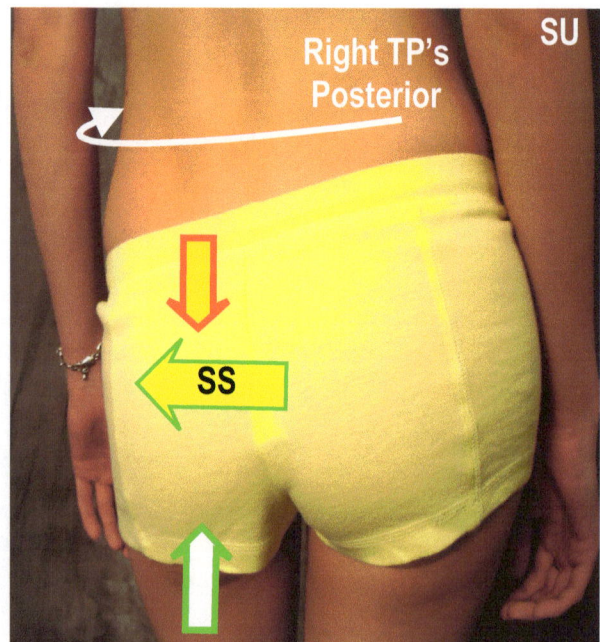

SU

Right TP's Posterior

SS

Rotation Right in Lumbar Flexion
Pelvic Mechanics

It should help to read this page in conjunction with page 40, Chapter 3.

As we come to the end of this chapter on the sacroiliac joints it needs be fully understood how the combination of weight bearing, knee flexion and side-shift tie in with the lumbar facet shape and their articulation. .

When weight is placed on the flexed left knee, because it is weight bearing the posterior facets come into play and facet alignment is directed to the left '**D**' facet which causes the pelvis to lift on the left and rotate right. This is shown in **figure SMRSSL** and below as **pelvis A**.

When pelvic side-shift to the left takes place the facet alignment is directed to the left '**E**' facet. This is shown in **figure SMRSSL** and below as **pelvis B**. At the far end of its lateral trajectory the pelvis makes a small radial arc posteriorly as the weight and side-shift transfer to the fully weight bearing '**F**' facets. This is illustrated in **figure SMRSSL-a** and below as **pelvis C**. The cause of this small but important arc is shown by the medially indented '**F**' sacral facet shown in **figure SMRSSL- b.**

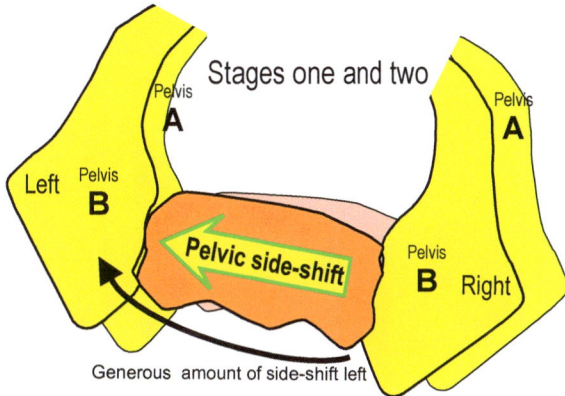

Figure SMRSSL Lumbar Flexion

View from above of pelvis and sacroiliac joints. This illustration shows the pelvis before and after pelvic side-shift is applied to the left. Note that the pelvis rotates right moves as forces transfer from facet 'D' to 'E' along a lateral trajectory.

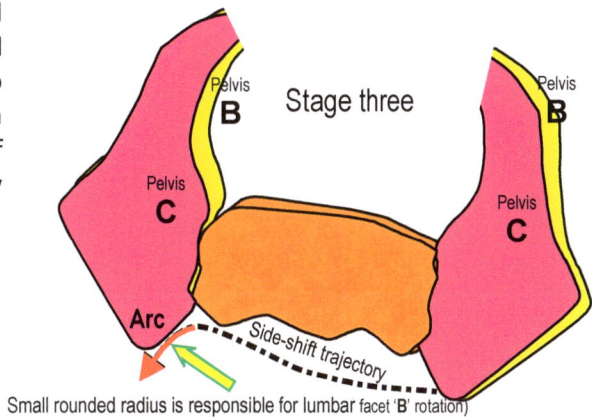

Small rounded radius is responsible for lumbar facet 'B' rotation)

Figure SMRSSL-a Lumbar Flexion

View from above of pelvis and sacroiliac joints. This illustration shows the pelvis in the final stage of pelvic side-shift to the left. Note that the left side of the pelvis arcs posteriorly in a small radius at the end of its lateral trajectory. This is because of the transfer to the more lateral 'F' facet.

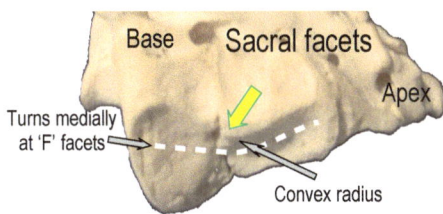

Figure SMRSSL- b

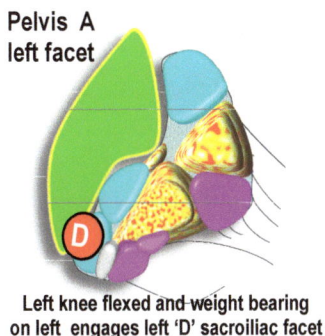

Pelvis A
left facet

Left knee flexed and weight bearing on left engages left 'D' sacroiliac facet

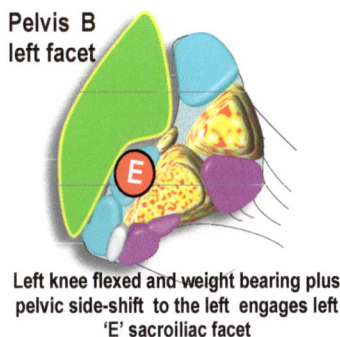

Pelvis B
left facet

Left knee flexed and weight bearing plus pelvic side-shift to the left engages left 'E' sacroiliac facet

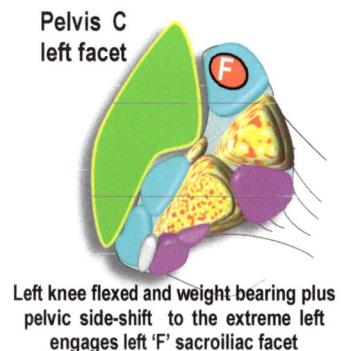

Pelvis C
left facet

Left knee flexed and weight bearing plus pelvic side-shift to the extreme left engages left 'F' sacroiliac facet

Rotation Right in Lumbar Extension
Pelvic Mechanics

It should help to read this page in conjunction with page 41, Chapter 3.

When weight is placed on the straight right leg with left knee flexion, facet alignment is confined to the right weight bearing 'F' facet which in turn causes the pelvis to lift on the right and generally rotate right. This is shown in **figure SMSSSR** and **pelvis D**.

Weight bearing combined with pelvic side-shift to the right is confined to the 'F' facets and the pelvis rotates further to the right. This is also shown in **figure SMSSSR** and **pelvis D** .

At the end of its lateral side-shift trajectory the pelvis makes a large radial deviation posteriorly as weight and side-shift are fully taken on the weight bearing 'F' facets (as in walking). At this point the reactive upward force from below lifts the right side of the pelvis still further. This is illustrated in **figure SMSSSR-a.**

Translation to vertebral joint articulation
In a lumbar vertebral joint the lower vertebra (in the case of L4 -L3 it would be L4) is forced along the same side-bending, side-shift and rotational arc trajectory as the pelvis.
See **figure SMSSSR-b.**

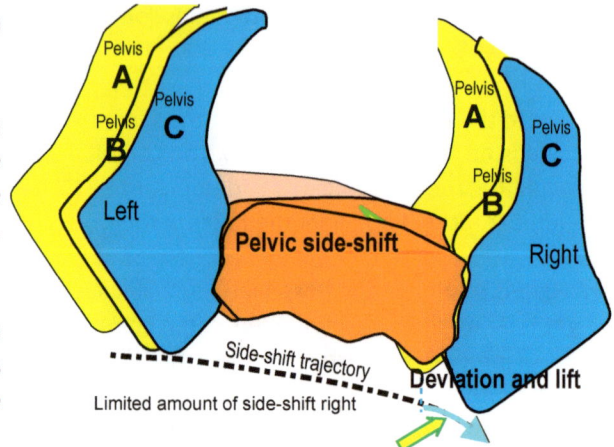

Figure SMSSSR Lumbar Extension
View from above of pelvis and sacroiliac joints. This illustration shows the pelvis before and after pelvic side-shift is applied to the right. Note that the right side of the pelvis lifts and deviates posteriorly in a minimal curve at the end of its lateral trajectory.

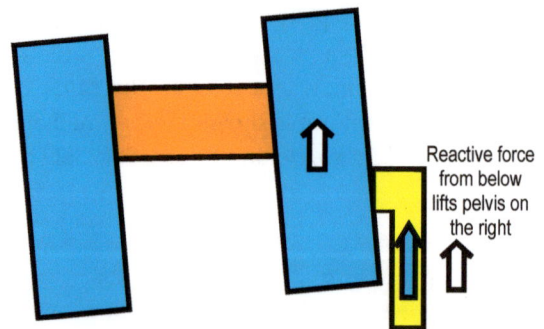

Figure SMSSSR-a Lumbar Extension posterior view
With the right 'F' sacroiliac facets engaged and pelvic side-shift is taken to the extreme right right the reactive force from below lifts pelvis on right.

Translation of pelvic trajectory reflected in passage of L3

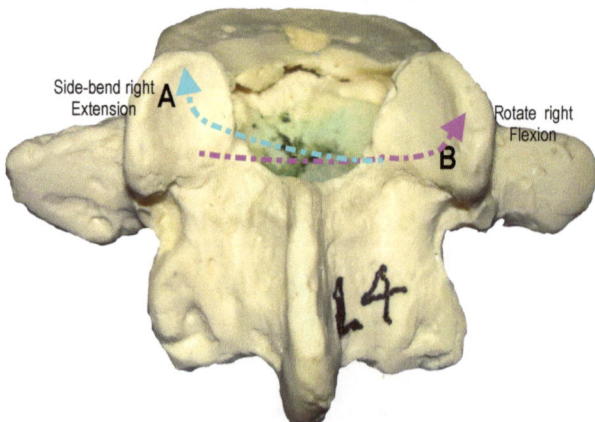

Figure SMSSSR-b

Pelvis D right facet

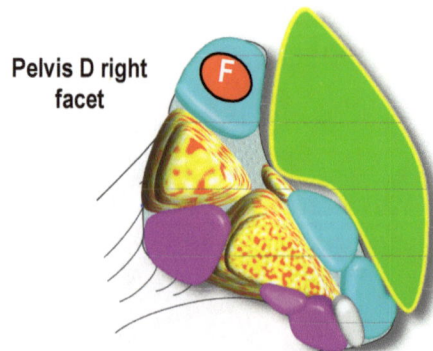

Right leg straight and weight bearing plus pelvic side-shift to the from minimal to the extreme right see the right 'F' sacroiliac facet engaged. At the most lateral the reactive force from below lifts pelvis on right.

Chapter Three

Physiology of the Lumbar Joints

Terminology

Before we go into any detail about the bio-mechanics, we need to co-ordinate our lumbar vertebrae terminology. See page 19.

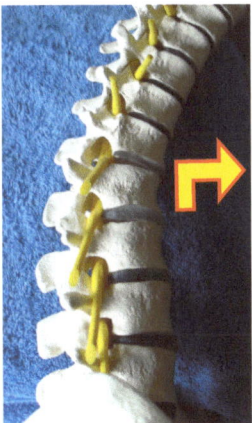

Lumbar extension
Forward bending

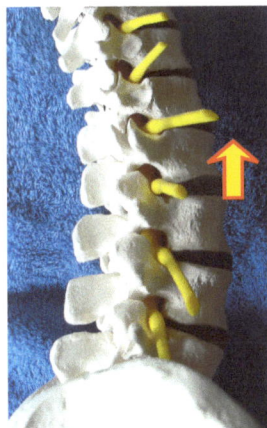

Lumbar in neutral
Standing vertically

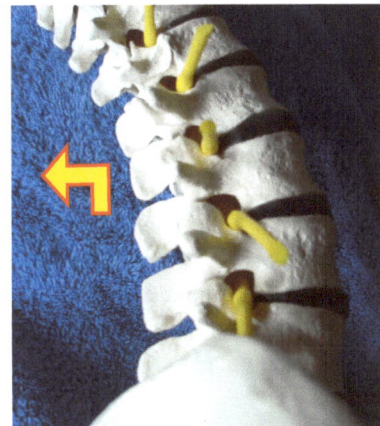

Lumbar in flexion
Backward bending

Lumbar vertebral function

All the lower vertebrae namely L5, L4, L3 and L2 are designed for weight bearing, flexion, extension, side-bending and rotation. For stability reasons, S1-L5 and L5-4 have less mobility than the lumbar vertebrae above.

The L1 vertebra is designed to rotate, flex and extend and to block pelvic side-bending and side-shift passing up into the thoracic spine in lumbar flexion. In lumbar extension, the forces of pelvic side-bending and side-shift are allowed to pass L1, which enables them to effect the thoracic spine. L1 also acts as a form of shock absorber and level base to keep the thoracic vertebrae in a vertical position. This will be explained

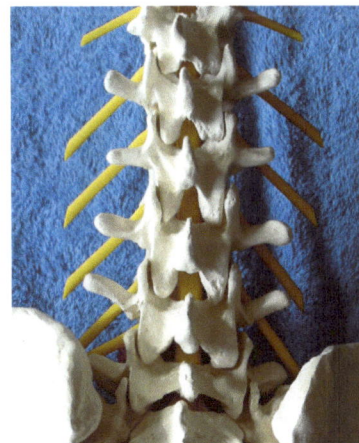

Lumbar
L4 Facet Anatomy

Overview of L4 upper facets

The L4-L3 joint is built for weight bearing. Their mating facets allow for movement in a vertical plane to facilitate lumbar flexion and extension whilst providing a furrowed path for simultaneous rotation and side-bending when required.

Figure LA is a posterior view of a typical L4 vertebra. It has two sets of facets; two at the top that face posteriorly (upper)and two at the bottom that face anteriorly (lower).

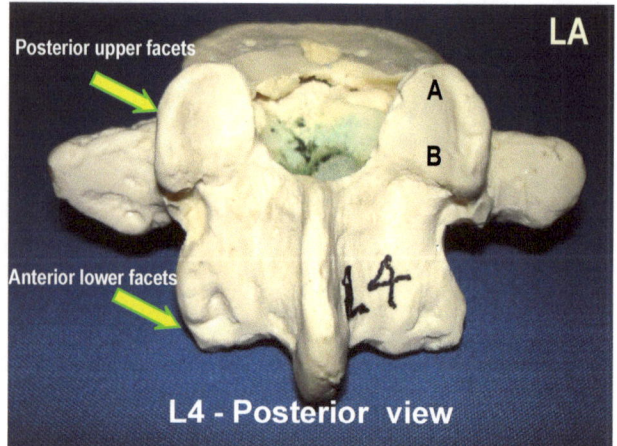

Posterior upper facets

A
B

Anterior lower facets

L4 - Posterior view

The L4 upper facets are petal shaped with their surface rounded at the inferior end shown as 'B'. This is to accommodate simultaneous side-bending and rotation in lumbar flexion. Rotation is driven by the 'G' and 'M' shearing force and is the local dominant movement.

The L4 upper facets are flatter at their superior end, shown as 'A'. This is to accommodate simultaneous rotation and side-bending in lumbar extension. Side-bending is driven by the 'G' and 'M' shearing force and is the local dominant movement.

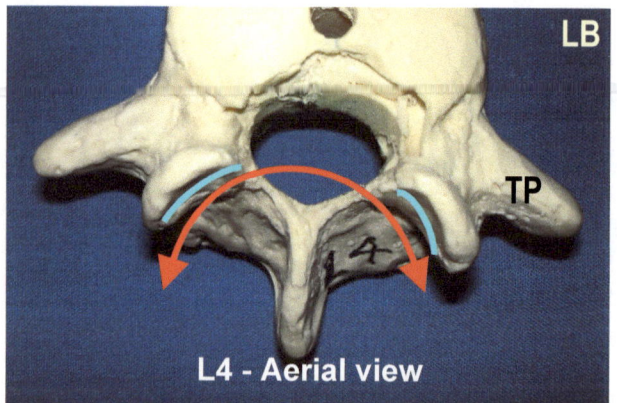

TP

L4 - Aerial view

The superior L4 facets shown in **figure LC** are convex vertically.

The L5-L4 joint has a very similar design and function, though the superior facets are more spade-like and heavy duty.

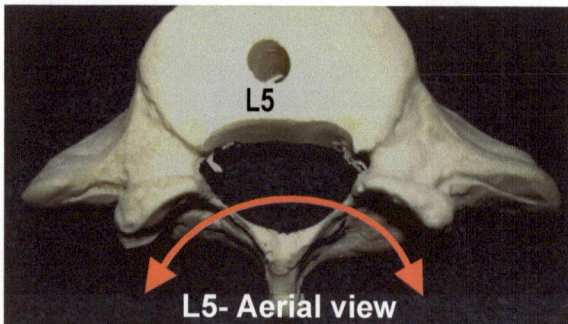

L5

L5- Aerial view

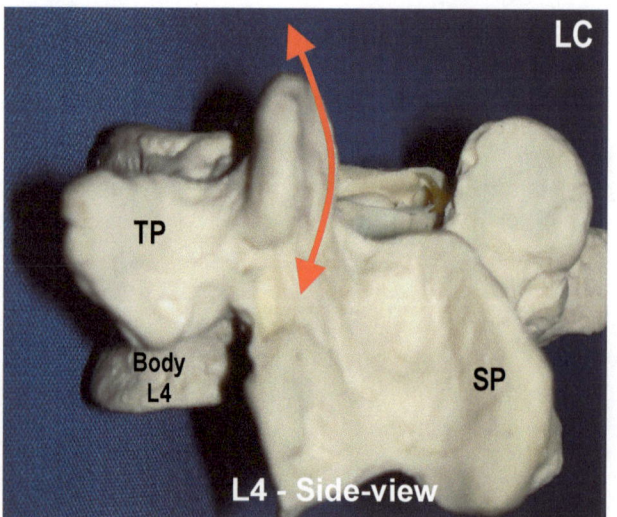

TP

Body
L4

SP

L4 - Side-view

Lumbar
L3 Facet Anatomy Inferior Facets

Overview of L3 lower facets

The lower L3 facets mate with the upper facets of L4 and allow for movement in a vertical plane to facilitate lumbar flexion and extension. They follow the furrowed petal shaped path set into the L4 facets to accommodate simultaneous L3 rotation and side-bending.

Figure LD is a side-view of an anterior L3 lower facet. The facets are concave vertically to accommodate flexion and extension movements.

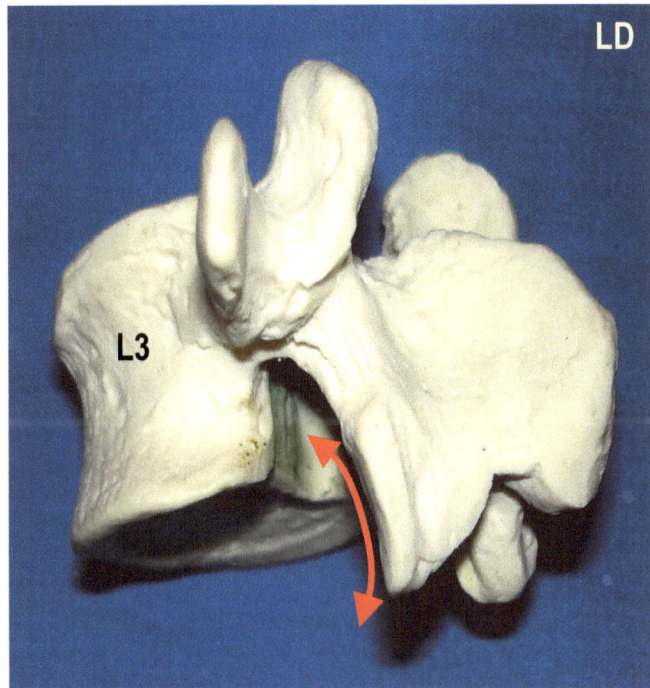

Figure LE illustrates how the L4-L3 vertebral facets accommodate lumbar flexion and extension.

The L3 lower facets have a design similar to a pair of skis and are convex horizontally, as shown in **figure LF**.

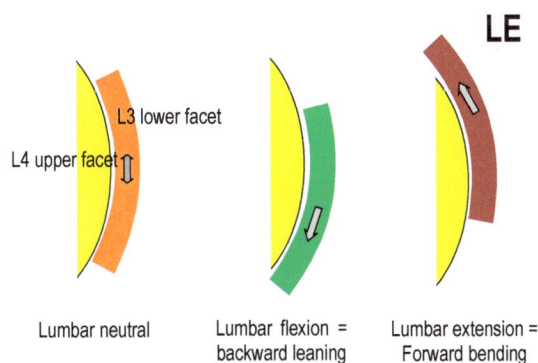

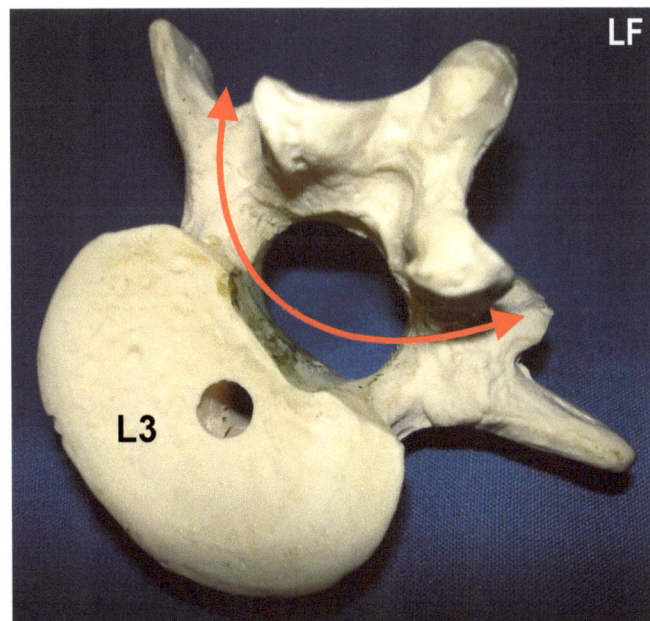

L3 side-view

L3 lower facet

L4 upper facet

Lumbar neutral

Lumbar flexion = backward leaning

Lumbar extension = Forward bending

L3 view from below

The Importance of the Nucleus Pulposus

Before the physiology of the lumbar joints is discussed further, a couple of words about working movements out on a cheap commercially manufactured plastic spine. For me the rubber discs between the vertebrae were a real hindrance because they do not simulate the arcing effect provided by a nucleus pulposus. The nucleus pulposus is important because it acts as a point of pivot for vertebral facet movements.

Nucleus pulposus shape

Figure LG shows a typical medical capsule. It is being used to represent the nucleus pulposus because it is spongy and pliable. The ideal shape would be oval.

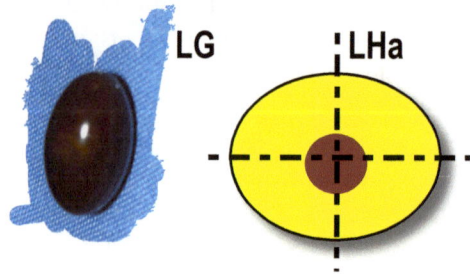

To get the best results, place the nucleus on the body of the lumbar vertebrae, as shown in **figures LHa** and **LHb**. Note that the nucleus pulposus is positioned towards the posterior half of the body.

The three drawings below show the horizontal and vertical benefits of a spongy nucleus pulposus, together with the horizontal and vertical orbits that are possible.

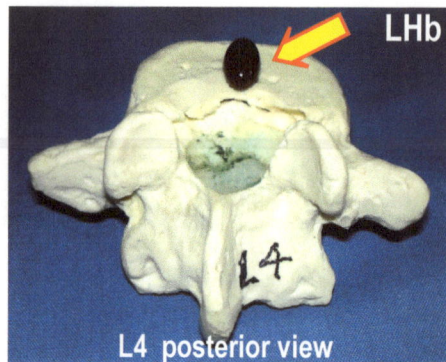

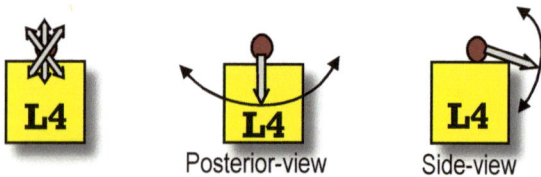

LG | LHa

LHb

L4 posterior view

L4

L4

L4
Posterior-view

L4
Side-view

Extension and flexion of the L3-4 joint

When the nucleus is in place and L3 is positioned over L4, the vertical arc of the facets can be illustrated as shown in **figures LHc, LHd** and **LHe**.

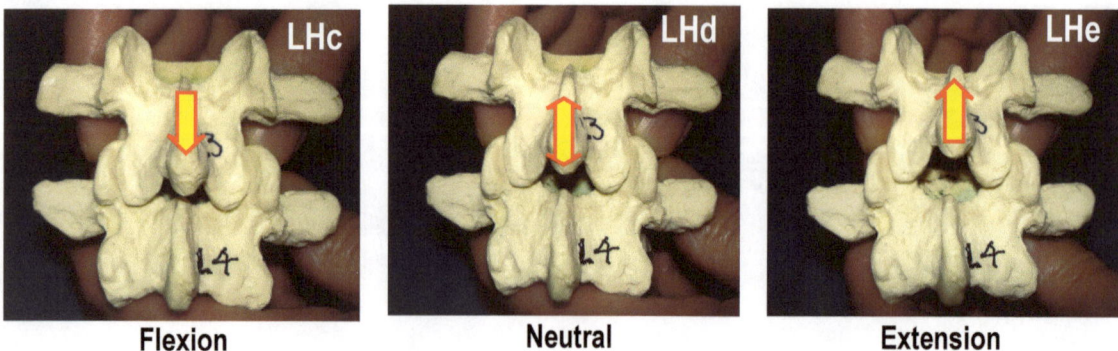

LHc

Flexion

LHd

Neutral

LHe

Extension

Why L3 Rotates Right in Flexion and Side-Bends Right in Extension

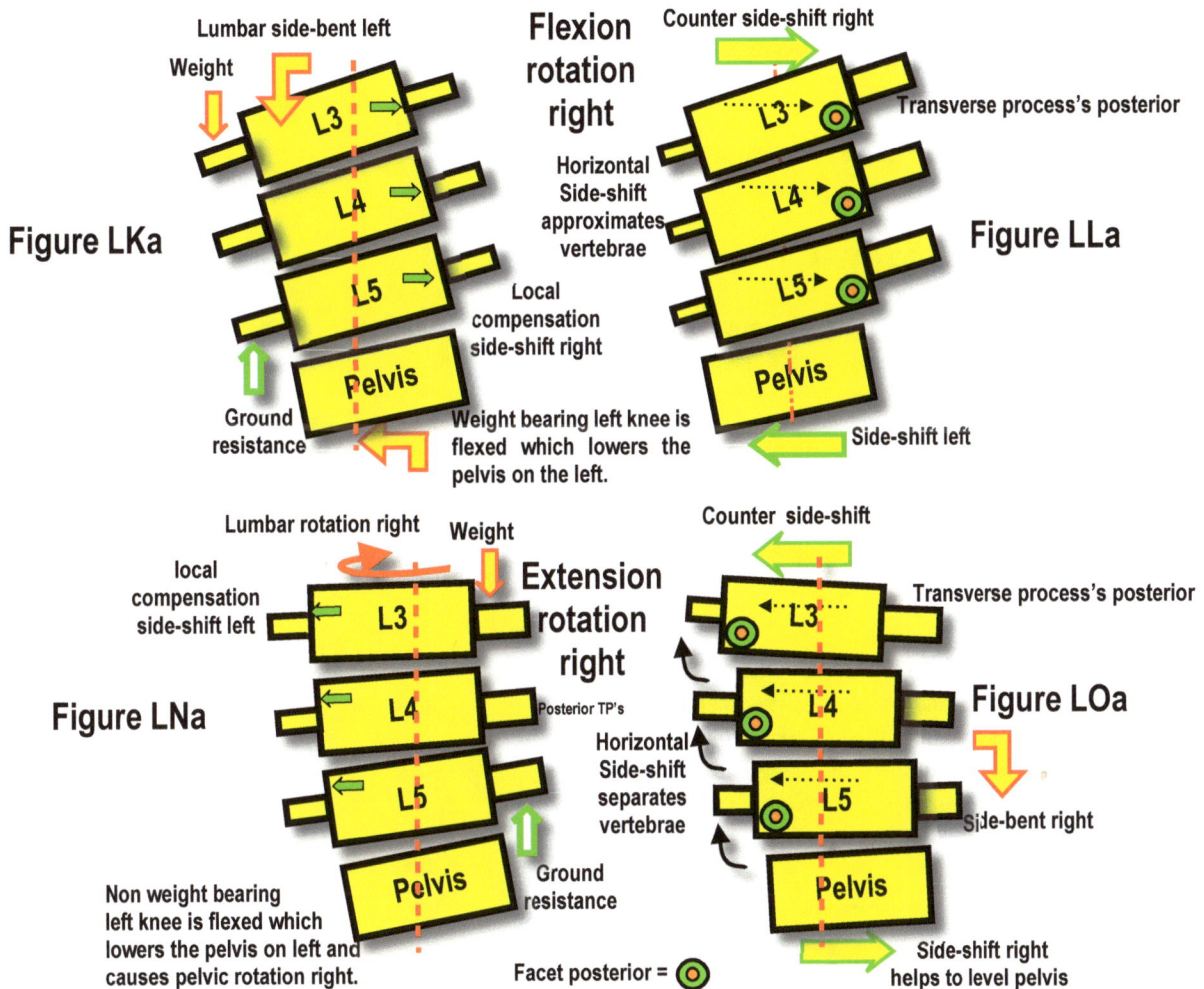

Figure LKa

Lumbar side-bent left

Weight

L3

L4

L5

Pelvis

Ground resistance

Flexion rotation right

Horizontal Side-shift approximates vertebrae

Local compensation side-shift right

Weight bearing left knee is flexed which lowers the pelvis on the left.

Figure LLa

Counter side-shift right

L3

L4

L5

Pelvis

Transverse process's posterior

Side-shift left

Figure LNa

Lumbar rotation right

local compensation side-shift left

Weight

L3

L4

L5

Pelvis

Non weight bearing left knee is flexed which lowers the pelvis on left and causes pelvic rotation right.

Extension rotation right

Posterior TP's

Horizontal Side-shift separates vertebrae

Ground resistance

Facet posterior = ◉

Figure LOa

Counter side-shift

L3

L4

L5

Pelvis

Transverse process's posterior

Side-bent right

Side-shift right helps to level pelvis

Figure LKa illustrates the effect flexing the left knee on the weight bearing left leg has on the lumbar vertebrae. **Figure LLa** illustrates the next stage. The side-bent pelvis side-shifts to the left. This has two effects; 1) As the lumbar vertebrae side-shift right the disc spaces approximate on the left and 2) The facets of the vertebrae above bank across the right facet of the vertebrae below and rotate right.

Figure LNa illustrates the effect of weight and ground resistance on the right side when the left knee is flexed. This initially side-bends the pelvis left. However, because of the counter force of balance from above the pelvis levels and rotates to the right. Due to the meeting of ground resistance (the reactive force) and body weight on the right there is a small amount of local lumbar vertebral side-bending to the right. **Figure LOa** shows the next stage and illustrates how pelvic side-shift to the right causes the disc spaces between the lumbar vertebrae to separate on the left. It is this that causes the facets of the vertebrae above to bank up the left facets of the vertebrae below and side-bend to the right.

L4-L3:
Rotation Right in Flexion

L3 rotation right in lumbar flexion

This page should be read in conjunction with page 33 in Chapter 2.

The lumbar is flexed (backward bent) as shown in **figure LJ.**

Weight bearing is focused on the left leg. The left knee is flexed and made weight bearing and this engages the left 'D' sacroiliac facets. This **'G'** force causes the pelvis and lumber to generally rotate right and side-bend left.

See **figure LK**. Within the L3-4 joint, the weight bearing left facet of L3 glides down the left facet of L4 which is pushed up by the reactive force from below. This creates the correct side-bending starting position for local rotation to the right to follow.

When the pelvis side-shifts to the left the sacrum articulates along the iliac facets and engages facet 'E'. This generally increases knee flexion and therefore pelvic and lumbar side-bending to the left. The **'G'** force side-shift takes L4 with it and side-shifts the facets of L4 to the right.

Within the L3-4 joint the resistant **'M'** force from above subject the facets of L3 to shear force in the opposite direction (left)on the L4 facets.

As the pelvic side-shift increases the sacrum continues to articulate along the iliac facets and engages facet 'F' in a posterior arc. L4 follows this posterior arc and causes the right L3 facet which is moving in the opposite direction to arc up the right L4 facet and rotate right. This is shown in **figure LL.**

It can be seen that the right transverse process of L3 is posterior and superior. Conversely, the left side is anterior and inferior. The spinous process of L3 is approximated and to the right of the L4 spinous process. The concavity is on the left side.

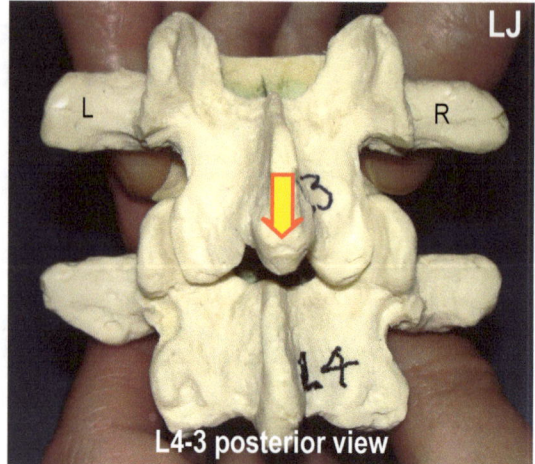

L4-3 posterior view

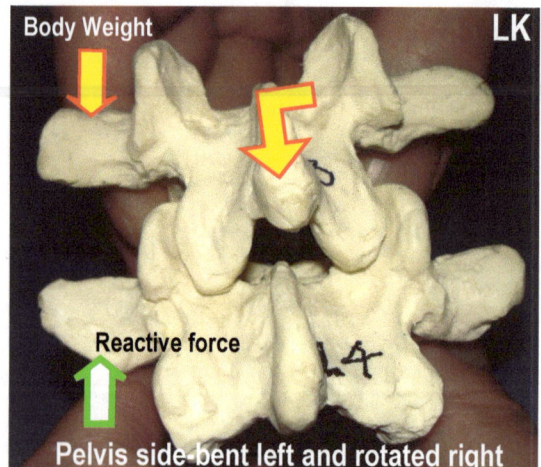

Body Weight

Reactive force

Pelvis side-bent left and rotated right

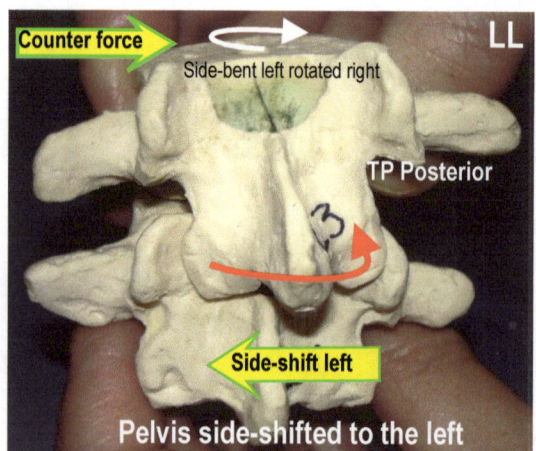

Counter force
Side-bent left rotated right

TP Posterior

Side-shift left

Pelvis side-shifted to the left

L3 Rotation Right in Extension

L3 rotation right in lumbar extension

This page should be read in conjunction with page 34 in Chapter 2.

The lumbar is extended (forward bent) as shown in **figure LM.**

Weight bearing is focused on the right leg. The left knee is flexed and the right leg made weight bearing and this engages the right 'F' sacroiliac facets. In this position the pelvis and lumber generally rotate to the right.

Within the L3-4 joint, the weight bearing right facet of L3 glides down the right facet of L4 whilst the upward reactive force from below slides the right L4 facet superiorly up the L3 facet. This is shown in **figure LN.** This position aligns the L3-4 joint facets in a side-bent right position for further local side-bending to the right to follow.

The pelvis side-shifts to the right in a posterior arc and the 'G' force side-shift takes L4 along with it. The L4 facets slide under the L3 facets in a downward posterior journey to the right. At the same time the shearing counter 'M' force from above levers L3 in the opposite direction, to the left.

When pelvic side-shift reaches the far right where the posterior large radial pelvic deviation occurs the right side of the pelvis becomes lifted by the reactive force from below and this approximates the weight bearing right L3-4 facets. The left L3 facet caught in a side-bending trajectory ride up the left L4 facets to complete their rotation and side-bending to the right.

The left transverse process of L3 is posterior and superior, while the right side is anterior and inferior. The spinous process of L3 is separated and to the left of the spinous process of L4. The concavity is on the right side.

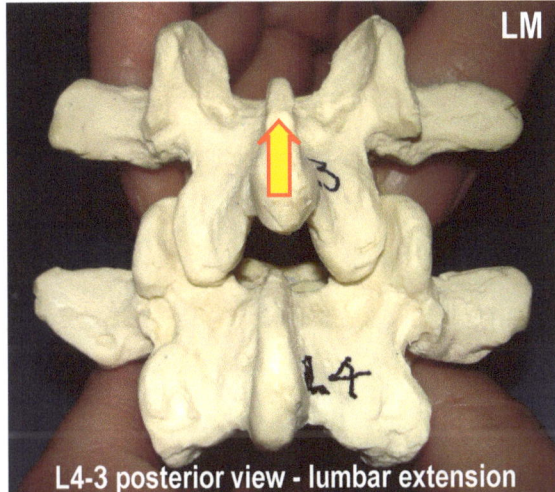

LM

L4-3 posterior view - lumbar extension

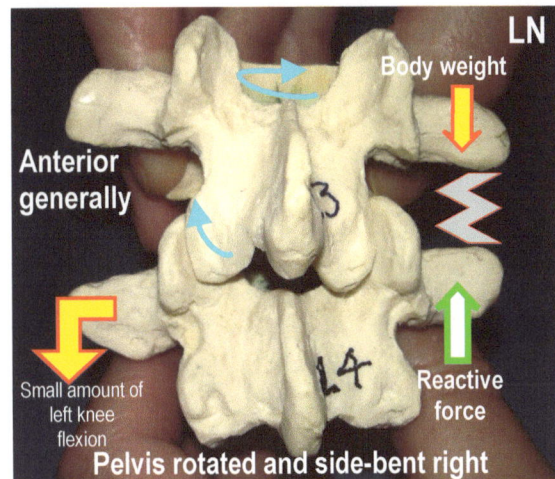

LN

Body weight

Anterior generally

Small amount of left knee flexion

Reactive force

Pelvis rotated and side-bent right

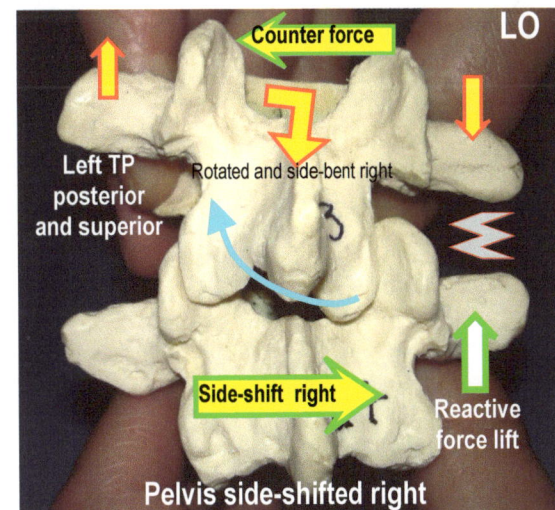

LO

Counter force

Rotated and side-bent right

Left TP posterior and superior

Side-shift right

Reactive force lift

Pelvis side-shifted right

In Lumbar Flexion the Thoracic Vertebrae Cannot Rotate or Side-bend

L1 the flexion gravity blocker

Figure 1 opposite is an illustration of the gravity line when L1 attempts rotation right in lumbar flexion. Notice that the gravity line passes directly through L1. This is not accidental, it is designed to block the pelvic side-shift driving force passing up the left side of the thoracic column. With no side-shift taking place above L1, the extended thoracic vertebrae are deprived of the necessary 'G' force side-shift required to make rotational movements.

In backward bending (lumbar flexion) the thoracic vertebrae are placed in thoracic extension.

Do this self test

See **figure 1a** opposite.

Stand up straight with your feet approximately two inches (5 cm) apart.

Place your weight on your left leg and then flex your left knee.

This sets up the precursor position for flexion lumbar rotation to the right, to follow.

Now side-shift your pelvis to the left and notice that the pelvic side-shift becomes blocked very quickly.

To confront the validity of this test, repeat the test on the other side. I.e. body weight on the right leg, right knee flexed and side-shift right.

You will get the same result.

Summary

Thoracic rotation is blocked in lumbar flexion (backward bending).

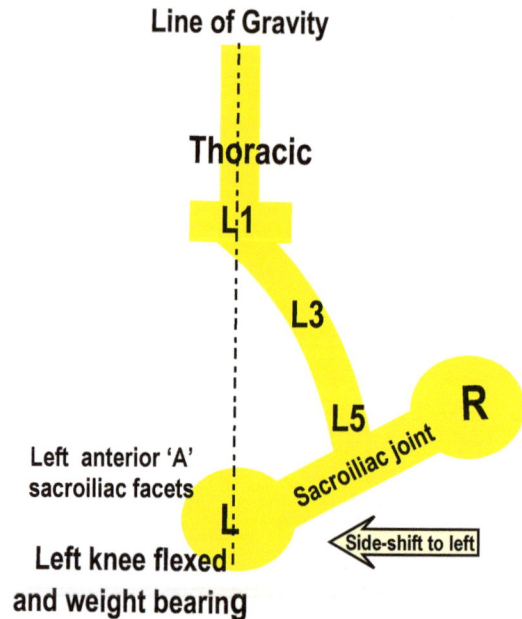

Line of Gravity
Thoracic
L1
L3
L5
R
Left anterior 'A' sacroiliac facets
Sacroiliac joint
Side-shift to left
L
Left knee flexed and weight bearing

Figure 1

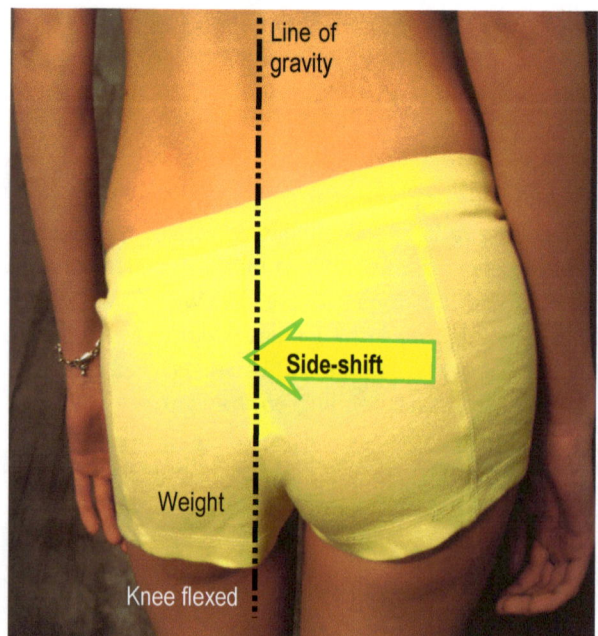

Line of gravity
Side-shift
Weight
Knee flexed

Figure 1a

42

In Lumbar Extension the Thoracic Vertebrae are Able to Rotate

L1, the extension gravitational gateway

Figure 2 is a drawing of the gravity line when L1 rotates right in extension.

When pelvic side-shift takes place to the right, the line of gravity passes to the right of L1. This is to allow the side-shift driving force to continue upwards to the thoracic vertebrae. This is the driving 'G' force that the thoracic vertebrae require to physiologically rotate right in thoracic flexion.

In forward bending (lumbar extension) the thoracic vertebrae with an increased AP curve, are placed in thoracic flexion.

Do this self test

See **figure 2a** opposite.

Stand up straight with your feet approximately two inches apart.

Place your weight on your right leg and then flex your left knee.

This sets up the precursor position for extension lumbar rotation to the right, to follow.

Now side-shift your pelvis to the right and notice that the pelvic side-shift moves a far greater distance to the right before the movement is blocked.

To double prove the validity of this test, repeat the test on the other side. I.e. body weight on the left leg, right knee flexed and side-shift right.

You will get the same result.

Summary

Thoracic rotation is allowed to take place in lumbar extension (forward bending).

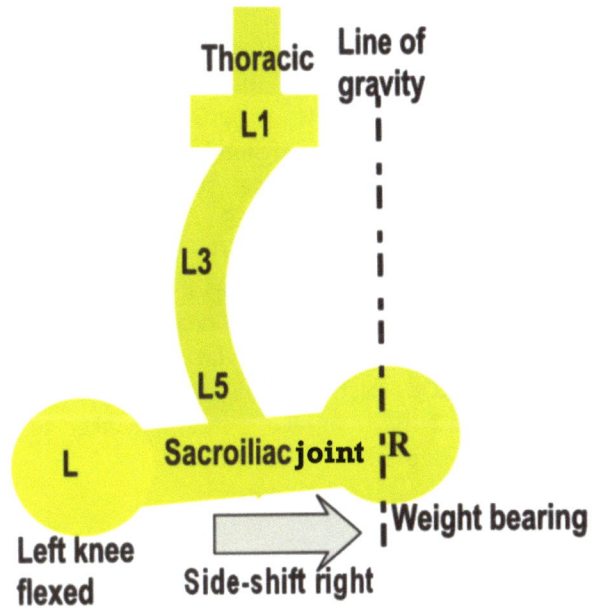

Figure 2

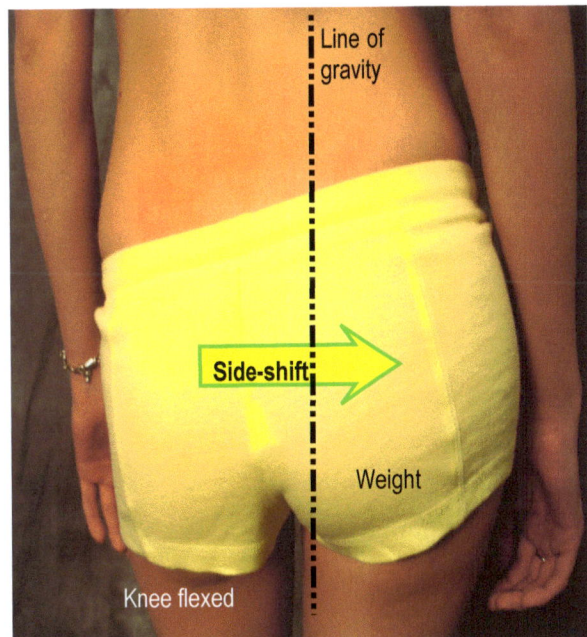

Figure 2a

L2-L1
Facet Surface Anatomy

L2 facet shape

Figure LP is a photograph of the upper posterior facets of a typical L2 vertebra. The primary function of the upper facets of L2 is to provide a surface that allows L1 to accommodate lumbar side-bending and rotation. Their vertical facet surface is offset posteriorly, as illustrated in **figure LPa**. The shape of the medial border of the facet surface is convex superiorly and concave inferiorly, as shown in **figure LPb**. From above, the facet shapes appear rounded, as shown in **figure LQ** but they have a flat quality to their surface. **Figure LQa** illustrates this shape in cross section. The L2 facet surface is steeply banked to prevent excessive rotation.

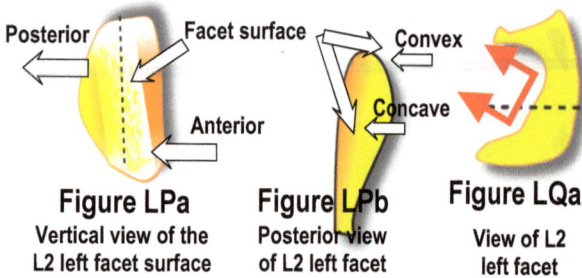

L2 posterior view

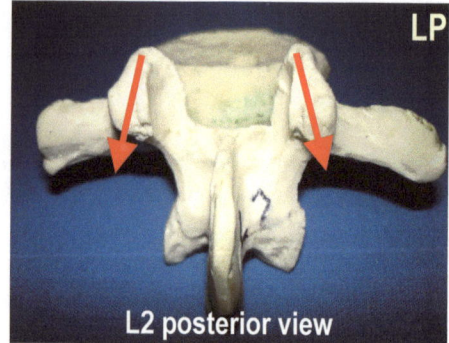

L2 view from above

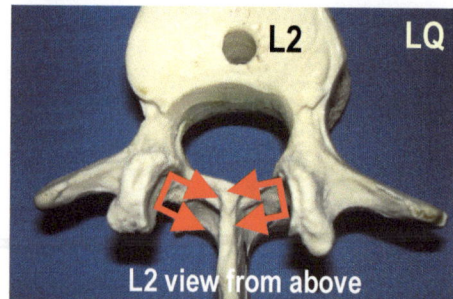

Figure LPa
Vertical view of the
L2 left facet surface

Figure LPb
Posterior view
of L2 left facet

Figure LQa
View of L2
left facet

L1 facet shape

Figures LR and **LS** show the concave and convex facet surface of the L1 vertebra. To make it easier to understand, this shape has been exaggerated and illustrated in **figure LRa**.

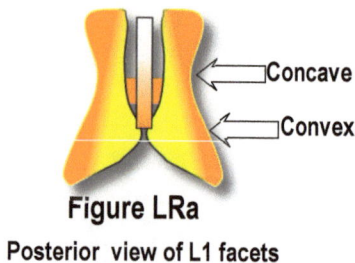

L1 view from below

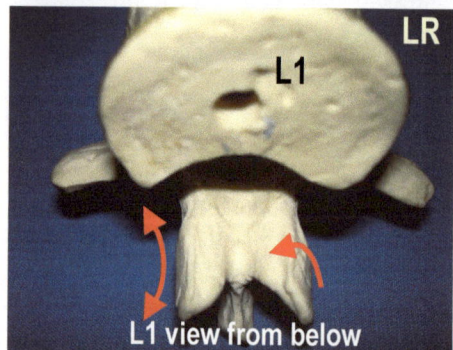

Figure LRa
Posterior view of L1 facets

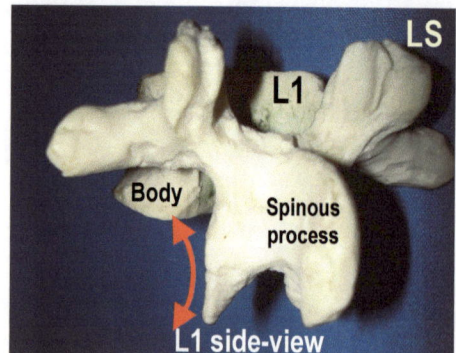

L1 side-view

L1
The Plateau Base

Figure LT shows the position of the nucleus pulposus on the body of L2. **Figure LUa** is a cross section and illustrates how the facet surfaces of the L1 and L2 vertebrae engage. **Figure LUb** is an illustration of the joint in neutral.

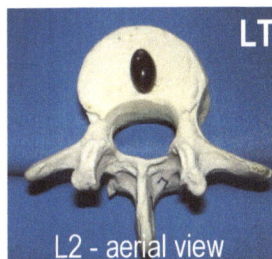

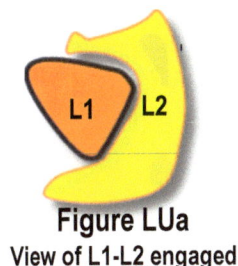

L1 the plateau base overview

To recap, the purpose of the L1 vertebra is to create a stable and level base for the thoracic column. L1 acts as a form of shock absorber that shields the thoracic column from the lumbar side-bending and rotation that takes place during walking. L1 also creates a level base for the thoracic column during rotation. L1 is also capable of making flexion and extension movements, as illustrated in **figures LUc** and **LUd**.

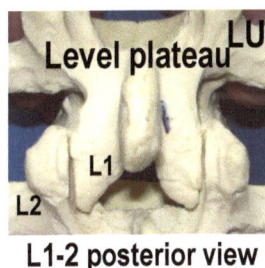

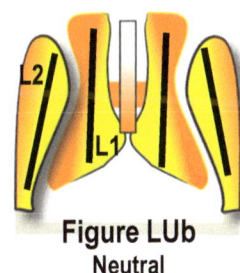

L2 side-bending and rotation

When L1 and L2 are placed together the first thing to notice is the amount of 'play' in the joint. This is illustrated in **figures LV** and **LW**. This amount of 'play' would appear to be a deliberate design feature because it allows L1 to efficiently absorb small amounts of side-bending and rotation without touching the facets of L2.

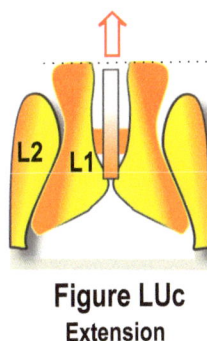

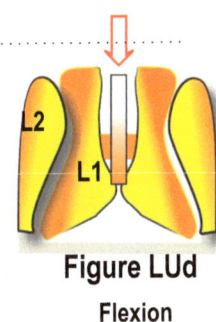

Due to the oblique angles of the L2 facet shape, see **figure LPa**, rotation from the lumbar vertebrae below is dissipated when the L1 facets travel this line.

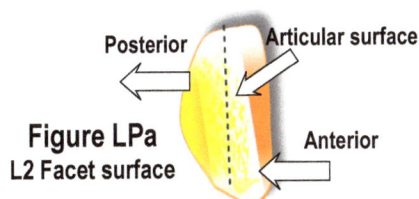

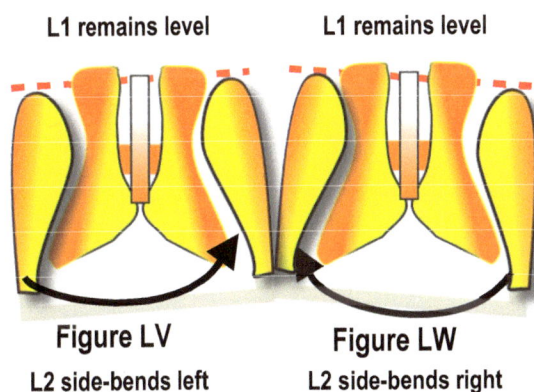

LT

L2 - aerial view

Figure LUa
View of L1-L2 engaged

Level plateau LU

L1-2 posterior view

Figure LUb
Neutral

Figure LUc
Extension

Figure LUd
Flexion

L1 remains level

L1 remains level

Figure LV
L2 side-bends left

Figure LW
L2 side-bends right

Posterior   Articular surface

Figure LPa
L2 Facet surface   Anterior

45

L1
Rotation Right in Lumbar Flexion

L1 flexion-rotation right

When the intention of a vertical person is to rotate to the right whilst leaning backwards, the following movements take place:

Figure LU on the previous page shows the L1 - L2 joint in the neutral starting point for the attempted flexion rotation to follow. (Be aware that the facets of the L1 mould are asymmetrical, which is what you would find in real human bones).

Weight bearing is taken on the left flexed knee through the anterior left 'A' sacroiliac facets. This causes L2, along with the lumbar vertebrae below, to side-bend to the left. **Figures LY** and **LYa** show the left L2 facet side-bending against the left LI facet.

Side-shift left in lumbar flexion is deliberately cancelled out for logistical reasons at L1. The mechanism of cancellation is illustrated in **figure 1** on page 42 and **figures LZ** and **LZa** .

When pelvic side-shift to the left takes place, the lumbar vertebrae including L2 are forced to the right. This causes L2 to cross over and engage against the right L1 facet, as shown in **figure LZa.**

Due to the vertical offset angle of the L1-L2 facets, as shown in **figure LZb,** the posterior aspect of the rotation of L2 is blocked.

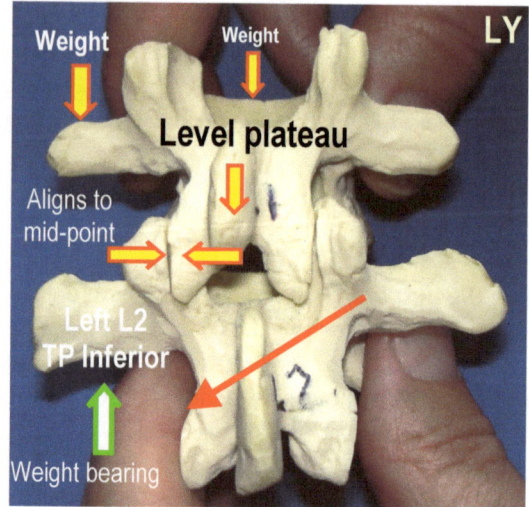

Figure LY

Weight — Weight — **LY**
Level plateau
Aligns to mid-point
Left L2 TP Inferior
Weight bearing

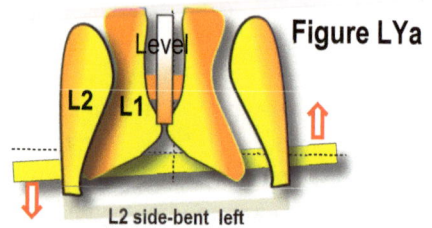

Figure LYa
Level
L2 L1
L2 side-bent left

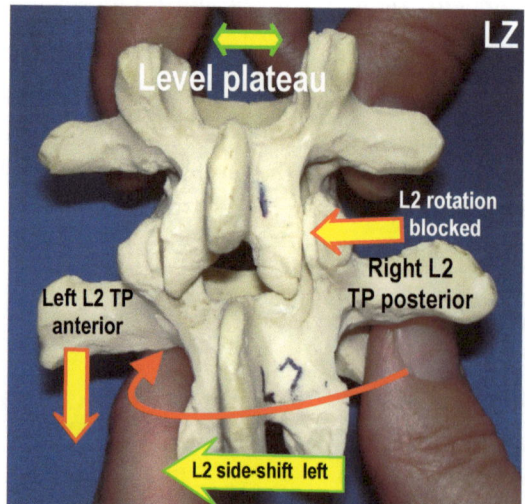

LZ
Level plateau
L2 rotation blocked
Right L2 TP posterior
Left L2 TP anterior
L2 side-shift left

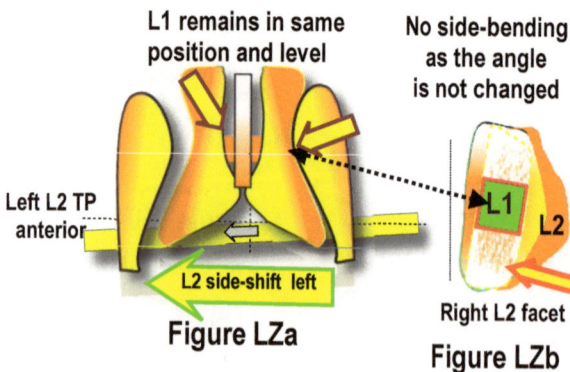

L1 remains in same position and level

No side-bending as the angle is not changed

Left L2 TP anterior
L2 side-shift left

Figure LZa

L1
L2
Right L2 facet

Figure LZb

Lumbar rotation is absorbed by the offset vertical angle of the L2-L1 joint.

L1
Rotation Right in Lumbar Extension

L1 extension, rotation right

When the intention of a vertical person is to rotate to the right whilst leaning forwards, the following movements take place.

Figure LU shown on page 45 is the neutral starting point for this movement.

Figures LBB and **LBBa** show L2 and L1 with rotation to the right. To cause this to happen, the left knee is flexed with the body weight taken on the right leg through the right sacroiliac 'F' facets. This action causes the pelvis and all the lumbar vertebrae, including L2-L1 to rotate right. The side-bending of the pelvis causes L2 to side-bend left fractionally, though the counter bodyweight and ground resistance on the right side make the side-bending considerably less than that caused in the flexion movement. L1 remains vertical throughout.

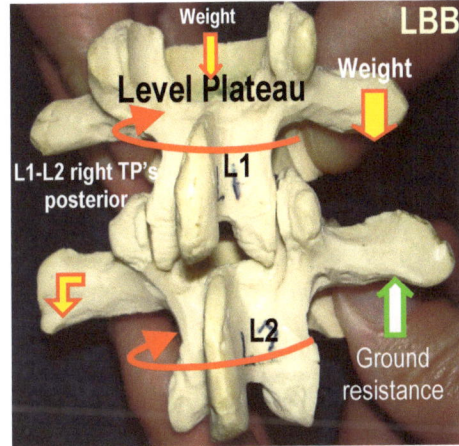

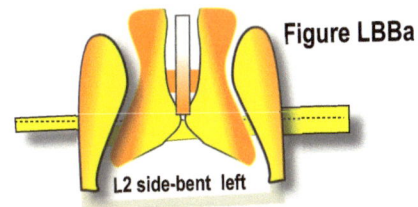

Figure LBBa

L2 side-bent left

The pelvis then side-shifts right and in turn all the lumbar vertebrae along with L2 side-shift right. In doing this the middle of the L2 facet engages with the middle of the left L1 facet, as shown in **figure LCCa.**

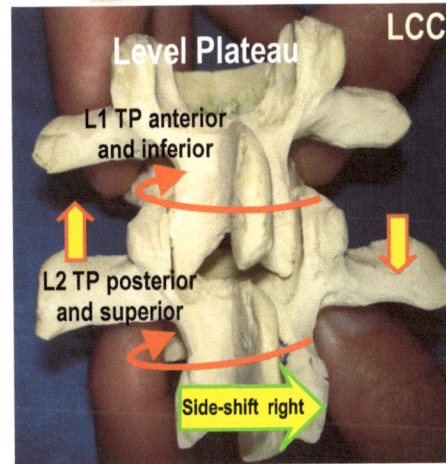

The side-bending to the right that takes place in the lumbar vertebrae below causes the left facet of L2 to move up the left L1 facet, as shown in **figure LCCb**. In doing this L1 remains vertical as L2 side-bends right. In relation to L2, L1 is rotated right and side-bent left.

With continued contact on the left facets of L1, pelvic side-shift can be passed upwards.

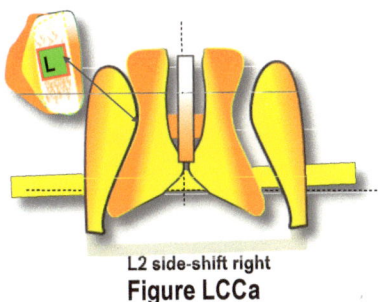

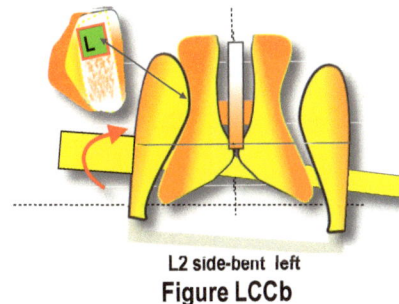

L2 side-shift right
Figure LCCa

L2 side-bent left
Figure LCCb

L1-T12
Anatomy

As was shown in the L2-L1 joint, rotation is limited. This shortcoming is corrected in the L1-T12 joint by some additional side-bending. The main function of L1-T12 though, is rotation.

L1 facet shape

Figures LCD and **LCDa** show the upper posterior L1 facets of a typical L1 vertebra. The upper facets of L1 are parallel vertically and marginally concave.

Figure LCE and **LCEa** show the concave and rounded shape of the upper L1 facets.

Figure LCEb illustrates the angle of the facet trajectory.

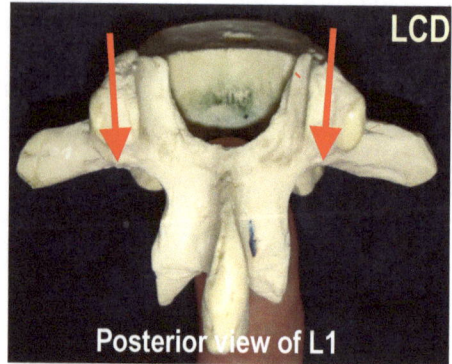

Posterior view of L1

LCD

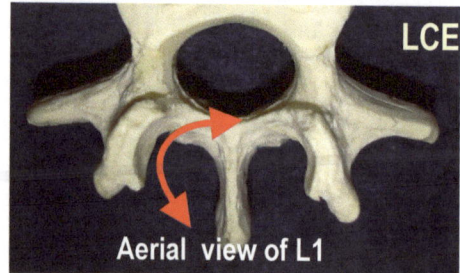

Aerial view of L1

LCE

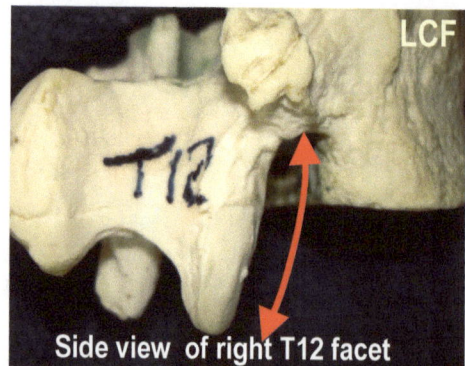

Figure LCDa

Figure LCEa
Cross section of L1 facet

Posterior

Articular surface

Figure LCEb
Angle of left L1 facet surface

Anterior

T12 facet shape

Figure LCF and **LCG** show the long marginally rounded shape of the inferior posterior facets of T12.

These shapes are made clearer by the illustrations shown in figures **LCFa** and **LCGa.**

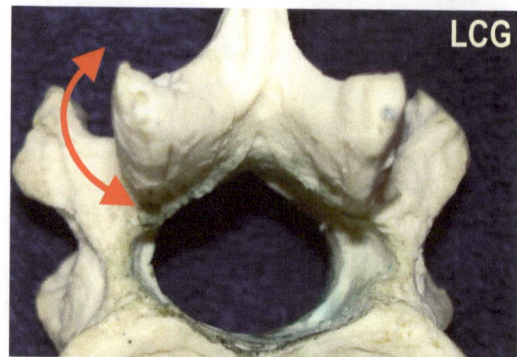

Side view of right T12 facet

LCF

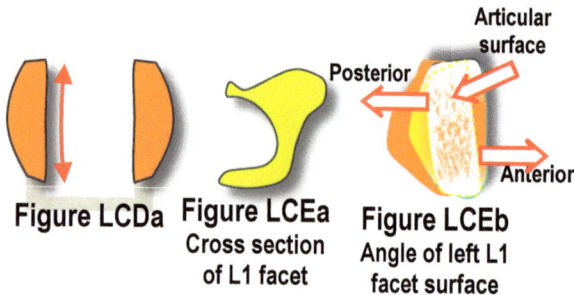

Vertical

Articular surface

Figure LCFa
Side view of left T12 inferior posterior facet

Figure LCGa
Cross section of inferior T12 facets

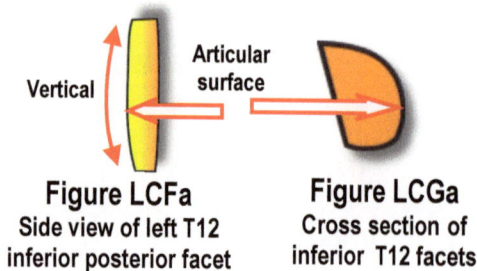

View from below of T12 facet

LCG

L1-T12
Physiology

Like the L2-L1 joint the first thing to notice when the L1-T12 facets are placed together is the amount of 'play' in the joint. This is illustrated in **figures LCH** and **LCHa.** The rounded facet shapes and the amount of play in the joint, are illustrated in the cross section **figure LCHf**.

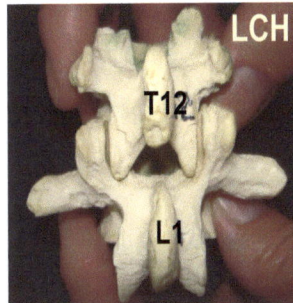

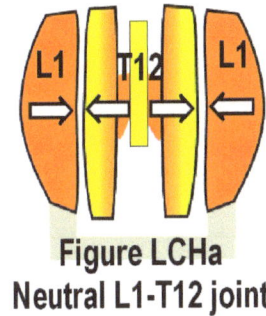

Due to the amount of 'play' in the joint, L1 has the ability to side-bend left and right without making contact with the sides of the T12 facets. This is illustrated in **figures LCHb** and **LCHc.** The 'play' in the L1-T12 joint and that found in the L2-L1 joint, act synergetically as a shock absorber during walking. Their purpose is to shield the thoracic column, neck and head from jerks, rotation and side-bending with minimal effort.

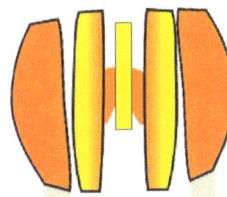

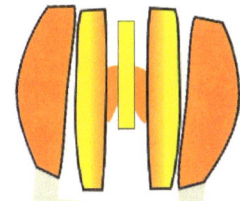

To further illustrate the versatility of the way the L1 facets move around the T12 facets **figure LCHbb** illustrates rotation singularly, and **figure LCHcc,** when rotation and side-bending are combined. Notice again that the sides of the L1 facets do not touch the sides of the T12 facets. **Figures LCHg** and **LCHh** illustrate this in cross section and show the way L1 rotates around T12 to take up the side-bending and rotation caused by the walking action without contact.

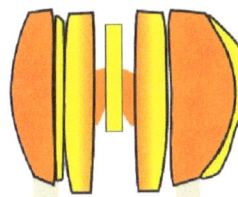

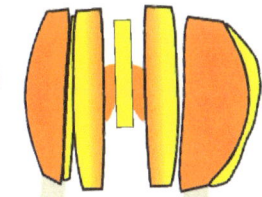

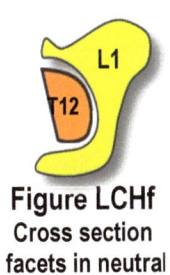

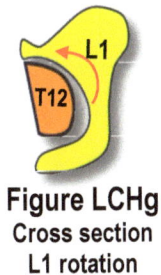

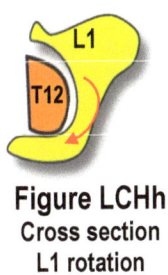

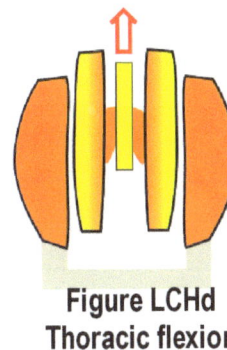

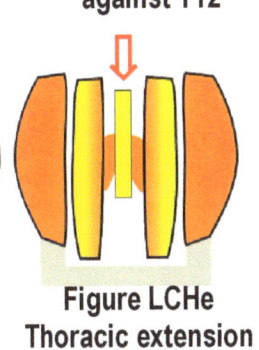

Figure LCHf
Cross section facets in neutral

Figure LCHg
Cross section L1 rotation

Figure LCHh
Cross section L1 rotation

The joint is also able to flex and extend as shown in **figures LCHd** and **LCHe.**

Figure LCHa
Neutral L1-T12 joint

Figure LCHb
L1 side-bending left against T12

Figure LCHc
L1 side-bending right against T12

Figure LCHbb
L1 rotating right against T12

Figure LCHcc
L1 rotating and side-bending right against T12

Figure LCHd
Thoracic flexion

Figure LCHe
Thoracic extension

49

T12 when Side-Shift is to the Right

Rotation left in thoracic flexion

When the L2-L1 joint rotates right as described on the previous pages, L1 should be level and rotated to the right in relation to L2. With side-shift and weight to the right, the gravity line will pass to the right of L1 and the thoracic column. This was shown in **figure 2** on page 43.

At the joint of L1-T12, two possible actions take place. **Figures LCHa** and **LCJ** show neutral.

Figure LCHa
Posterior view
L1-T12 facets in neutral

Figure LCJ
Cross section
left facets in neutral

Thoracic rotation right

1) When the intention is for the thoracic vertebrae to rotate right, the right side facets of L1 side-shift right and engage squarely against the left T12 facets. In doing this T12 follows the general pelvic rotation to the right. This is illustrated in **figures LCK** and **LCL**.

Side-shift right

Figure LCK
L1 side-shift right

Figure LCL
L1 side-shift right

T12 rotation left

2) If side-shift is taken further to the right, along with increased left knee flexion, there would be an excessive amount of rotation to the right in the upper torso. This would cause de-stabilization.

To compensate for this, T12 limits the amount of rotation to the right that originated from the pelvis by rotating to the left. The mechanics work like this, when excessive side-shift to the right continues unchecked, as shown in **figures LCM** and **LCN**, the left T12 facet banks up the left L1 facet and causes T12 vertebra to rotate left.

This brings stability back to the spine and limits thoracic rotation right. This is illustrated in **figures LCO** and **LCP.**

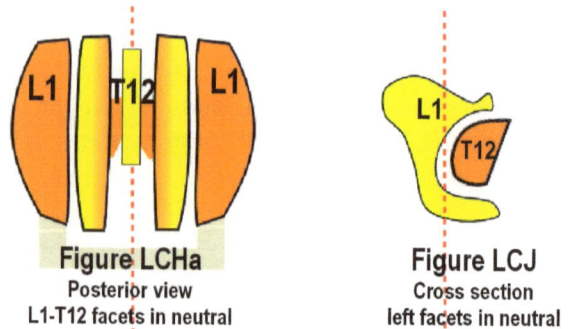

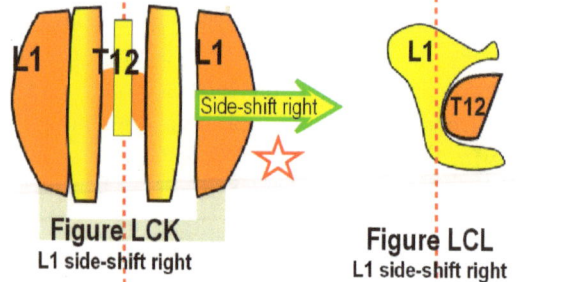

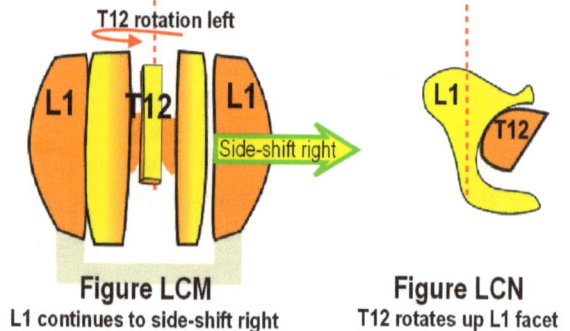

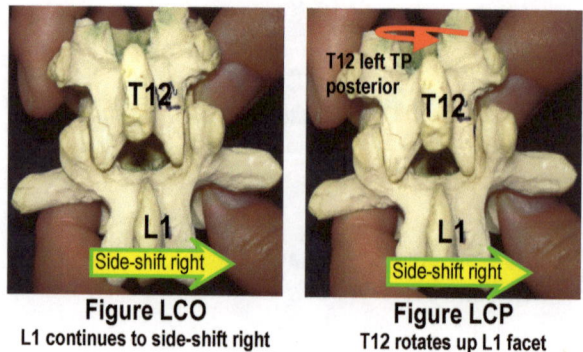

T12 rotation left

Side-shift right

Figure LCM
L1 continues to side-shift right

Figure LCN
T12 rotates up L1 facet

T12 left TP
posterior

Side-shift right

Figure LCO
L1 continues to side-shift right

Side-shift right

Figure LCP
T12 rotates up L1 facet

50

Chapter Four

Physiology of Walking

For a sacroiliac theory to be proved, it must satisfy working criteria. It must be capable of applying forward and backward bending, side-bending, rotation and most important of all, locomotion.

Ambulation overview

The photograph in **figure WA** demonstrates the first stage of the walking action.

It can be seen that Lisa's pelvis has side-shifted to the right and that her right leg is posterior, lateral and weight bearing.

Reciprocally her left leg is lifted medially, superiorly and anteriorly.

From the front, the sacroiliac joints would look like the illustration in **figure WAa**.

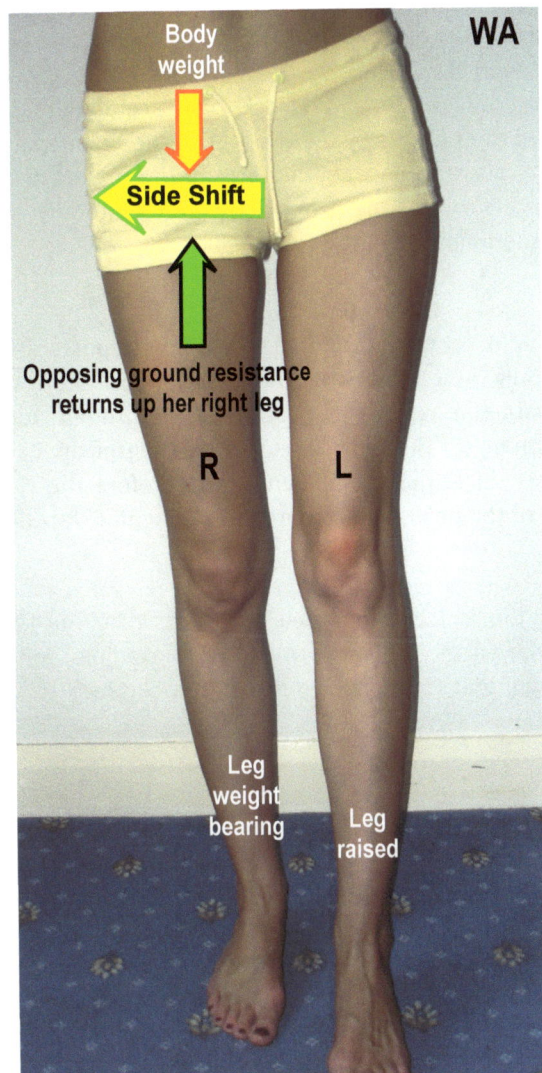

Figure WAa

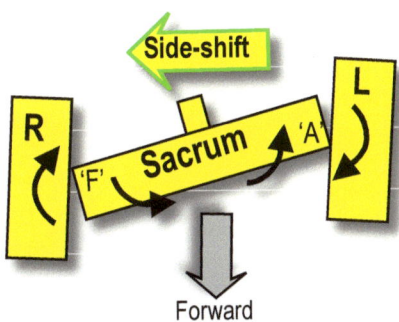

Walking Stage One
Weight Bearing

Stage one of the pelvic and transitory stage shown on the previous page illustrated the position of the pelvis. This position prepares the lumbar vertebrae to work in harmony.

To initiate the walking action, body weight must be directed to one leg. In our example, the right leg is being demonstrated. It is physiologically impossible to stand on one leg without toppling over so the pelvis side-shifts to the right leg to compensate for the redistribution of body weight. We start from here.

Figure WB shows the weight bearing right sacroiliac joint with the 'F' facets engaged. Resistant ground force passes up through the right acetabulum and levers the right 'F' posterior facet of the Ilium against the 'F' posterior facet of the sacrum. This mating of the 'F' facets rotates the right Ilium posterio-laterally and the sacrum to the left. See page 34.

The right acetabulum would be positioned posteriorly, laterally and inferiorly. The inferior position of the acetabulum is met by the reactive ground force returning up the right leg. This meeting of opposing forces lifts the acetabulum and therefore the right side of the pelvis and compresses the right 'F' facets.

With the 'F' facets engaged and weight bearing, the lumbar vertebrae (using L4-L3 as an example) follow the general rotation of the pelvis and rotate to the right.

The body weight and opposing ground counter force on the right side approximate the right L3-L4 facets. This aligns the left facets of L3 in the correct starting position for side-bending to the right to follow when side-shift right is applied, as shown in **figure WC**.

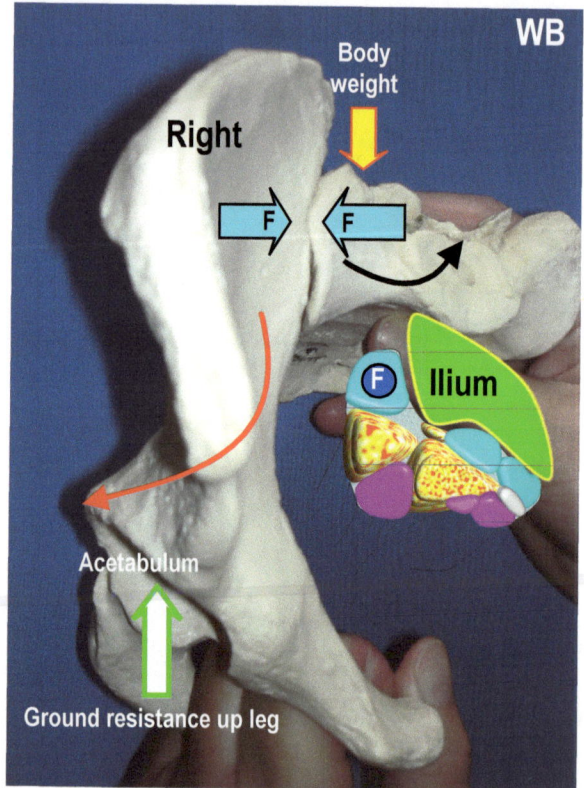

Anterior view of right sacroiliac 'F' posterior facets engaged

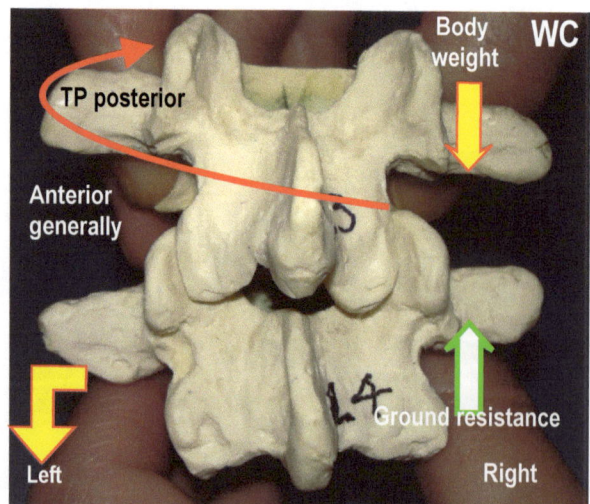

Posterior view of L4-L3 rotation right from pelvis

Walking Stage One
Joint action

In **stage one** of the pelvic transition to full side-shift to the right, shown in **figures WB** and **WBa** the sacrum would be rotated right with weight directed down the right leg. This initial rotation is shown for completeness in **figure WBa**.

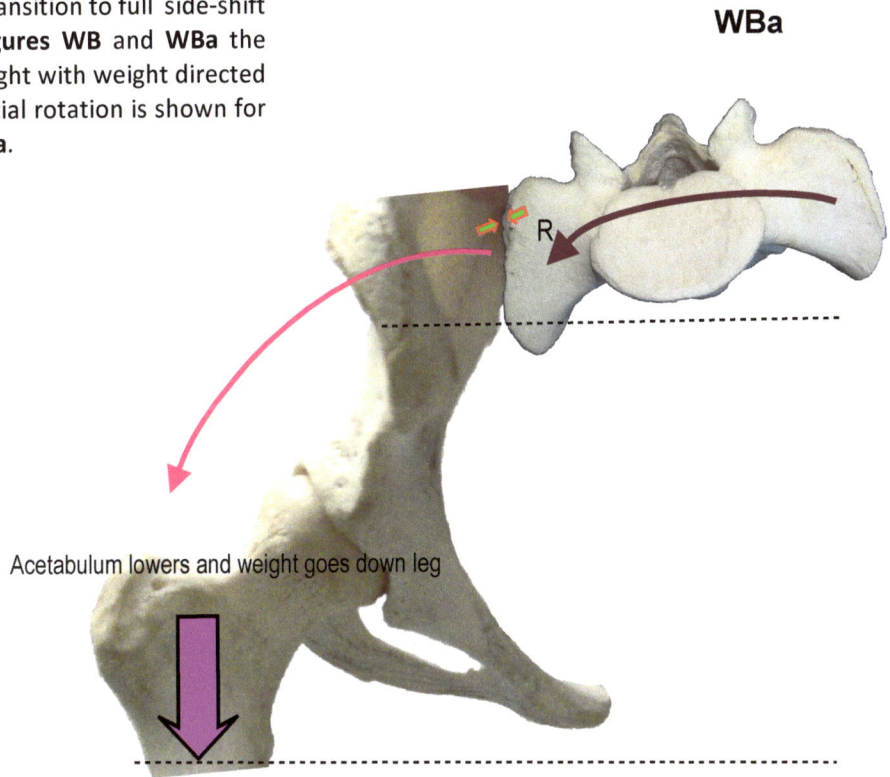

WBa

R

Acetabulum lowers and weight goes down leg

In **stage two,** full pelvic side-shift to the right is shown in **figures WDa** and **WD**. The sacral rotation to the right is countered by the reactive ground resistance returning up the right leg. By raising the acetabulum the side-shift compressing the 'F' facets blocks extreme sacral rotation and pelvis side-shift to the right, as shown in **figure Wdb**.

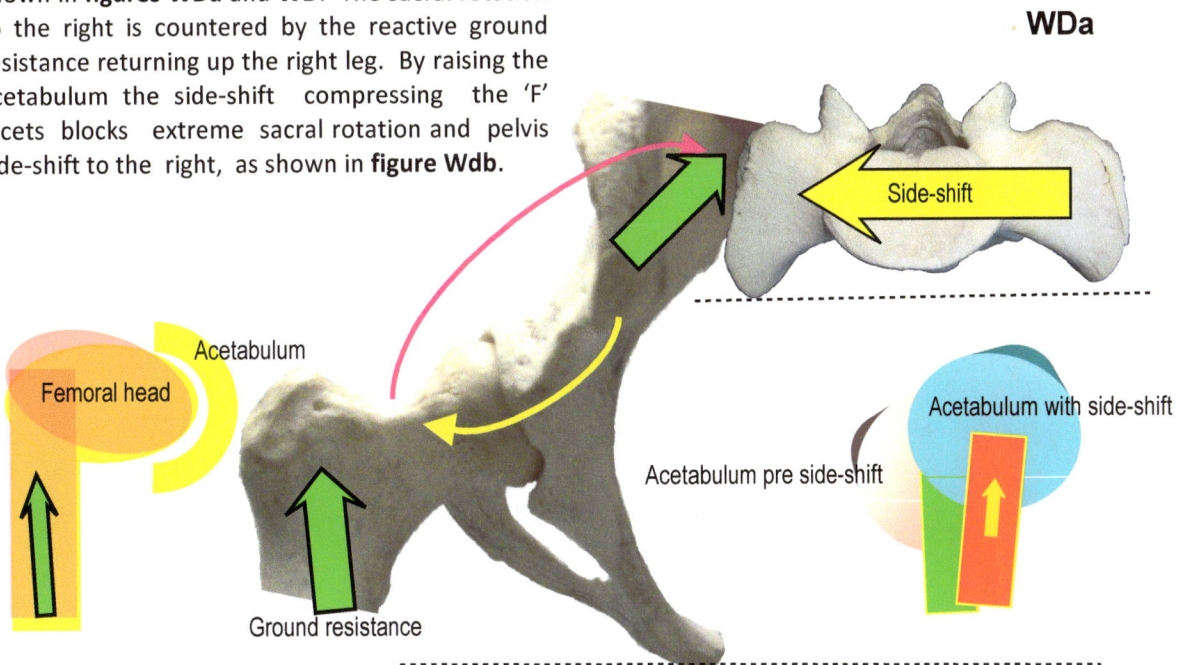

WDa

Side-shift

Acetabulum

Femoral head

Acetabulum with side-shift

Acetabulum pre side-shift

Ground resistance

Walking Stage Two
Side-Shift and Ground Resistance

When pelvic side-shift to the right is applied, as shown in **figure WD,** the right 'A' facets are forced apart still further and the sacrum rotates left and directs left side of the pelvis to lift. This was shown in **figure WAa** at the start of this chapter and in **figure Wfa** on the next page. The acetabulum and femur are thus levered anterio-medially.

On the left, this lever action lifts the anterior thigh muscles attached to the anterior of the part of the Ilium posterio-laterally and angles the left leg forward. The posterior thigh muscles attached to the posterior ischial tuberosity are also pulled posterio-laterally and cause the knee to flex. This kick starts the muscle action to follow.

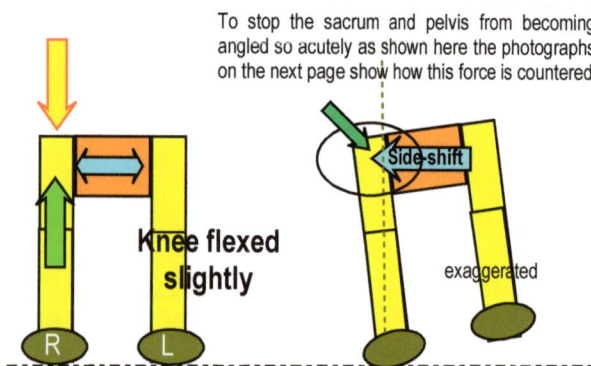

WD

Body weight

Right

F   F

Side-shift

A   A

Reactive ground Resistance

Anterior view of right innominate

To stop the sacrum and pelvis from becoming angled so acutely as shown here the photographs on the next page show how this force is countered

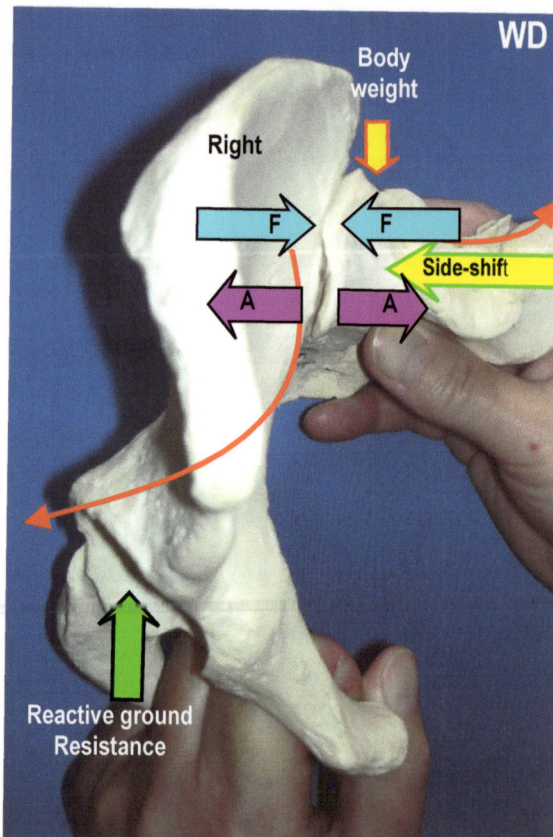

Side-shift

Knee flexed slightly

exaggerated

R   L

**Figure WDb
Anterior View**

The pelvic side-shift continues up the spine and in turn L4 side-shifts to the right. With counter resistance to the left from above, the left facet of L3 banks up the left facet of L4. In doing this L3 becomes side-bent to the right, as shown in **figure WE.**

Therefore, in the walking lumbar movement, rotation and side-bending are to the same side, which is lumbar extension.

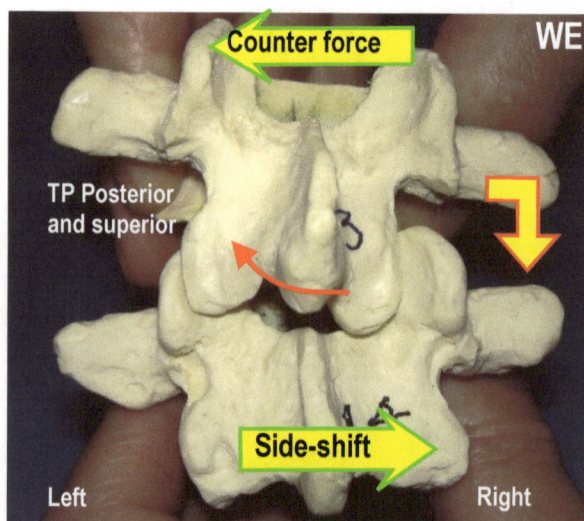

WE

Counter force

TP Posterior and superior

Side-shift

Left   Right

**Posterior view of L4-L3
L3 side-bending right**

Walking Stage Three
Reciprocal Facet Action

When the right weight bearing 'F' sacroiliac facets are engaged and pelvic side-shift is to the right, the reciprocal action of the sacrum is to engage the left 'A' sacroiliac facets, as shown in **figures WF and WFA**.

When the left non-weight-bearing 'A' sacroiliac facets are engaged, the left acetabulum is levered anteriorly, medially and superiorly. This is described in more detail in **figure SK**. This force, with the aid of the left leg muscles, lifts the left leg forward as shown in **figure WA** on page 51 and **illustration A** below.

The right leg shown in **illustration B** is straight and weight bearing. The line of the body weight is taken through the load bearing 'F' sacroiliac facet.

If you watch an athlete run you will see that their left shoulder and arm move anteriorly when their body weight is to be taken on their right leg. This is an efficient way of transferring body weight without having to lean forwards and backwards.

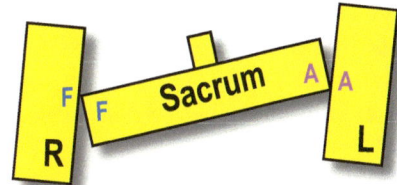

Figure WF
Anterior left facets engaged

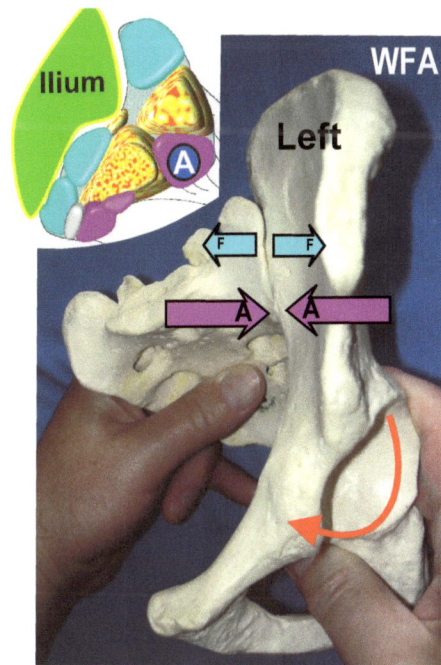

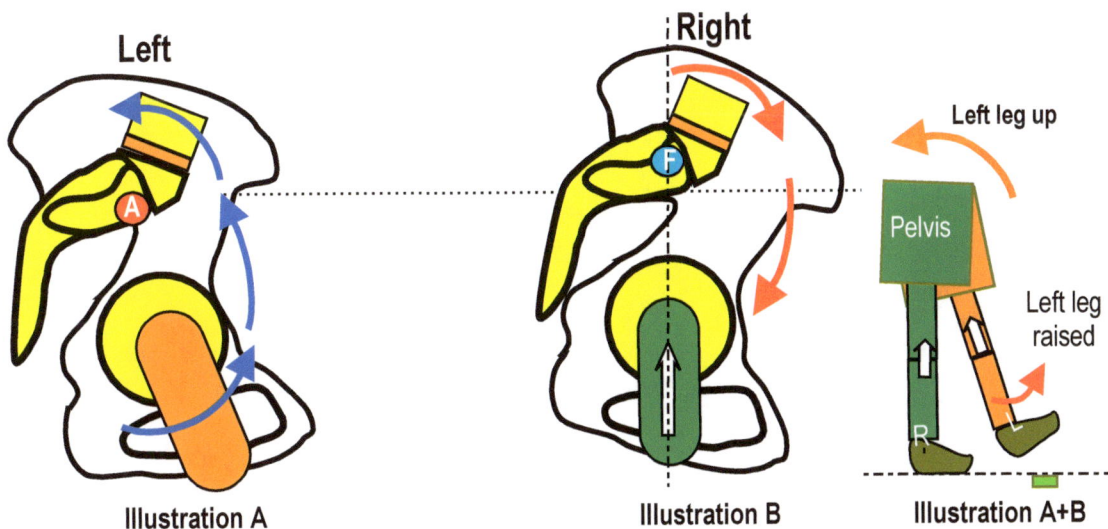

Ilium

Left

WFA

Left

Illustration A

Right

Illustration B

Left leg up

Pelvis

Left leg raised

Illustration A+B

Walking
Reciprocal Facet Action

In our illustration, to move forward the upper body inclines anteriorly on the left. This changes the weight focus and pushes the left leg downwards and levers the transitory 'B' sacroiliac facets on the left to engage and guide the left leg laterally. The heel of the left foot is the first to touch the ground. However, at this point the leg is still not fully weight bearing. Body weight is still taken on the right leg, though at this point, through the transitory right 'E' facets.

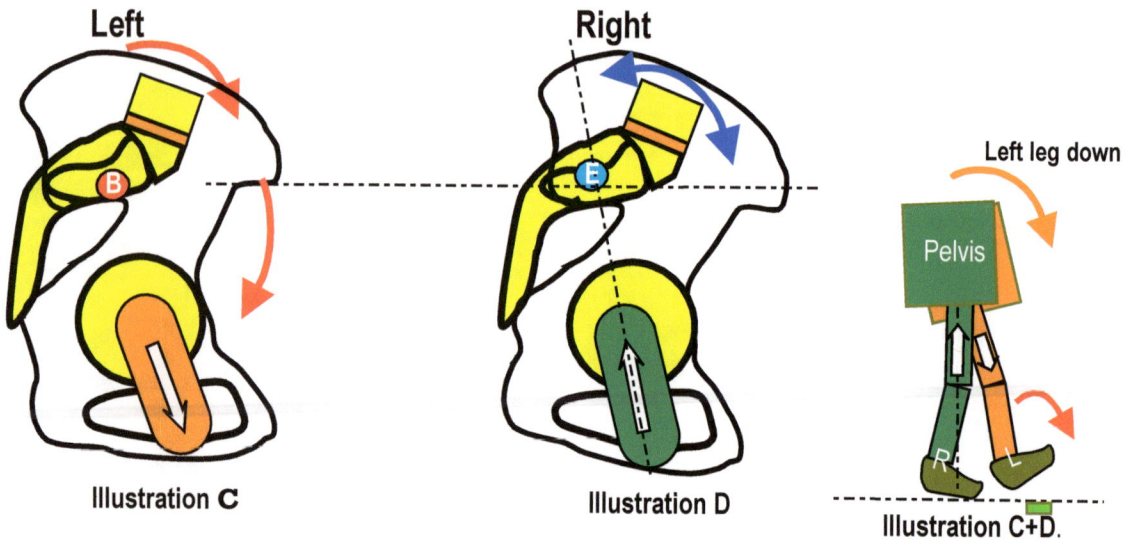

Left

Right

Left leg down

Pelvis

Illustration **C**

Illustration D

Illustration **C+D**.

As the body weight continues to focus down on the left leg, the sacroiliac fulcrum changes from the left 'B' sacroiliac facets to the transitory 'C' sacroiliac facets, as shown in **illustration E.** Reciprocally, the right sacroiliac 'E' facets transfer to the right transitory 'D' sacroiliac facets, as shown in **illustration F.** At this transitory point, weight is evenly distributed down both legs, as shown in **illustrations E** and **F.** Side-shift is marginally to the left.

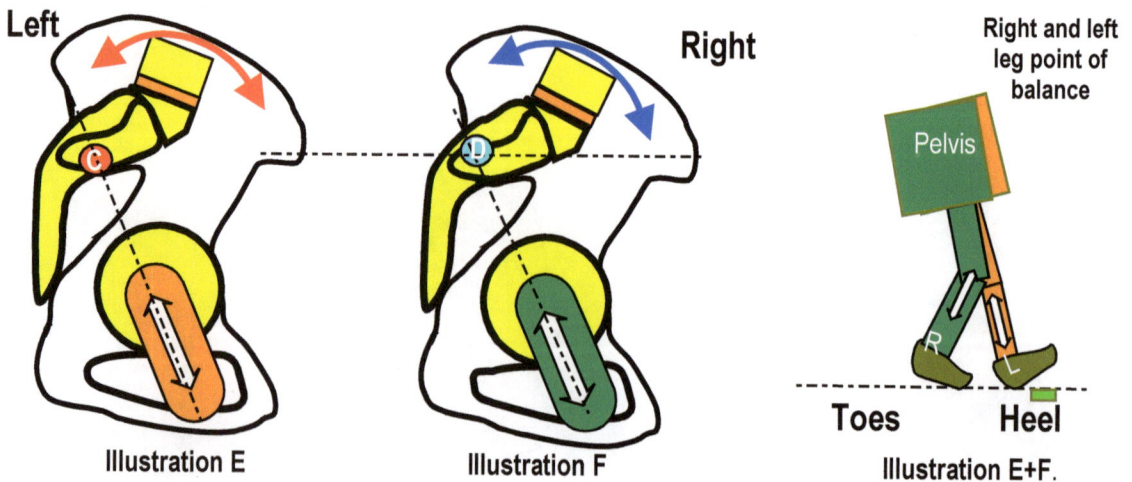

Left

Right

Right and left leg point of balance

Pelvis

Illustration **E**

Illustration **F**

Toes   **Heel**

Illustration **E+F**.

56

Walking
Reciprocal Facet Action

As the upper body weight continues to bear down on the left leg, the fulcrum applied to the left sacroiliac facet transfers to the opposite side against the weight bearing 'E' sacroiliac facets, as shown in **illustration E.** Reciprocally on the right, the facets transfer to the transitory non-weight-bearing 'B' sacroiliac facets, shown in **illustration F.** The left knee flex's to accommodate the transfer of body weight onto the left leg, shown in **illustrations E** and **F.**

Left

Right

Left leg becomes fully weight-bearing

Pelvis

Illustration E

Illustration F

Illustration E+F

And finally we have come full circle. The left leg becomes the true weight bearing leg with the weight taken through the left 'F' facet. When pelvic side-shift to the left takes place, the right 'A' facets engage and the right leg is levered forward.

Left

Right

Left leg up

Pelvis

Illustration G

Illustration H

Illustration G+H

Walking
Backwards

The principles shown previously within this chapter refer specifically to walking forward. These principles can be equally applied to the actions of running or climbing stairs. Forward motion is mainly governed by the lower limbs of the body interacting on the Ilia. Within this action the sacrum plays a secondary role. Therefore, walking forward is an **iliosacral movement**.

These principles however, cannot be applied to the action of walking backwards. This involves a much less complicated procedure and is described next. Backward motion is governed by the top half of the body placing a rotational force on the sacrum. Within this action the Ilia play a secondary role. Therefore, walking backwards is a **sacroiliac movement**.

Figure WQ shows Sam taking a step backwards with her right leg. In order to complete this movement she had to focus her body weight through her left sacroiliac joint and leg.

Her torso had to be inclined forward with her muscles braced, in order to act as a long lever. Her pelvis then had to be side-shifted to the left to engage the 'F' sacroiliac facets.

The combination of the side-shift and weight focus on the left side of her pelvis and leg caused her right leg to lift. The side-shift also caused her sacrum and therefore her torso to rotate to the right and thereby guide her right leg backwards, with minimal effort.

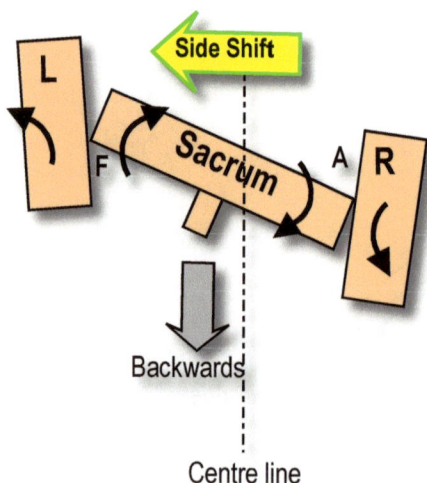

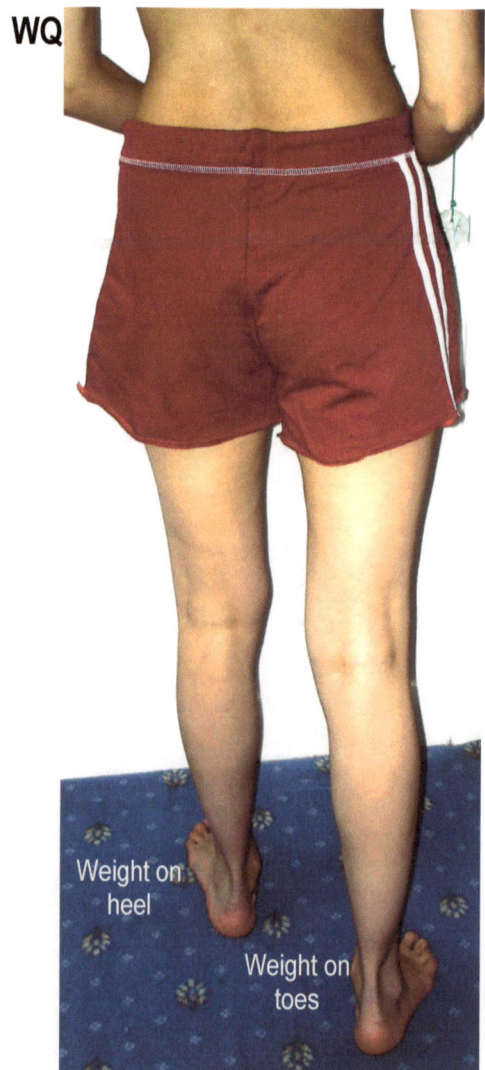

Walking
Backwards Left Side Facet Action

Figure WO shows the left side of the sacroiliac joint when weight bearing is on the left. The sacrum is rotated to the right by the engagement of the left 'F' sacroiliac facets.

It is important to remember that the sacrum is moving against the Ilium.

Figure WM is a picture of the L4-L3 joint. With body weight pivoting through the left leg, the levering lumbar vertebrae work as one with the sacrum and rotate to the right.

When pelvic side-shift takes place to the left and compress the 'F' sacroiliac facets, L3 as shown in **figure WP** side-bends to the left.

This means that when walking backwards, lumbar rotation and side-bending are to opposite sides.

Below for information, **figure WPa** shows the line of gravity passing to the left of L1. This line of gravity causes the thoracic vertebrae which will be in thoracic flexion, due to the leaning forward, to rotate to the left.

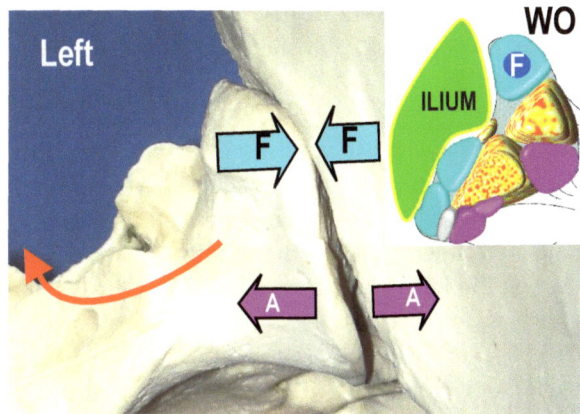

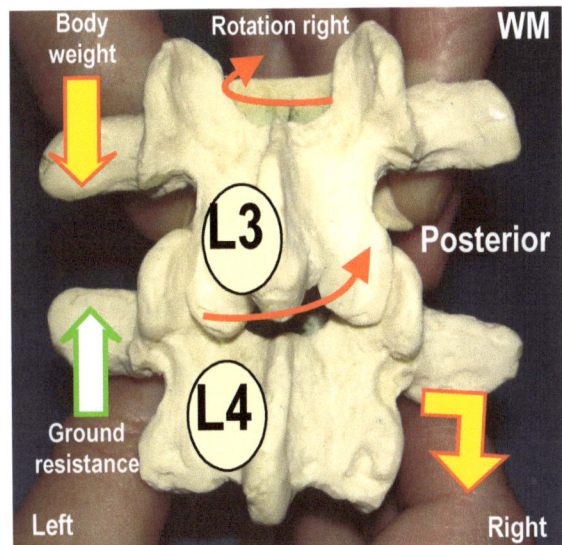

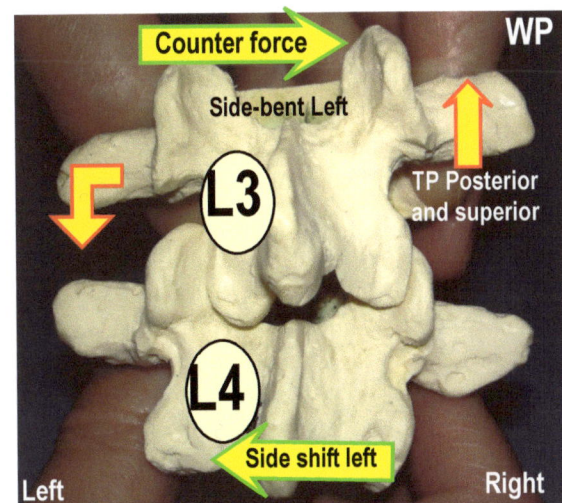

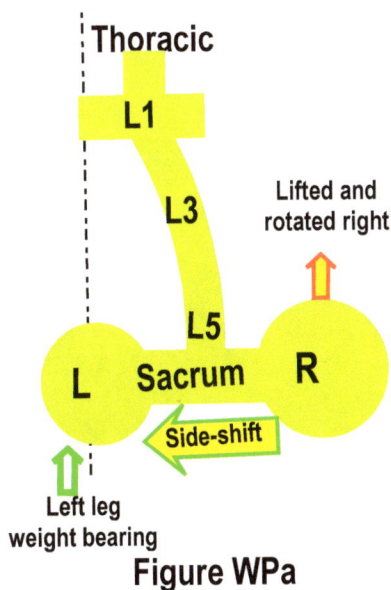

Figure WPa

59

Walking
Backwards Right Side

When the right leg rotates backwards, the right 'A' sacroiliac facets engage, as shown in **illustration WR**.

To continue moving backwards, side-shift transfers to the right and the torso rotates to the left. This causes the weight bearing 'F' sacroiliac facets on the right to engage and reciprocally, the guider 'A' facets to engage on the left. This is shown in **figure WRa**.

Because the guiding rotation originates from the torso/vertebrae, the torso rotates from side to side as the person walks backwards.

This is because backward walking is governed by the forward bent rotation of the torso acting on the sacrum. This limits the articulation of the sacrum to two facets of the Ilia only; the 'F' facets on one side and the 'A' facets on the other.

With only two facet engagements, walking backwards is uneven and jerky when compared to the smooth motion of walking forward.

Figure WRa

Direction of Rotation

During backward walking, when backward rotation to the left takes place, the torso rotates along with the sacrum to the right. This is illustrated in **figure WRb**.

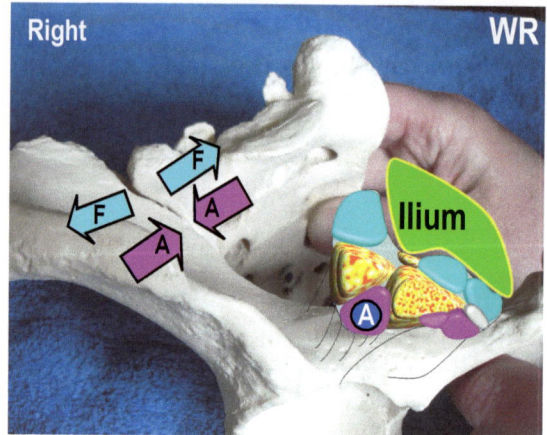

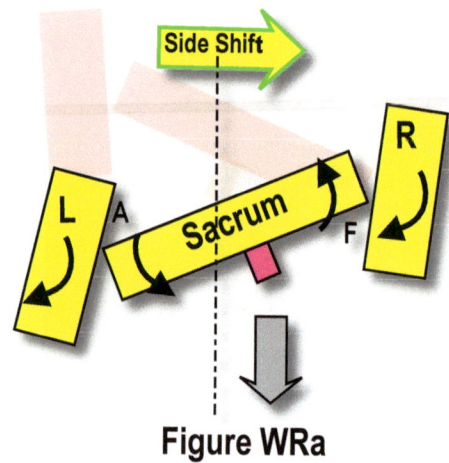

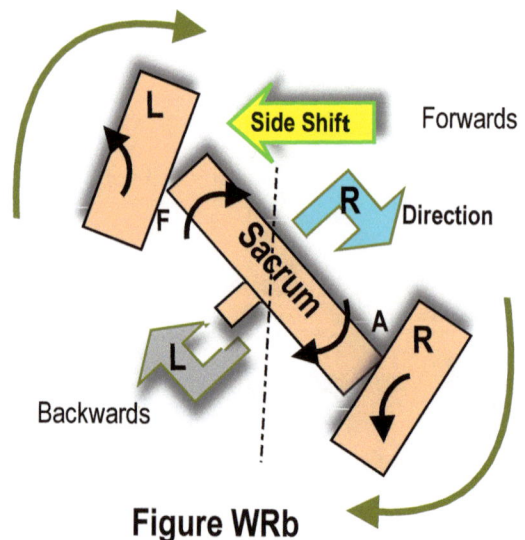

Figure WRb

60

Chapter Five

Physiology of the Thoracic Joints

Overview

Attached to the thoracic vertebrae are ribs. For the rib bucket handle mechanism to work efficiently the ribs need to be kept parallel at all times. To take account of this, nature developed a facet shape for the thoracic vertebrae, that not only enabled this to happen when the thoracic vertebrae are vertical, but also when rotation and side-bending takes place.

The overall shape of the thoracic spine is convex posteriorly. This is an opposite curve to the cervical and lumbar vertebrae.

Like the lumbar vertebrae thoracic articulation is governed by the **G** and **M** forces. In **figure 1** on page 42 it was shown that the **G** and **M** forces become blocked in thoracic extension (backward bending) and encouraged in thoracic flexion (forward bending), see **figure 2** page 43.

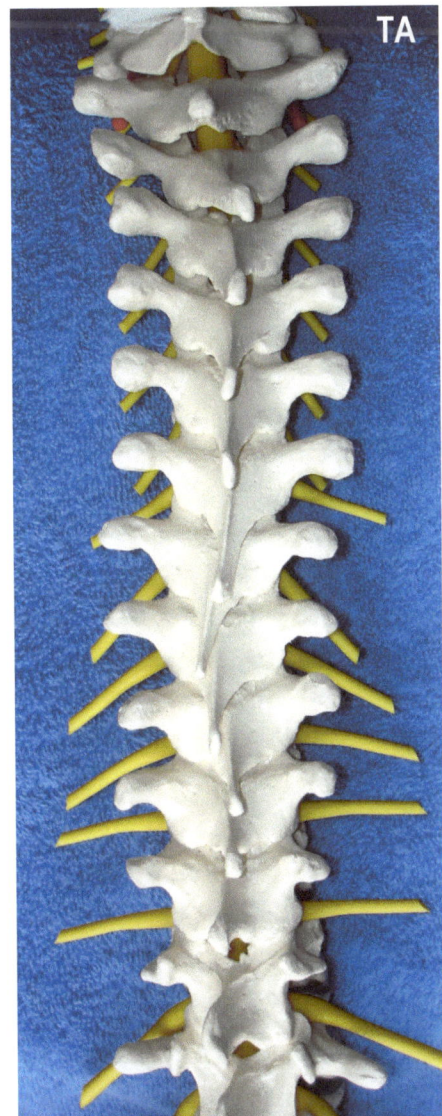

61

Thoracic Reference

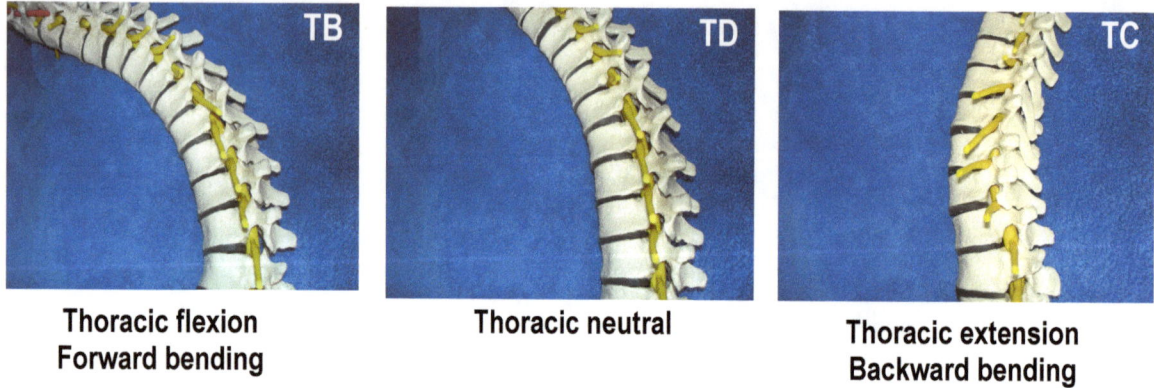

Thoracic flexion
Forward bending

Thoracic neutral

Thoracic extension
Backward bending

Figure TB shows the thoracic spine in flexion. Flexion is forward bending.

Figure TC shows the thoracic spine in extension. Extension is backward bending.

When neither flexion or extension is present, the thoracic spine is in neutral, as shown in **figure TD**.

There are twelve thoracic vertebrae. The facet shapes are not all the same. Some of the facets are obviously rounded in their horizontal plane and others flat. However, in the examples I have seen they are all rounded in such a way as to allow the joint above some degree of rotation. The T2-T1 joint facets are concave and work in a vaguely similar way to the lower lumbar facets. The list below compares the facet shapes of my plastic bones with real bones:

Thoracic Vertebrae	Plastic Bones Facet shape	Real Bones* Facet shape
T1	Convex	Convex
T2	Concave***	Concave***
T3	Convex	Convex
T4	Convex	Convex
T5	Convex	Convex
T6	Convex	Convex
T7	Flat -Convex**	Convex
T8	Flat -Convex**	Convex
T9	Flat-Convex**	Convex
T10	Flat -Convex**	Convex
T11	Flat -Convex**	Convex
T12	Flat -Convex**	Spacer

* The real bones originate from Asia. I think the skeleton is that of an unfortunate boy who must have died somewhere between the age of ten and thirteen years of age.

** Flat-Convex, is shown on the next page. Convex facets would provide greater rotation than those that are flatter yet angle convexly in relation to each other.

*** At T2-T1 there is a change in the thoracic curve from flexion to extension.

Thoracic
T7 Facet Anatomy

TE — T7 — Posterior view

TEa — T4 — Posterior view

Thoracic joints

Figures TE and **TEa** show the posterior superior facets of T7 and T4 in overview. T4 has been added for facet comparison purposes.

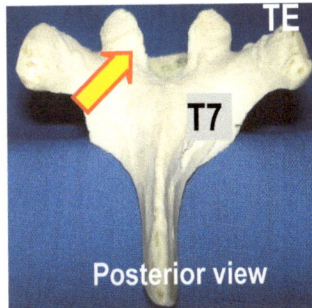

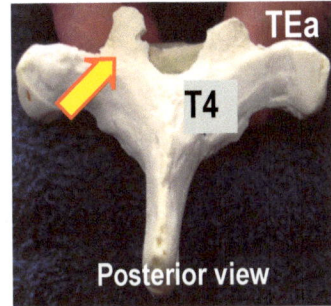

TF — T7 — Right side view

TFa — TX — Right side view

Figures TF and **TFa** show side views of the T7 and T4 facets. Both are marginally convex along their vertical plane.

Note that the T7 facets are more upright and less convex vertically.

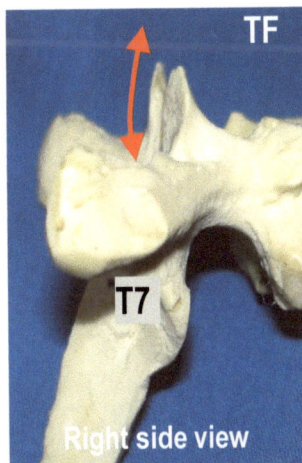

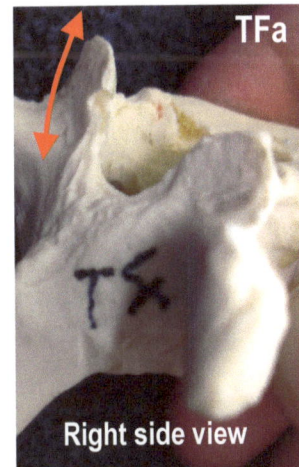

TG — T7 — Flat-Convex — View from above

TGa — T4 — Convex — View from above

Figures TG and **TGa** show aerial views of the T7 and T4 facets. It can be seen that both are convex horizontally. The T4 facets form a more rounded circumference. This is illustrated more clearly in **figures TGb** and **TGc**.

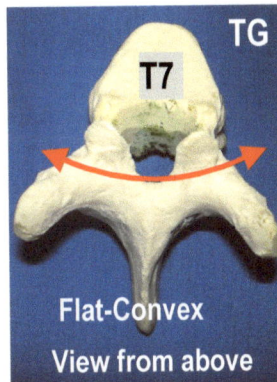

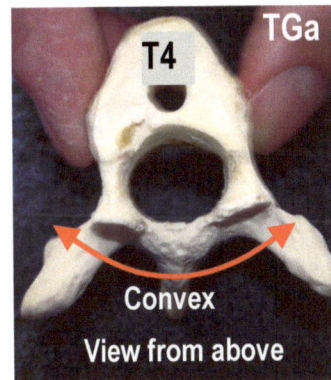

Figure TGb
Flat-Convex

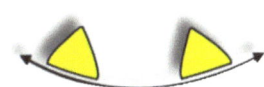

Figure TGc
Convex

Thoracic
T6 Facet Anatomy

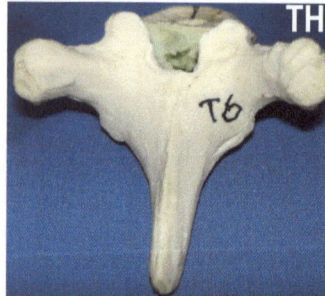

TH

Posterior view
of T6

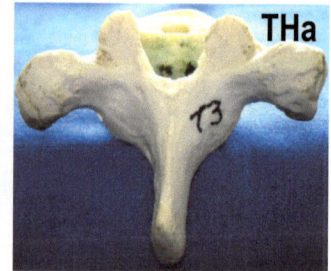

THa

Posterior view
of T3

Figures TH and **THa** show for reference the T6 and T3 vertebrae in overview**.** Again, T3 has been added for facet comparison.

Figures TJ and **TJa** show views from below of the T6 and T3 facets. It can be seen that both sets of facets are concave horizontally. The T4 facets are more rounded.

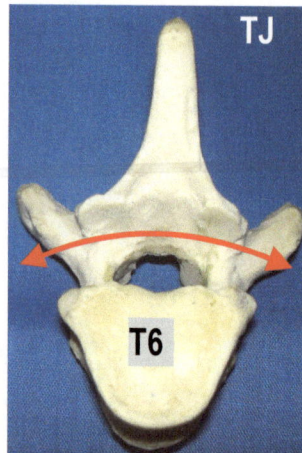

TJ

T6

View from below
of T6 facets

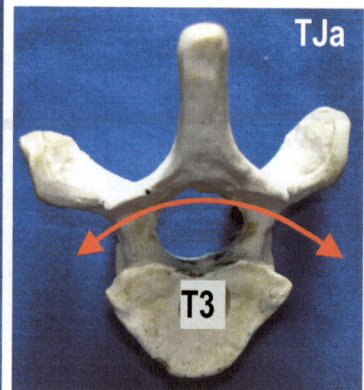

TJa

T3

View from below
of T3 facets

Figures TK and **TKa** show side-views from below of the T6 and T3 inferior facets. It can be seen that both sets of facets are marginally concave in their horizontal axes. The vertical concavity provides the facets with the ability to flex and extend.

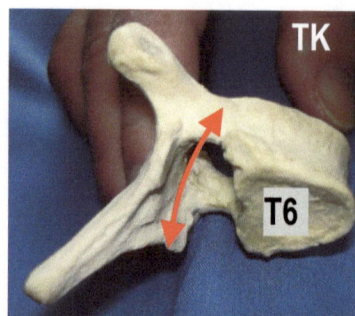

TK

T6

Right side view
from below of T6

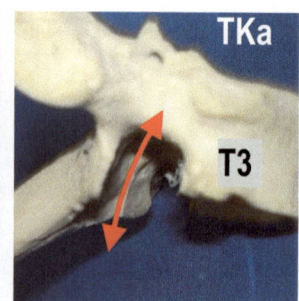

TKa

T3

Right side view
from below of T3

Thoracic Flexion and Extension

There are two reasons why thoracic vertebrae flex and extend:

1. To aid the rib breathing mechanism with very small amounts of flexion and extension.

2. To achieve forward and backward bending of the thoracic spine.

Figure TL shows the position of the facets when the T7-T6 joint is in neutral.

Figure TM shows the position of the facets when the T7-T6 joint is placed in flexion or when breathing out; expiration.

Figure TN shows the position of the facets when the T7-T6 joint is placed in extension or breathing in; inspiration.

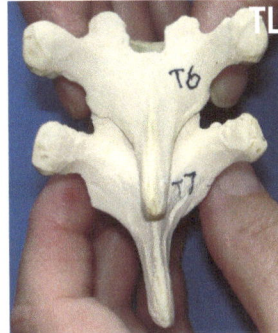

Posterior view Neutral

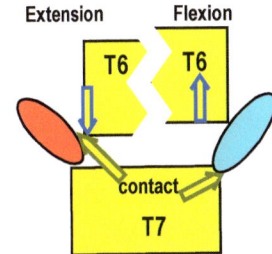

Figure TOc
Exaggerated side-views showing how each side of the demi-facets connect with the ribs

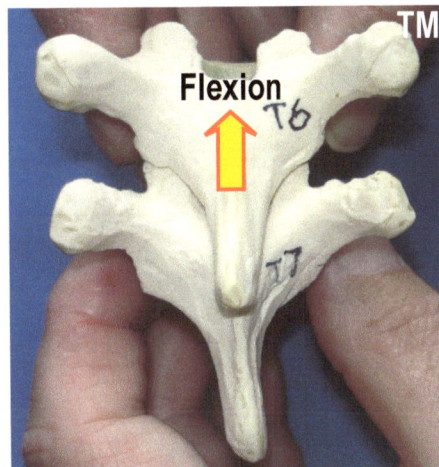

Figure T0a
Anterior view of left side of T6-T7 joint

Refer to **figures TOa** and **TOc.**

Extension: During inspiration the inferior demi-facets of the T6 vertebra travel inferiorly and engage against the superior facet heads of the T6 ribs. Shown in red.

Flexion: During expiration the superior demi-facets of the T6 vertebra travel superiorly, and leave the inferior facet heads of the T6 ribs against superior demi-facets of T7. Shown in blue.

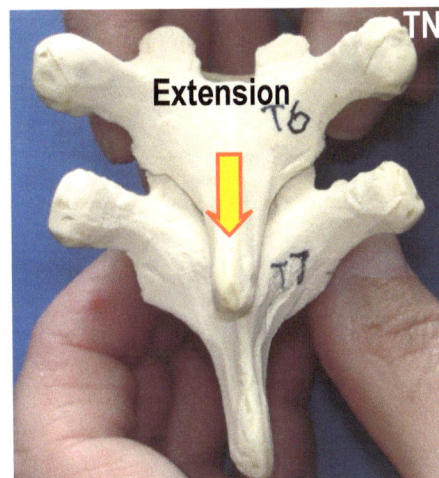

Expiration

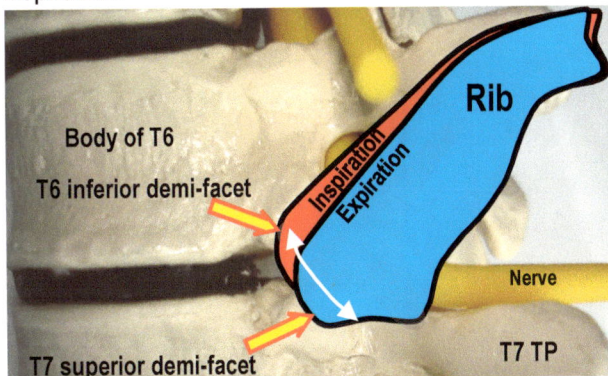

Inspiration

Thoracic Rotation and Side-bending Problems

Working rib theory overview

For a rib theory to be proved, it must satisfy working criteria. It has to account for the way ribs remain level and parallel at all times to complement efficient breathing. The theory must also make allowance for vertebral articulation in flexion, extension, side-bending and rotation.

The thoracic joints **do not** rotate and side-bend as shown in **figure TOb.** This is because if they moved like this the ribs, which need to be kept in parallel on either side to function efficiently, would be compromised.

For arguments sake, if the side-bending shown in **figure TOb** were to occur, the left transverse process of T6 would be raised superiorly. This would angle the conical apex of the attached 6th rib superiorly by several degrees and thereby seriously hinder the ribs ability to function normally.

Side-bending followed by rotation are necessary for the normal physiological movement of the thoracic vertebrae. Via moving X-rays, I was able to observe how the thoracic spine side-bent and rotated in a way that kept the ribs parallel. The method is very simple and is demonstrated below.

Imagine the line of cards shown in **figure TP** represents the thoracic column and each card an individual vertebra.

If the cards are moved into a stepping sequence, as shown in **figure TQ,** it can be seen that a general pseudo side-bending pattern emerges that keeps the cards in horizontal alignment.

It is this principle that the thoracic vertebrae use when side-bending is required.

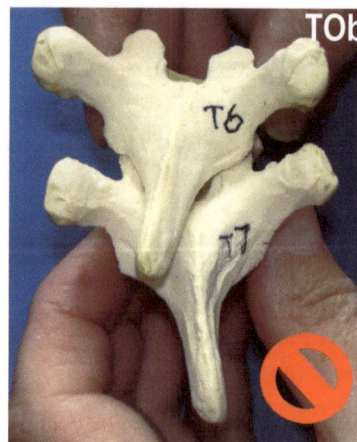
TOb

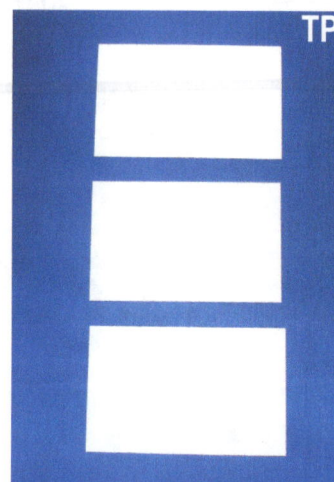
TP

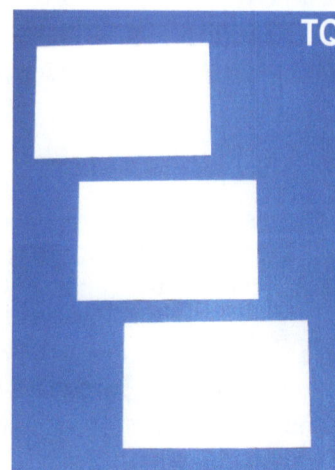
TQ

66

Thoracic
Nucleus Pulposus Placing

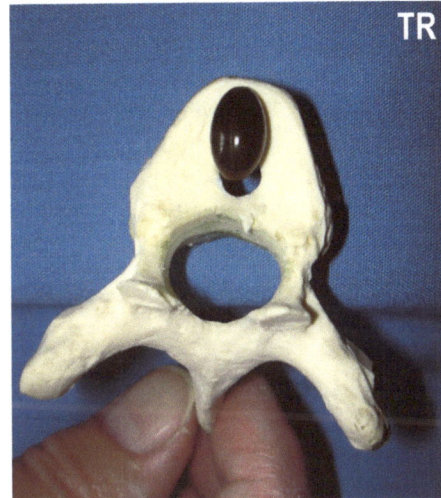

To allow the thoracic joints to articulate efficiently the nucleus pulposus needs to be positioned towards the anterior half of the T7 body, as shown in **figure TR.**

Figure 2b is an approximation of the arc taken by the T6 facets.

This convex arc is opposite to the concave arc produced by the more posterior positioned nucleus, found between the lumbar discs. **Figure 2a** shows for comparison an approximation of the more rounded arc taken by the L3 facets.

The anterior placement of the nucleus pulposus in the thoracic vertebrae probably explains why disc related problems are rare in the thoracic vertebrae.

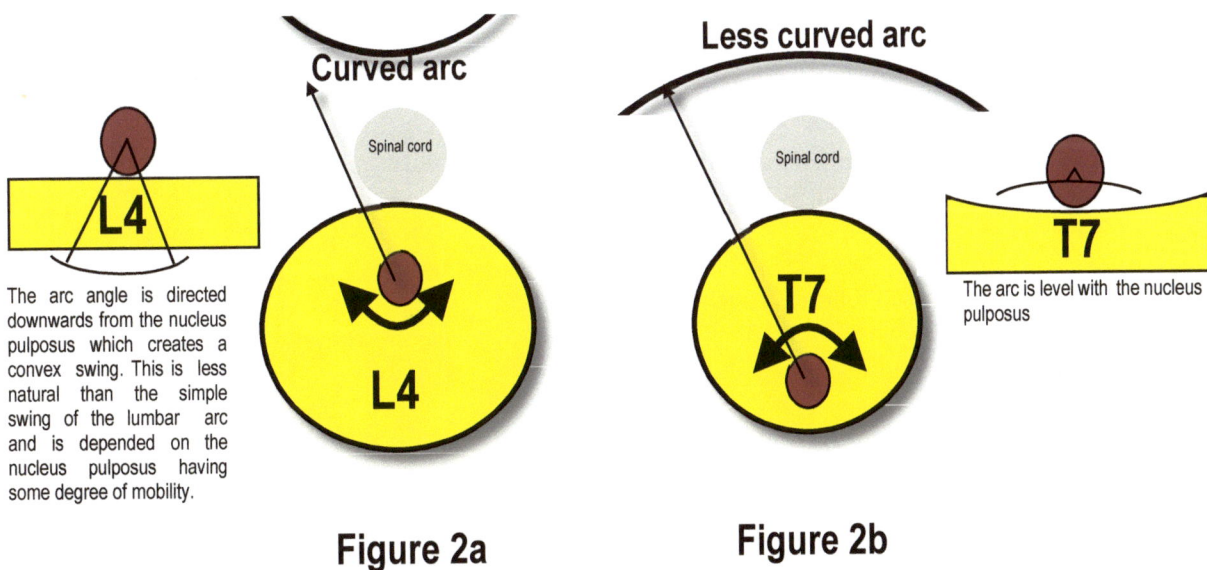

The arc angle is directed downwards from the nucleus pulposus which creates a convex swing. This is less natural than the simple swing of the lumbar arc and is depended on the nucleus pulposus having some degree of mobility.

The arc is level with the nucleus pulposus

Figure 2a

Figure 2b

Thoracic Rotation Right Flexion

Figure TS shows what would happen when T7 is side-shifted to the right in neutral or thoracic flexion. The nucleus pulposus arcs the facets of T6 like a pendulum to the left. This swings the facets superiorly and laterally to the left and creates side-bending and rotation to the right. That is side-bending and rotation to the same side in thoracic flexion which is invalid and would be a precursor to what the old Osteopaths termed a 'complicated lesion'.

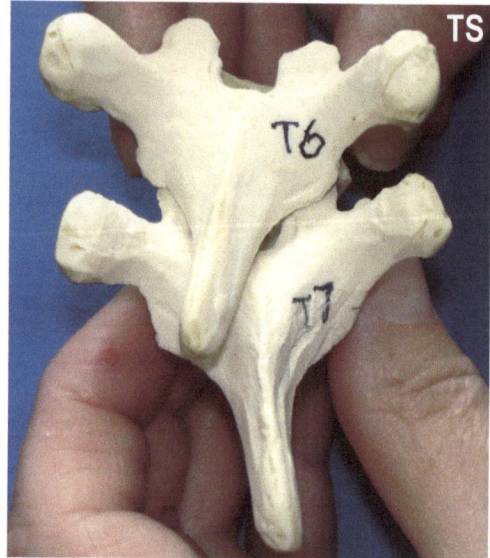

If we analyse this conundrum further, it can be seen that the left transverse processes have separated and the right approximated. This means that the transverse processes are no longer parallel and therefore unable to achieve the side stepping action required to keep the ribs parallel.

Figure TT is an aerial view showing the rib attachments either side of the thoracic vertebrae and shows the stabilizing effect the ribs have on either side.

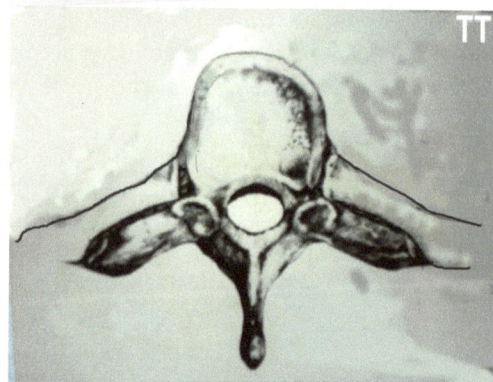

Articular surfaces for rib attachment

Figure TU is a side-view of T6 and shows the articular surfaces where the sixth and fifth ribs attach to the T6 vertebra.

The inferior head of the fifth rib articulates with the T6 body at the superior demi-facet, shown by arrow A.

The articular facet of the sixth rib tubercle attaches to the costo-transverse facet. Shown by arrow B.

The superior head facet of the sixth rib attaches to the inferior demi-facet of T6. Shown by arrow C.

More detailed information on how the ribs articulate with the thoracic vertebrae can be found in chapter 14.

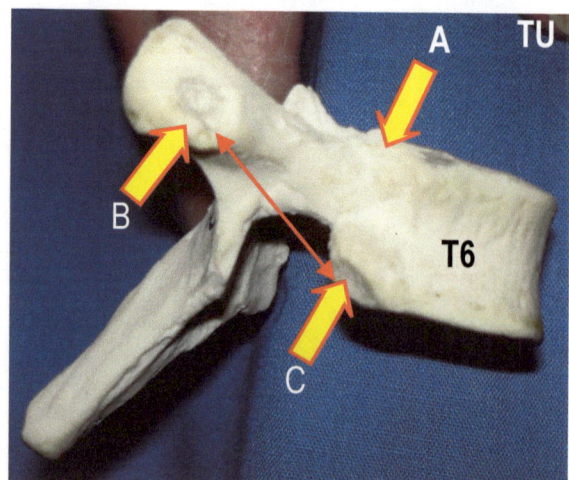

Side-view of T6 thoracic vertebra

Thoracic Rotation Right:
Stepping Action

When T7 follows the pelvic side-shift to the right, the movement of T6 is not only governed by the shape of the facets and nucleus pulposus, it has the additional stabilizing influence of the attached ribs.

In **figure TV** the action of rotating a thoracic vertebra to the right is shown again, only this time T6 is held in parallel to simulate the counter force of the ribs on either side. The facets still engage, provided that the nucleus pulposus has the ability to side-shift.

By observing the shape of the upper body of T7 it can be concluded that the thoracic nuclei pulposi have the ability to side-shift in a form of rocking. See **figure Twa.** This rotated side-shift is kept in check by the scooped design of the thoracic vertebra. This scooped shape is shown in **figure TW**.

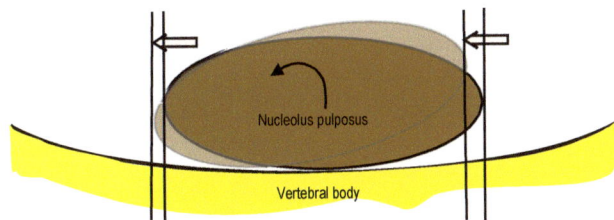

Figure TWa

With T7 and T6 held in parallel, the left lateral shift of T6 has no choice other than to conform to a stepping sequence, as was shown in **figure TQ**.

If the completed side-shift movement is examined, using **figures TV** and **TX** for reference, it can be seen that the left transverse process of T6 is marginally anterior and that the spinous process of T6 is separated and to the right of the T7 spinous process. This means that rotation to the right has also taken place.

This is thoracic flexion with side-bending and rotation to opposite sides.

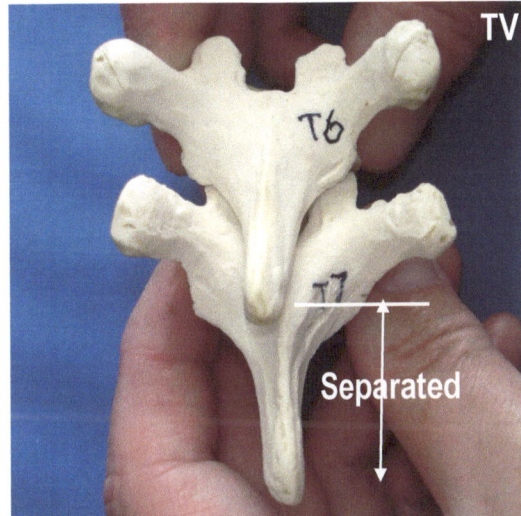

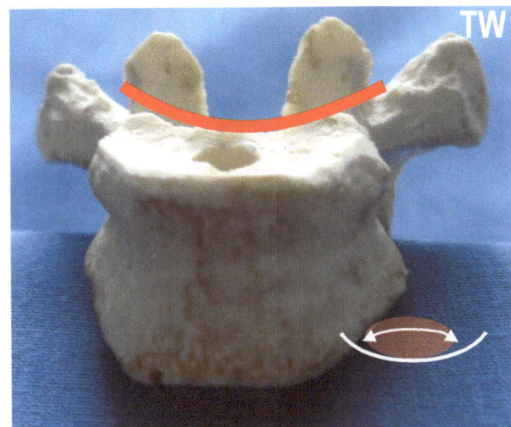

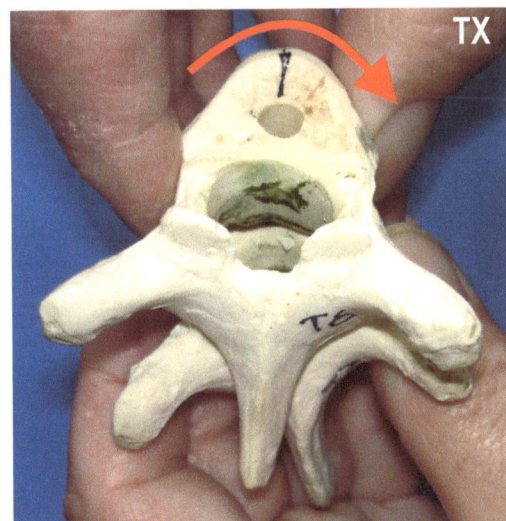

Rotation Right, Side-Bending Left in Thoracic Flexion

Recap on the articulation.

In thoracic flexion (forward bending), side-shift continues up the spine past L1, as shown in **figure 2.**

T6 is being used as an example. Thoracic flexion-rotation movements start with the T6 facets sliding up the T7 facets as shown in **figure TM.**

The left knee is then flexed as weight is directed to the right leg. This causes the pelvis to rise up and engage the right 'F' sacroiliac facets and rotate the pelvis to the right. If the intention is for the thoracic spine to rotate right, the thoracic column will generally follow the pelvic rotation.

When pelvic side-shift to the right takes place it passes to the right of L1. The pelvic side-shift causes the T7 facets to side-shift to the right. As can be seen from **figure TO**, the counter force of balance emanating from above causes the facets of T6 to slide left across the convex T7 facets. In doing this the body of T6 is forced to rotate to the right. This is shown from above in **figure TX.**

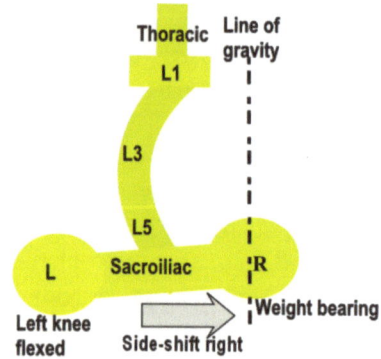

Figure 2

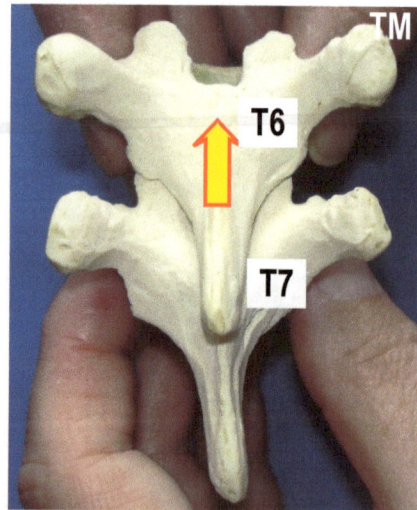

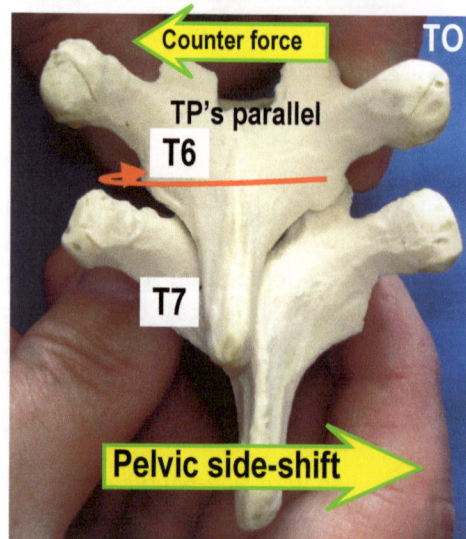

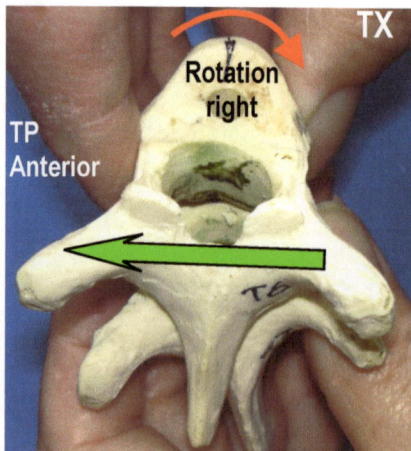

Blocked Rotation
in Thoracic Extension

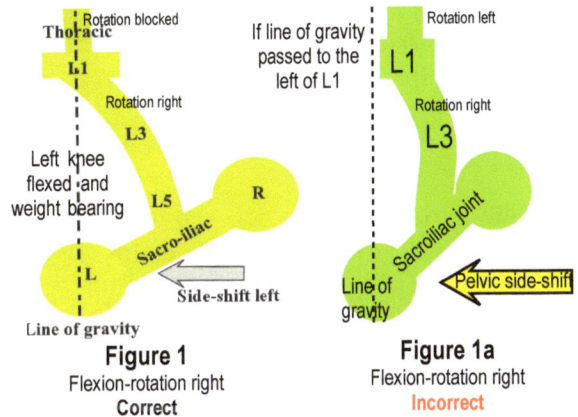

Figure 1
Flexion-rotation right
Correct

Figure 1a
Flexion-rotation right
Incorrect

When there is no side-shift to the left above L1, T6 has no driving force to rotate the thoracic vertebrae in extension.

In thoracic extension, rotation is prohibited

Figure TY shows T6 in thoracic extension (backward bending) the T6-7 joint becomes approximated. Only a very small amount of extension is possible in thoracic extension due to the likelihood of bone grinding against bone. In our example **figure TY**, the anterior surface of T6 makes actual bony contact with the posterior surface of the T7 spinous process and leaves no play within their meeting.

Should the 'G' force created by pelvic side-shift and weight bearing to the left pass to the left of L1, as shown in **figure 1a,** the 'M' counter force from above would attempt to rotate T6 to the **left**. With the proximity of the T6/7 bones they would be ground against each other. Note that **rotation** to the **left** is the opposite direction to the lumbar rotation and would create enormous tension.

Figure TZ is an example of what happens when the 'G' force pelvic side-shift and weight bearing pass to the left reaches T7. The T7 facets would follow the pelvic side-shift to the left. Conversely the 'M' counter force above would side-shift T6 to the right and the spinous process of T6 would be pushed against the transverse process of T7. This would cause T6 to buckle and be impacted by bone and against bone.

This is why L1 blocks the 'G' force, as shown in **figure 1.**

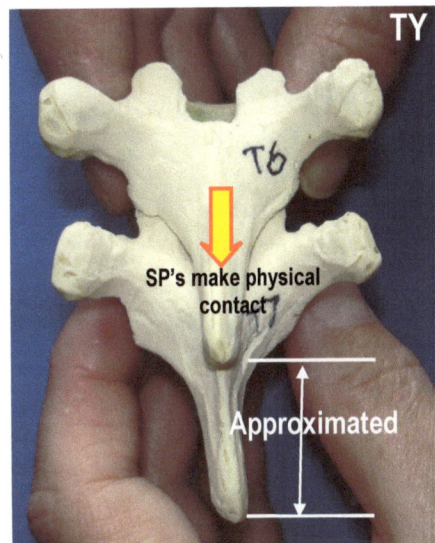

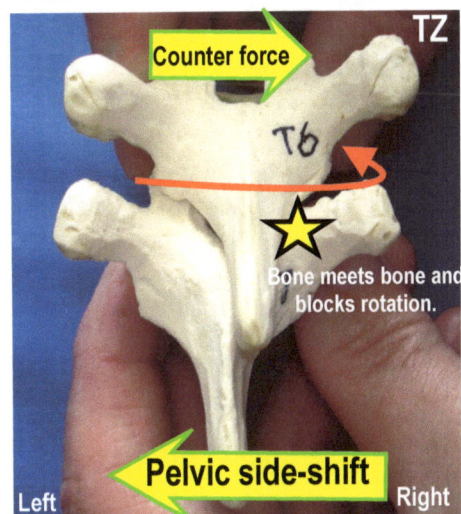

Thoracic Anatomy
T1 and T2

The T2-T1 joint is unique from the thoracic joints below, because it links the thoracic vertebrae with the cervical vertebrae and forms a reverse change in the vertical curve.

Figure TAB shows the superior posterior facets of a typical T2 vertebra. The facets of T2 follow the line of a swinging pendulum.

Figure TAC shows an inferior anterior view of the facets of a typical T1 vertebra. Like the T2 facets the T1 facets follow the line of a swinging pendulum.

Figure TAD shows the T2 superior posterior facets from above. The red arrow highlights the convex shape of the facets.

Figure TAE shows the inferior anterior facets of T1 from below. The red arrow highlights the concave shape of the facets.

Figure TAF shows the vertical slightly convex shape of the T2 superior facets from the right side.

Figure TAG shows the vertical slightly concave shape of the inferior T1 facets.

Figure TAH is a side view from the right of the T2-T1 joint in neutral. Notice that when the facets meet, T1 becomes backward leaning.

Figure TAJ is a posterior view of the T2-T1 joint in neutral. Again notice the backward leaning position of T1. Again note the scooped line of the facets, indicated in red. This would mean that the joint is capable of small amounts of pendulum swing.

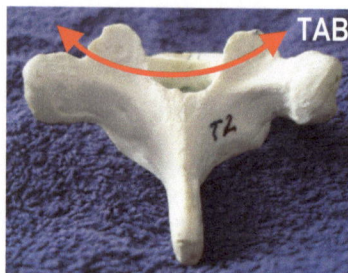

Posterior view of T2

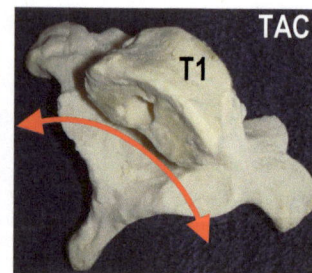

Anterior inferior view of

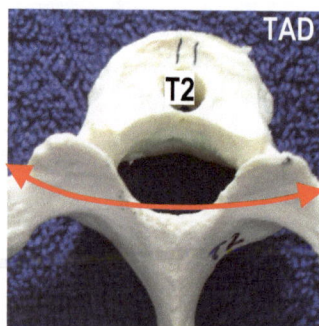

Posterior aerial view of T2 superior facets

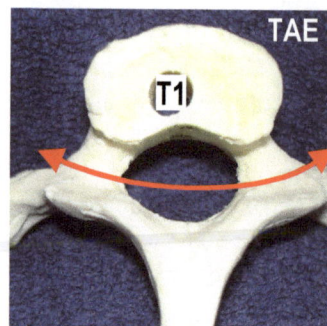

View from below of TI inferior facets

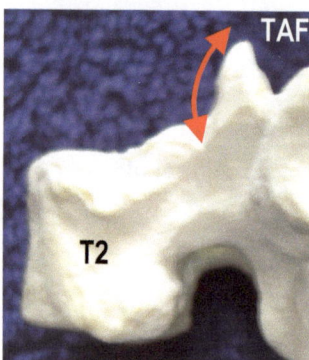

Right side- view of T2 superior facets

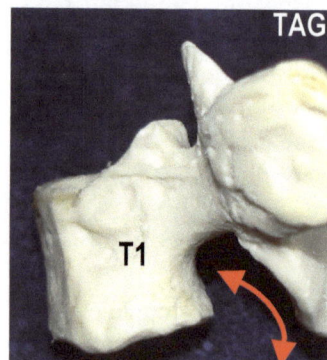

Right side- view of T1 inferior facets

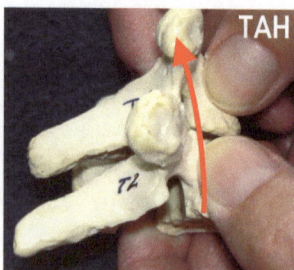

Right side- view of T1-T2

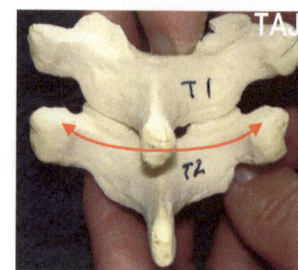

Posterior view of T1-T2

Thoracic Physiology
T1 and T2

Figure TAK is a posterior view of T2-T1 in thoracic extension (backward bending). T1 has approximated with T2. Because of the close proximity of the T1 and T2 facets, **no** rotation can take place.

Figure TAL is a posterior view of T2-T1 in thoracic flexion (forward bending). T1 has separated from T2.

Figure TAM shows T1 rotating right in thoracic flexion. T2-T1 rotation to the right works on a similar principle to the vertebrae below. Pelvic side-shift causes T2 to side-shift right. Whilst the counter balance from above causes T1, steadied by the ribs at either side to side-shift to the left. In doing this the T1 facets slide over the convex T2 facets and rotate right in a small pendulum arc that keeps T1 level. See illustration 'A' below.

There is probably slightly more side-shift allowed in this joint in neutral and extension than the other thoracic joints. This is because T1 has to counter the side-shift of the joints below.

The T2 -T1 joint has two main functions:

1) To change the direction of the anterio-posterior curve of the thoracic spine in order to align the neck in a upright and vertical position. See 'B' below.

2) To counter the side-bending (side-shift) of the thoracic vertebrae below to keep the neck vertical. See **figure TAM** and 'A' below.

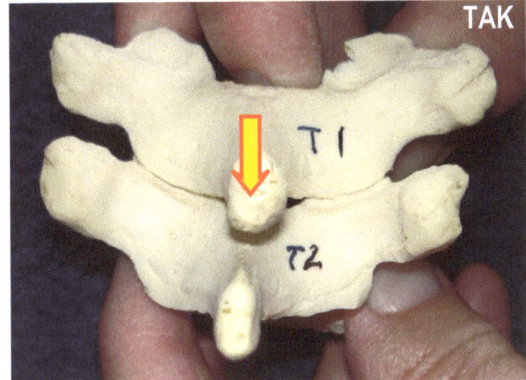

Posterior view of T1-T2
Thoracic extension

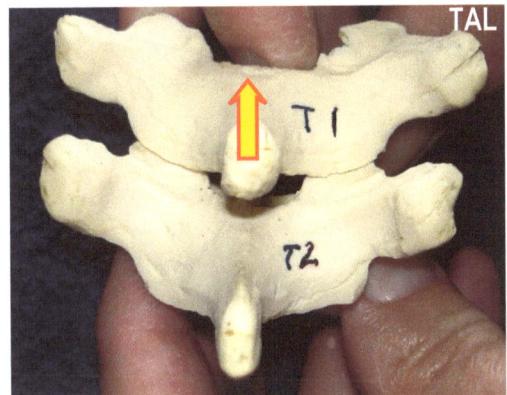

Posterior view of T1-T2
Thoracic flexion

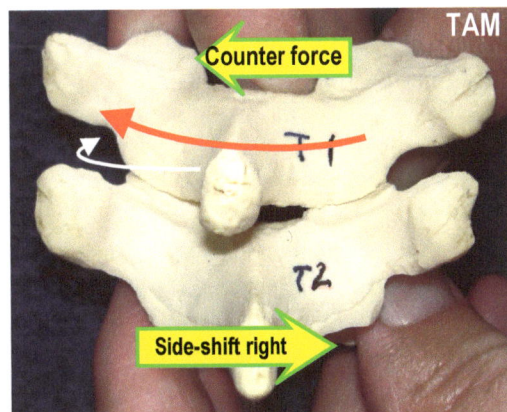

Posterior view of T1-T2
T1 rotating right

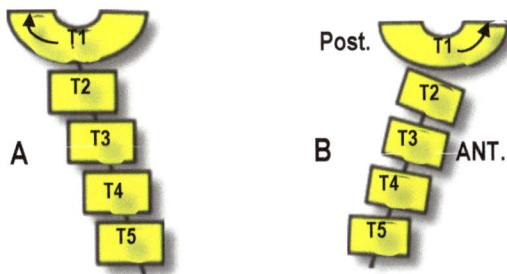

<u>Posterior view</u> showing how T1 compensates for side-bending

<u>Side-view</u> showing change of A-P curve

73

Thoracic Physiology: Rotation and Side-Shift

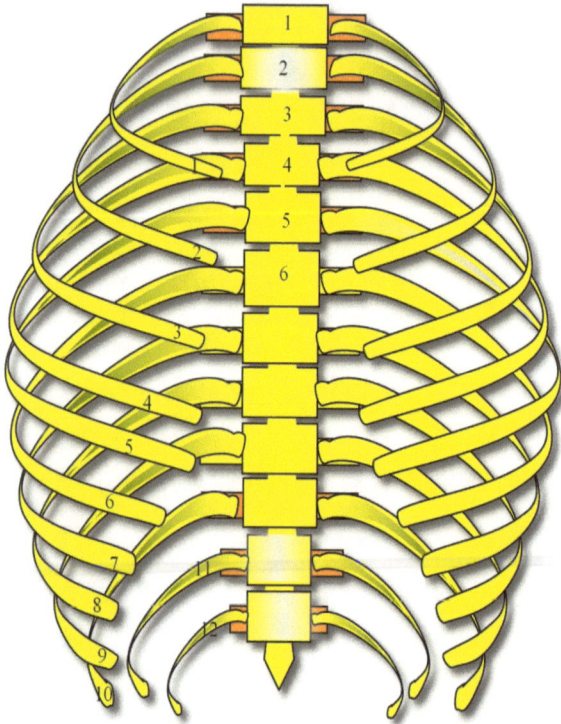

Figure TAN
Anterior view of the thoracic
spine and rib cage.

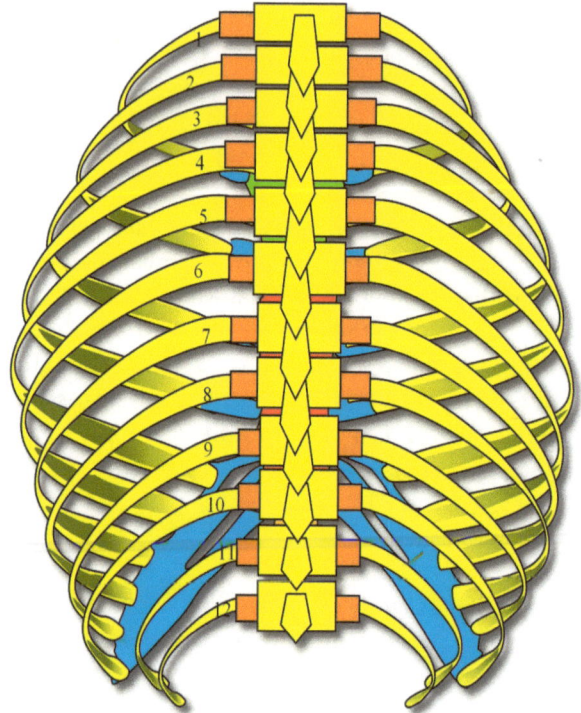

Figure TAP
Posterior view of the thoracic
spine and rib cage.

The rib cage and thoracic vertebrae are illustrated in **figures TAN** and **TAP** to help you visualize and contrast the differences in the amount of rotation and side-shift possible.

The upper five ribs allow for only small amounts of rotation but it is an important synergetic rotation as it aids neck rotation. This is due to the flatter shape of the vertebral facets and the short length of cartilage at their anterior attachment to the sternum. Their main role is side-shift, with a degree of rotation.

The middle five ribs allow for more side-shift and a greater amount of rotation. This is due to the increased flexibility of the suspended cartilage. Their flexibility allows for equal amounts of side-bending and rotation, though the lower ribs in this area should produce a greater rotation and side-shift.

The lower two ribs are not joined to the sternum and this allows them much greater freedom of movement. The more rounded facet shapes of their corresponding vertebrae and their freedom of movement dictate that their primary role is rotation with adequate flexibility to take up the side-shift overspill.

Chapter Six

Physiology of the Cervical Joints

The cervical vertebrae work in a different way to the thoracic and lumbar vertebrae. This is because pelvic side-shift does not initiate their rotational or side-bending movements. Their articulations are entirely dependent upon muscle energy. This provides them with an independence of movement.

For example, a person leaning forward can turn their head to the opposite side their body is facing. However, the rotation is limited.

The cervical spine is concave towards the posterior with a similar curve to that of the lumbar spine.

C7 to C2 have the ability to side-bend and rotate in extension. In flexion these same vertebrae are limited to singular flexion movements only.

C2 and C1 are rotators. Their function is to arc laterally.

The Occiput against C1 can flex and extend to a small degree. In neutral it has the ability to rotate.

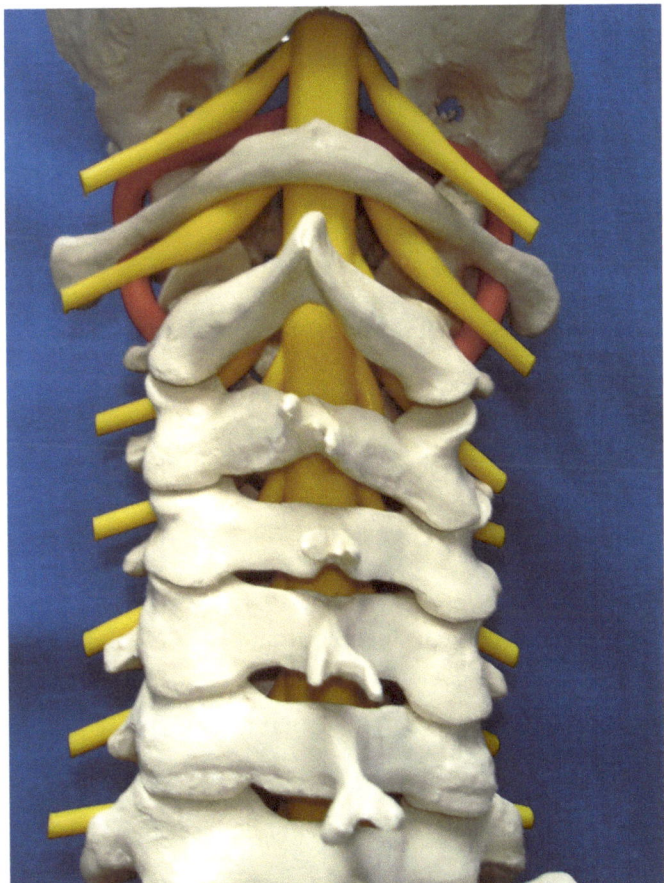

Cervical Reference

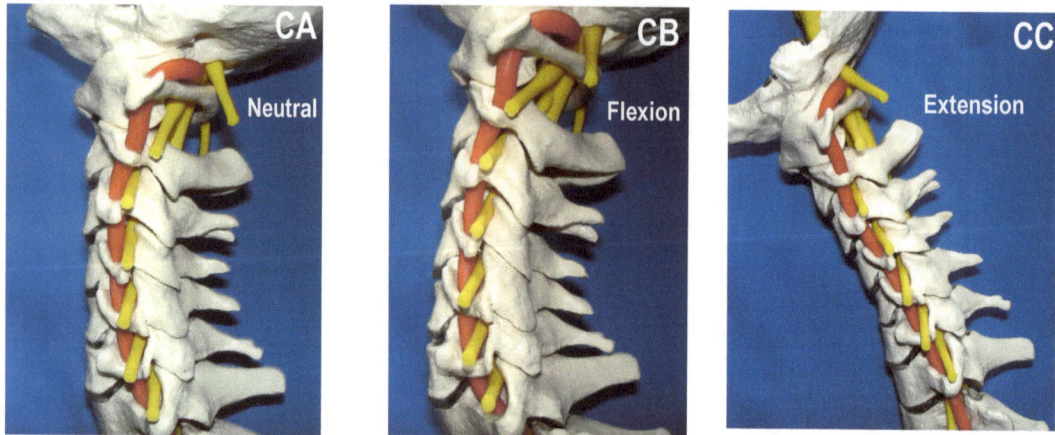

Figure CA is a side-view of the cervical spine in neutral. **Figure CB** is a side-view of the cervical spine in flexion. Cervical flexion is backward bending. **Figure CC** is a side-view of the cervical spine in extension. Cervical extension is forward bending.

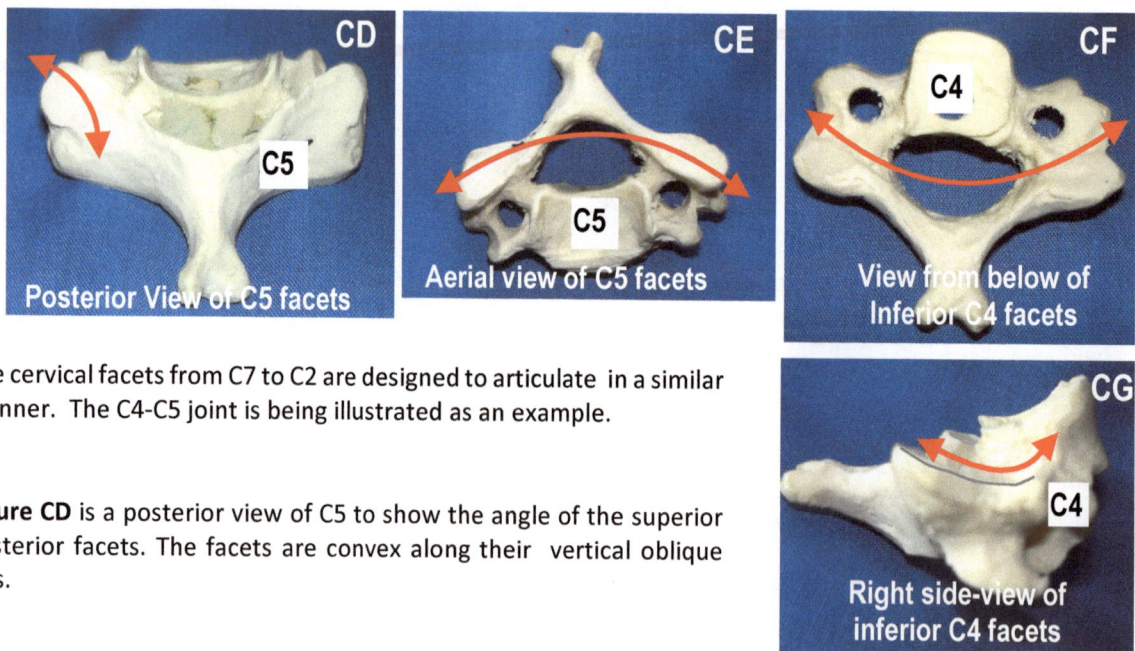

The cervical facets from C7 to C2 are designed to articulate in a similar manner. The C4-C5 joint is being illustrated as an example.

Figure CD is a posterior view of C5 to show the angle of the superior posterior facets. The facets are convex along their vertical oblique axis.

Figure CE is a view from above of the C5 facets and shows the convex shape of the facets along their horizontal axis.

Figure CF is a view of the inferior C4 facets across their horizontal axis and illustrates their concave shape.

Figure CG is a side-view of the inferior C4 facets, and shows the concave shape of the anterior facets along their vertical axis.

Cervical Flexion and Extension

Figure CH is a posterior view of C5. Note that the body of C5 is concave. This usually means the physiology should allow for limited side-shift. The capsule is placed in the centre of the body. There is little room between the nucleus and the spinal cord, which may explain why disc related problems have the potential to occur in the cervical spine.

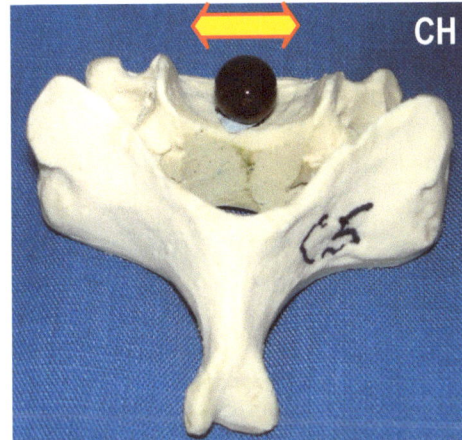

View of C5 nucleus placement

Figure CJ shows C4 in flexion. The facets and spinous process of C4 are approximated to those of C5.

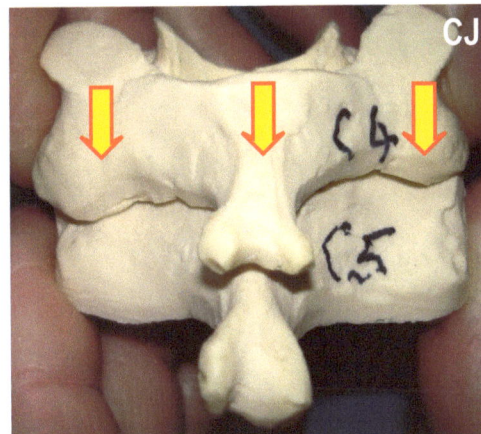

View of C4 in flexion

Figure CK shows C4 in extension. The facets and spinous process of C4 are separated from those of C5.

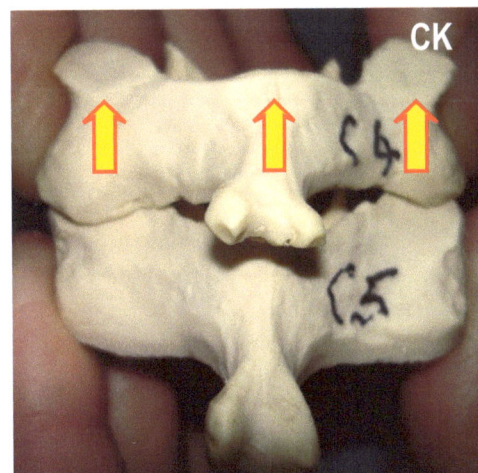

View of C4 in extension

Cervical Rotation
Flexion and Extension

Overview

The cervical facet shapes between C7 and C2 do not allow for rotation in flexion. This is because the horizontal axes of the facets are designed purely for rotation and side-bending to the same side; which is extension.

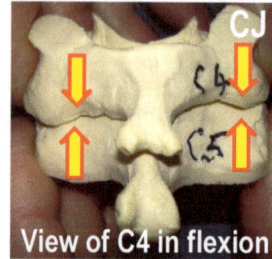

View of C4 in flexion

Rotation right in flexion

If flexion rotation was attempted, initially the inferior facets of C4 would approximate with the lamina of C5, as shown in **figure CJ.**

If rotation to the right was then attempted, the right inferior facets of C4 would grate against the lamina of C5 and prohibit movement. This is shown in **figure CL**.

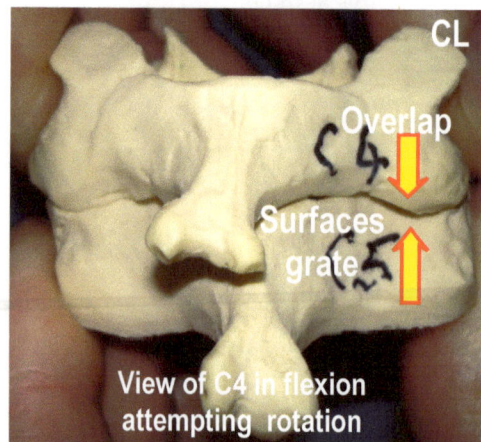

View of C4 in flexion attempting rotation

Rotation right in extension

Initially the facets of C4-C5 separate as shown in **figure CK.**

The neck muscles lever the right hand facet of C4 inferiorly, medially and posteriorly over the right C5 facet. On the left, the left C4 facet moves superiorly, laterally and anteriorly. This action causes C4 to rotate and side-bend to the right in extension, as shown in **figure CM.**

At the maximum point of this movement the C4 spinous process is separated and to the left of the C5 spinous process. The border of C4 on the left is superior, anterior and lateral. The right C4 facet is posterior. The convexity is on the right side.

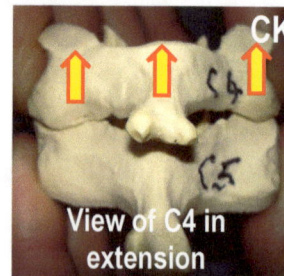

View of C4 in extension

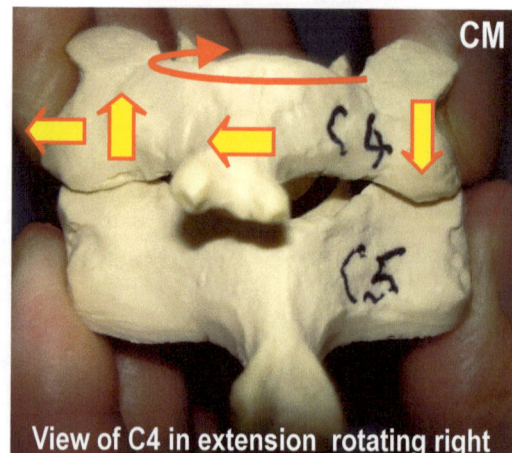

View of C4 in extension rotating right

Cervical
C2-1 Facet Anatomy

There is no disc or nucleus pulposus between the junction of C2 and C1. The odontoid peg of C2 replaces the nucleus pulposus as the point of pivot.

The facets of C1-C2 and the occiput, are designed specifically to rotate and side-shift in one movement, and allow for lateral arcing.

Figure CN is a posterior view of C2. The superior facets are convex across their horizontal medio-lateral axis.

Figure CO is a side view of C2. The facets are convex across their anterio-posterior horizontal axis. The anterior surface banks in a gentle superior slope that drops away inferiorly.

Figures CP and CQ show the rounded shape of the inferior facets of C1. The anterior surface of the facets bank in a gentle inferior slope so that they can fit snugly against the superior facets of C2. Together they act as a form of ball and socket joint. Notice that the width of the facet of dens is designed to allow the odontoid peg to slide along as it rotates.

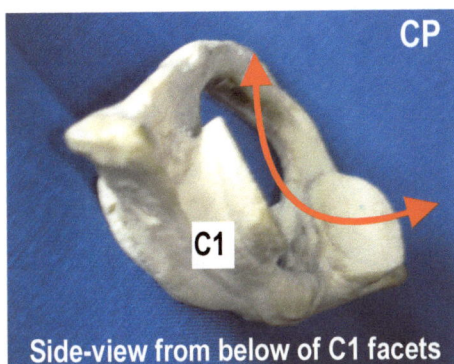

CN

View from above of C2 facets

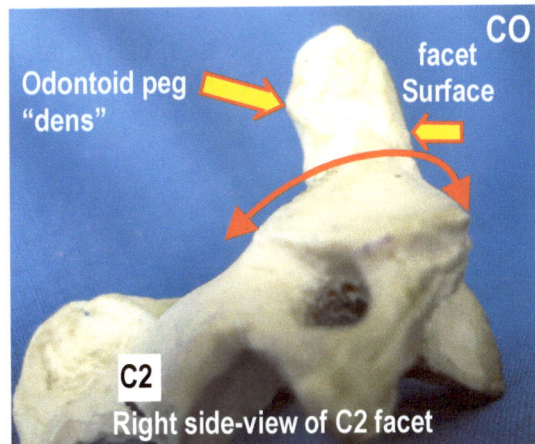

CO

Odontoid peg "dens"

facet Surface

C2

Right side-view of C2 facet

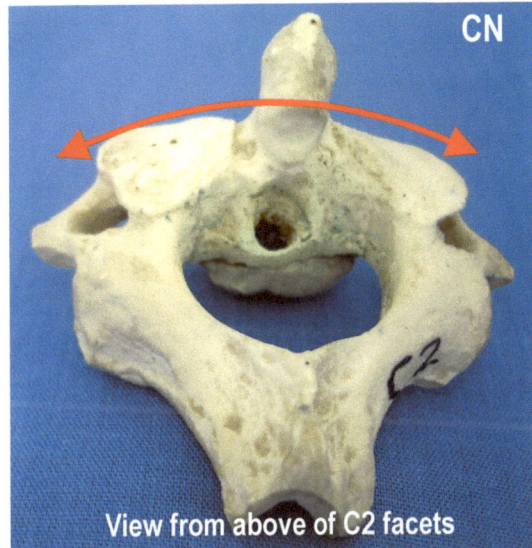

CP

C1

Side-view from below of C1 facets

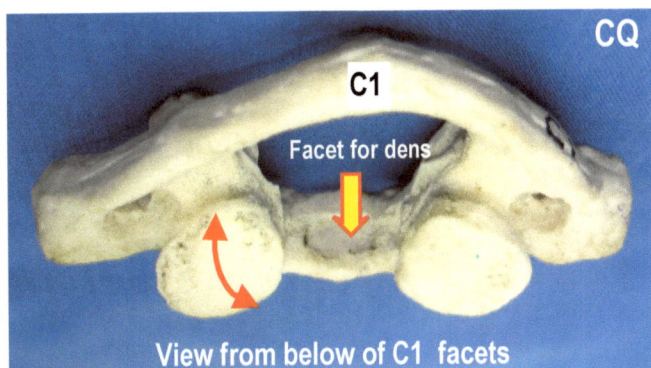

CQ

C1

Facet for dens

View from below of C1 facets

79

Cervical
Odontoid Peg

Figure CR is a posterior view of the C2-C1 joint. It shows the alignment of the facets which are angled inferiorly and laterally.

The odontoid peg at its articulation with C1 prohibits C1 from sliding posteriorly and injuring the spinal cord. This is an important safeguard to limit the effects of whiplash.

Figure CS is an aerial view of the C2-C1 joint. It identifies the position of the odontoid peg at its articulation with the anterior arch of C2. The joint is held firmly in place by the cruciform ligament. The joint is designed for the odontoid peg to simultaneously rotate and side-shift.

Figure CT is a side-view, taken from below, of the inferior anterior slope of the C2 body.

Figure CU is a side-view above C3 and shows the inferior anterior slope of the body.

Below is a side-view drawing of the C3-C2 vertebrae showing the way the C2 body is designed to resist posterior shift.

Figure CV is a superio-anterior view of the vertebral bodies of C3 and C2. It is the combination of the rounded shape of the bodies and the cruciform ligament that gives the odontoid peg its rigid stability.

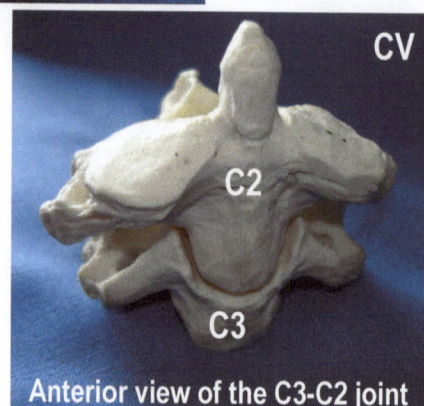

CR

C1

C2

Posterior view of the C2-1 joint

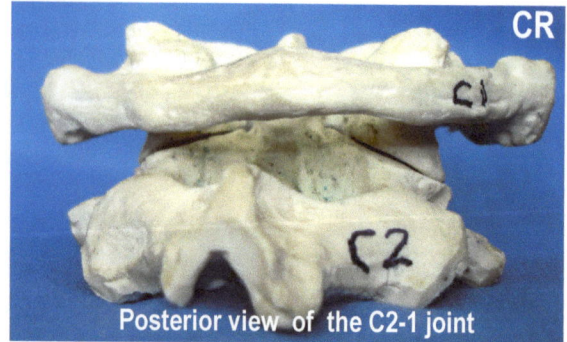

CS

C2 articular surface

Odontoid peg articular surface

Cruciform ligament

View from above of the C2-C1 joint

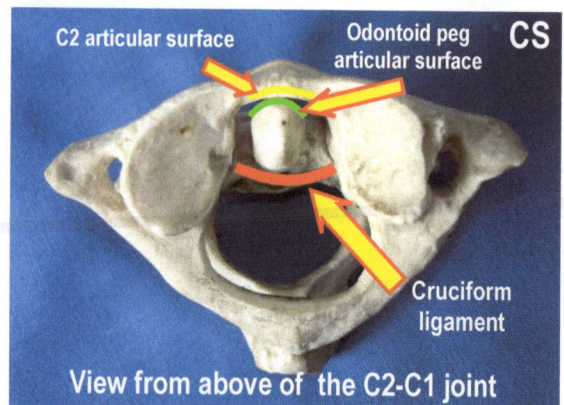

CT

C2

View from below of the C2 body

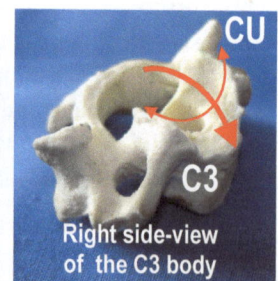

CU

C3

Right side-view of the C3 body

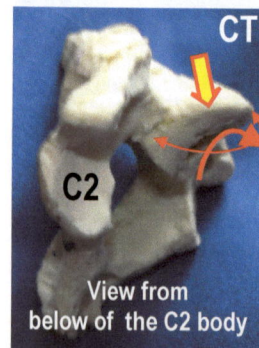

O Peg

Body C2

Disc

Body C3

Anterior

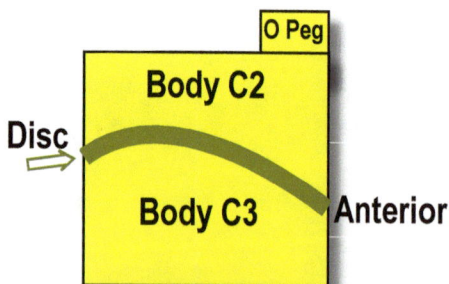

CV

C2

C3

Anterior view of the C3-C2 joint

Cervical Extension
Rotation Right at C1

Figure CR is a posterior view of the C2-C1 joint. Note that the spinous processes are in very close proximity when aligned correctly.

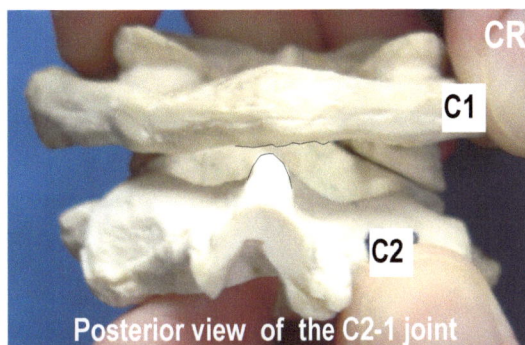

CR

C1

C2

Posterior view of the C2-1 joint

Figure CW is a view from above of the C2-C1 joint in neutral. Note that the spinous process of C1 is anterior to that of C2. This is to avoid collision when C1 rotates and side-shifts.

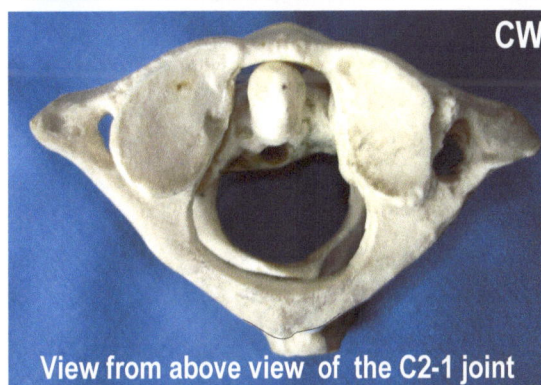

CW

View from above view of the C2-1 joint

Figure CX is a posterior view of C1 rotating to the right. The facet shapes of C2 dictate that C1 has to side-shift laterally to the left for rotation to take place.

Position-wise, the left transverse process of C1 is anterior, inferior and side-shifted to the left. The C1 spinous process is to the left of the C2 spinous process.

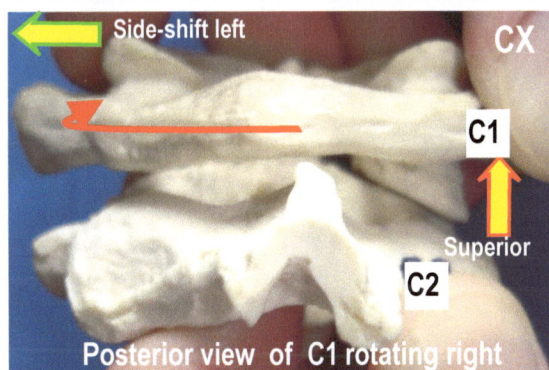

Side-shift left

CX

C1

Superior

C2

Posterior view of C1 rotating right

In order for the C1 facets to follow the line of sideways arcing, the odontoid peg has to side-shift left along the articular facet of C2. This is shown more clearly in **figure CY.**

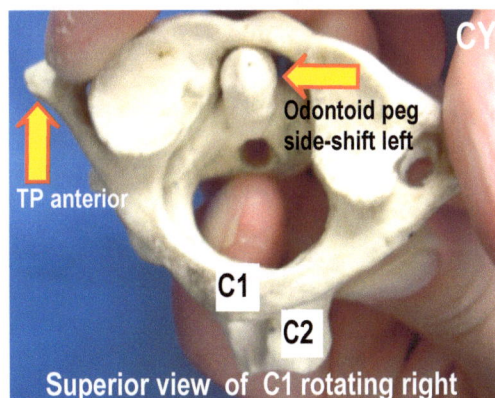

CY

Odontoid peg
side-shift left

TP anterior

C1

C2

Superior view of C1 rotating right

81

Cervical
C1 Facet Anatomy

Figure CY shows the superior facets of C1. Occipital rotation takes place against these facets in neutral, as illustrated by the circular movement of the arrows .

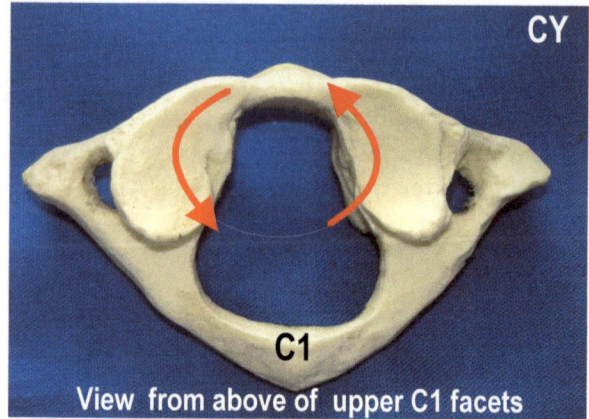

View from above of upper C1 facets

Figure CAA shows the varying concave shapes of the superior articular surfaces of C1. The arrow in green illustrates the more scooped shape at the anterior part of the facet. The red arrow shows the less scooped general concave shape.

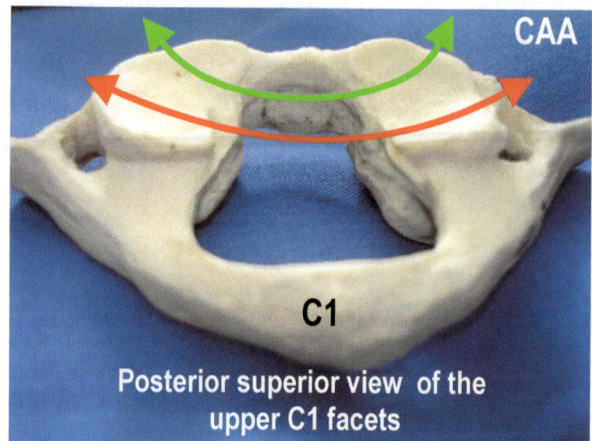

Posterior superior view of the upper C1 facets

Figure CAB is a side-view of the superior articular surface of C1. The facets are concave along their anterio-posteriorly axis. The anterior surface of the facet is angled more acutely than at the medial and posterior surface. The anterior shape allows for chin nodding to take place.

The socket shape of the upper C1 facets allow for extension and flexion movements, along with rotation in neutral. Rotation cannot take place when the occiput is positioned in either extension or flexion. Although it may be possible, movements laterally are very unlikely.

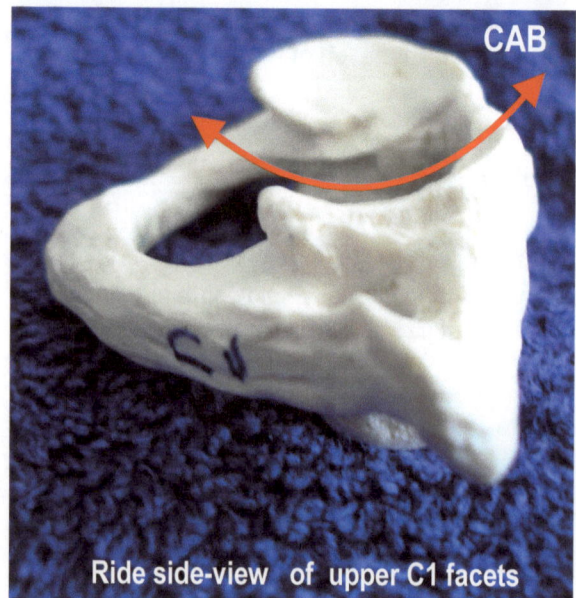

Ride side-view of upper C1 facets

Occiput
Facet Anatomy

Figure CAC is a posterior view of the occiput and shows the inferior convex shape of the facets. The styloid process is indicated for reference purposes only.

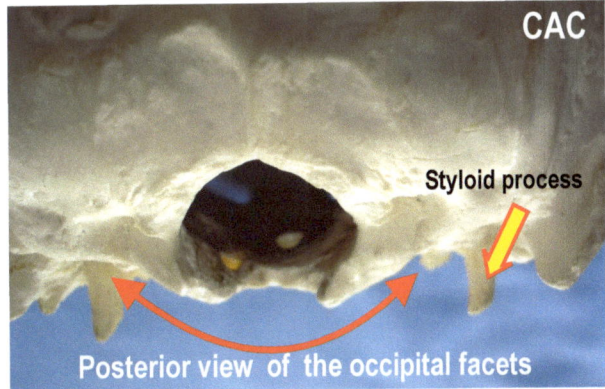

Styloid process

Posterior view of the occipital facets

CAC

Figure CAD is a side-view taken from underneath, of the occipital facets. The green arrow follows the anterio-posterior axis and highlights the change in articular curves. The red arrow shows the area where rotation takes place.

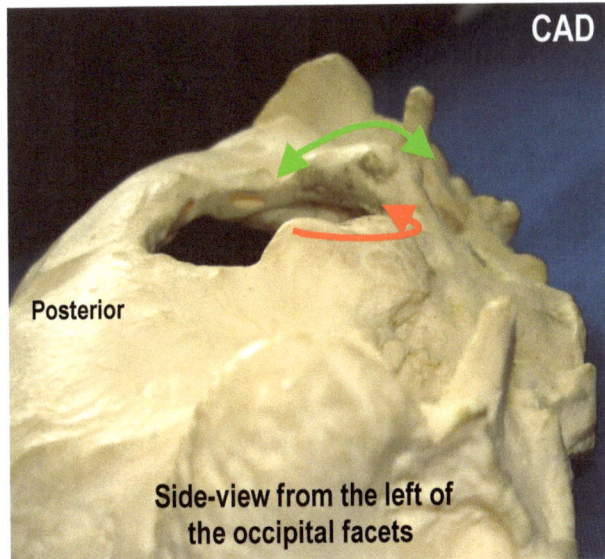

CAD

Posterior

Side-view from the left of the occipital facets

Figure CAE is a posterior view taken from underneath of the facets of C1 engaged against the occipital facets, in neutral. There is no disc between C1 and the Occiput.

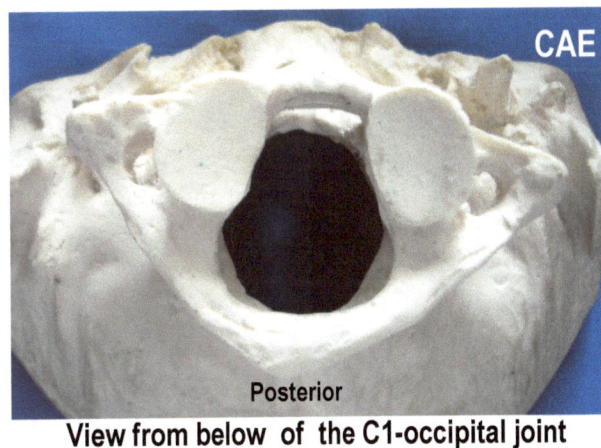

CAE

Posterior

View from below of the C1-occipital joint

C1-Occipital Articulation

Overview

The C1-Occipital joint allows the following movements:

- 1) Forward bending of the head
- 2) Backward bending of the head
- 3) Rotation of the head in neutral and slightly in extension

Figure CAF is a view from below of the C1 occipital joint in neutral.

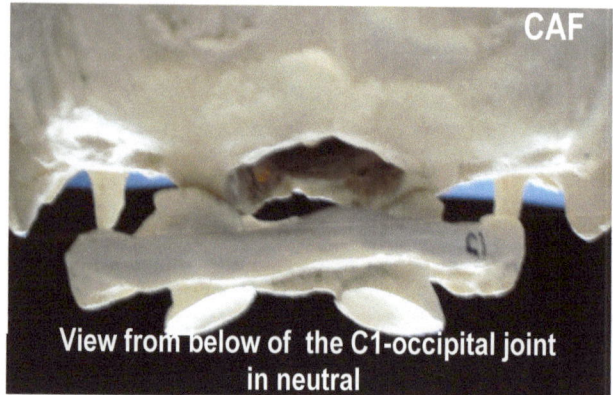

CAF

View from below of the C1-occipital joint in neutral

Figure CAG is a posterior view of the occipital bone in flexion (backward bending). The posterior surface of the C1-occipital articulation allows for a gentle decline of the head when backward leaning.

In cervical flexion, no rotation can take place.

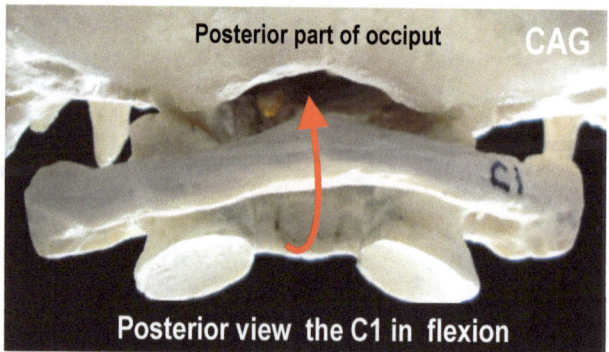

Posterior part of occiput

CAG

Posterior view the C1 in flexion

Figure CAH is a posterior view of the occiput in extension (forward bending). The anterior surface of the C1-occipital articulation dips down sharply, to accommodate the action of chin nodding.

In cervical extension, only minor rotation can take place.

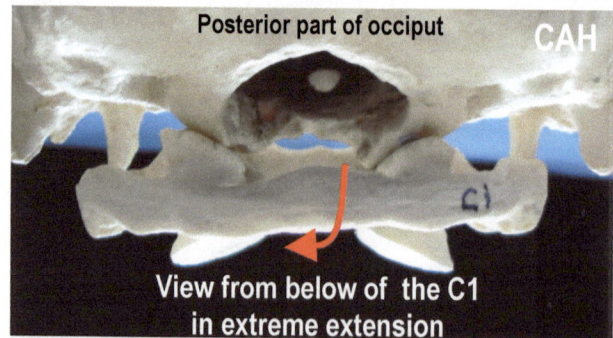

Posterior part of occiput

CAH

View from below of the C1 in extreme extension

Figure CAJ is a view from below of the occiput rotated to the left. For rotation to take place the C1 and occipital facets must be in neutral.

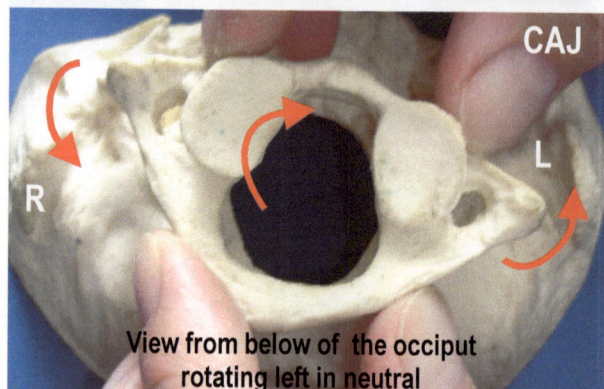

CAJ

R

L

View from below of the occiput rotating left in neutral

84

Chapter Seven

L3-Left-Right
Flexion Lesions of the Lower Back

Flexion subluxations in the lumbar vertebrae are caused in lumbar flexion (backward bending) in the absence of left knee flexion. This creates a misaligned starting position for normal lumbar rotation to follow. When weight bearing and side-shift are transferred to the left, the correct trajectory for the lumbar and sacroiliac facets is prohibited.

When forced rotation is applied from above using the 'M' force, the joint subluxates. This subluxation is compounded when weight and side-shift are transferred to the right leg and lumbar extension is attempted.

Figure 1 is an illustration of the lower back in lumbar flexion with rotation to the right.

It can be seen that L4-L3 takes the maximum side-bending and stress. The secondary areas of stress are taken above at L2-L1 and below in the L5-left sacroiliac joint.

L4-L3 is therefore the area of prime torsion.

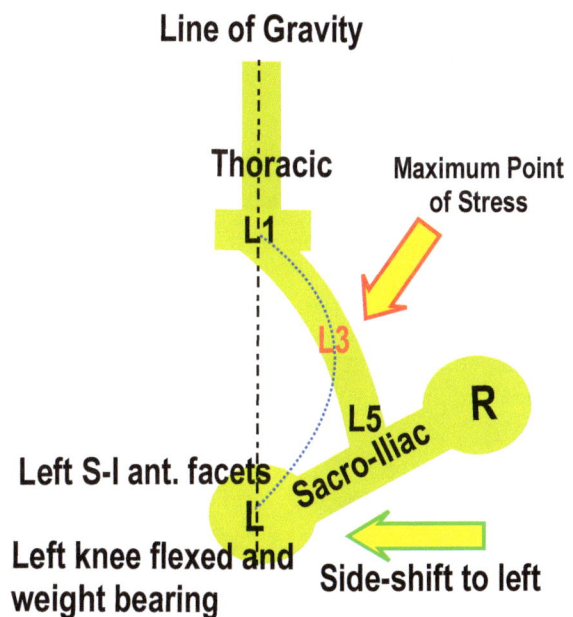

Line of Gravity

Thoracic

Maximum Point of Stress

L1

L3

L5

R

Sacro-Iliac

Left S-I ant. facets

L

Left knee flexed and weight bearing

Side-shift to left

Figure 1

The Principles of a Lumbar L3-L-R Flexion Lesion Part 1

This chapter specifically covers how lumbar flexion subluxations are created. A subluxation is a form of bony locking and is the precursor to an osteopathic lesion. To create an osteopathic lesion two additional forces are exerted on a subluxated joint. These forces tighten the joint to a point where local blood circulation is restricted, often to the point of pain. The two addition forces are general and hard to show by illustration with individual joints, so the principles are shown here.

It may help to refresh your memory of how normal lumbar flexion takes place by re-reading page 21 in Chapter One.

Do this self test:
By doing these hand movements yourself you will gain an understanding of the tightness and pain locked within a simple osteopathic lesion.

Lumbar flexion lesion with rotation to the right.
Figure 0041 is an illustration of the starting point. Make sure your hands are clasped tightly together. Your palms and the heels of hands should also be pressed into one another.

Joints have very little slack. In these illustrations think of your elbows as knees, the base of your hands as the pelvis and your interlaced fingers as the L3-4 joint.

To create a subluxation your knees must not be flexed, so make sure your elbows are level and on a flat surface and in line with each other as shown in **figure 0041A**.

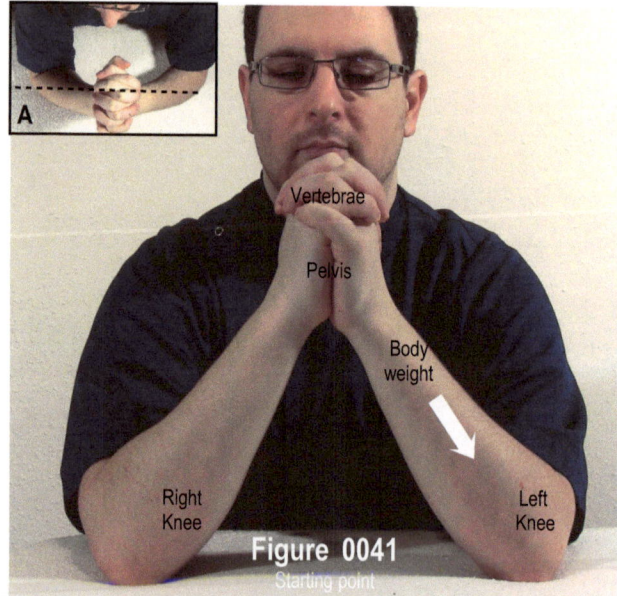

Figure 0041
Starting point

Labels: Vertebrae, Pelvis, Body weight, Right Knee, Left Knee, A

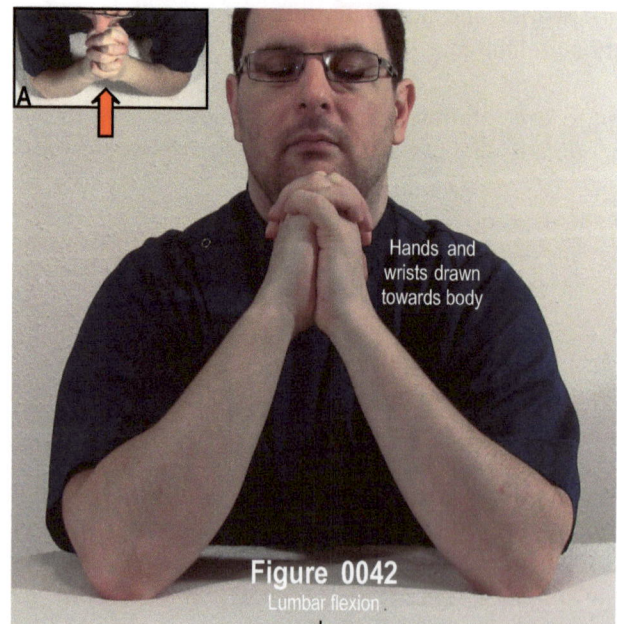

Figure 0042
Lumbar flexion

Labels: Hands and wrists drawn towards body, A

Place your body weight on your left elbow and try not to allow any play in your wrists.

To simulate lumbar flexion (backward bending) draw your hands towards your body. See **figure 0042** and **figure 0042A**.

The Principles of a Lumbar L3-L-R Flexion Lesion Part 2

With limited pelvic side-bending to the left due to the knees being in line, no general precursor pelvic rotation and side-bending takes place so the lumbar joint articulations are forced to start from a misaligned starting point.

Now, side-shift your right elbow towards your left to simulate pelvic side-shift left as per **figures 0043** and **0043A.** No side-bending or rotation takes place. Rotation to the right therefore, has to be forced on the sacrum by the 'M' force muscles above. So you need to rotate both hands to the right to simulate.

Push your hands away from your body to simulate a person attempting to straighten (extending) into spine neutral. The tightness in your fingers now becomes painful. See **figure 0043B**. If you are doing this correctly you will feel that you never quite reach an upright position, spine neutral. This is because the joint is locked in flexion. This is a lumbar flexion subluxation to the right.

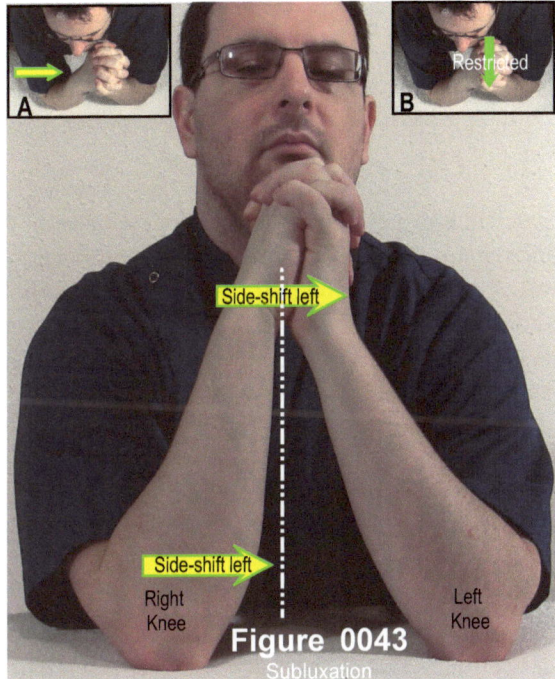

Figure 0043
Subluxation

Flexion lesion to the right

See **figure 0044**. To compound the subluxation side-shift your left elbow towards your right elbow to simulate pelvic side-shift to the right and push your hands away from your body to simulate lumbar extension as per **figure 0044D**. Notice that your fingers tighten and bite into each other and cause much discomfort or pain. Keep your weight on your right elbow. To ease the discomfort in your fingers you need to draw your hands back towards your body. Thus your hands are locked (lesioned) in backward bending which is lumbar flexion.

Note, the final position. Your hands are to the left of the mid-line and side-bent to the left. Also note as per **figure 0044C** that your right elbow is anterior.

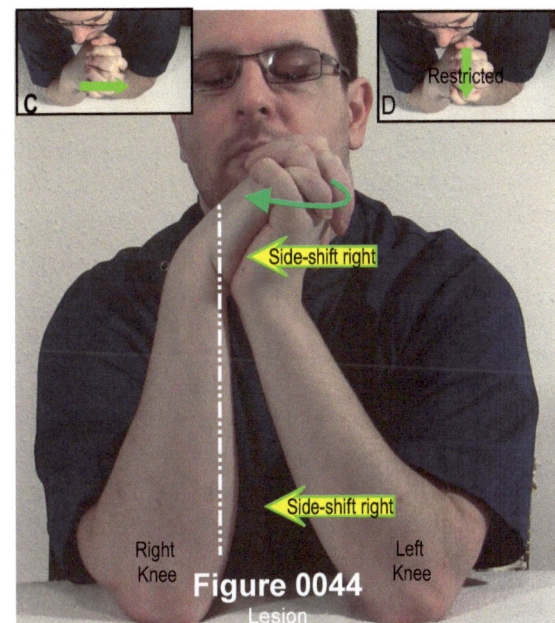

Figure 0044
Lesion

In normal physiology lumbar flexion is side-bending followed by rotation to the opposite side. But here we have rotation followed by side-bending to the opposite side. The 'old Osteopaths' called this a 'complicated lesion' and thought it was rare. However, worse is to come when the pelvis below lesions in flexion and forces the lesioned lumbar joint/s to generally rotate to the left.

L4-L3
L3-L-R Flexion lesion to the Right

Lumbar flexion subluxation side-bending left with rotation right

The person leans backwards as shown in **figure FSA** arrows **AA**. This approximates the L3-4 facets. There is no knee flexion.

Body weight is exerted on the left side of the pelvis and in the absence of left knee flexion the pelvis is unable to correctly rotate right or side-bend left. The restricted amount of side-bending at L3-L4 is shown in **figure FSA.** Without the correct lumbar rotation to the right and the necessary pre-side-bending to the left, L3 is set up to follow a misaligned trajectory.

When the pelvis side-shifts to the left as shown in **figure FSB,** the 'G' force takes L4 with it. While the 'M' force from above slides L3 to the right.

Destined on an incorrect trajectory the right L3 facet impacts into the side of the right L4 facet (instead of sliding up it) whilst the left L3 facet lodges into the L4 lamina. This causes the joint to buckle.

When the person attempts to straighten or forward bend the right L3 facet instead of moving up the L4 facet is forced further right into the side impaction and the joint binds. This is a subluxation. Any forced forward bending becomes uncomfortable and stretches the bound ligaments.

Subluxated

Compare the difference in rotation between the normal physiological movement shown at its limit in **figure FSC** with the subluxated version, shown in **figure FSB.** It can be seen from the illustrations in the top left hand corners of each photograph that the possible rotation to the right of the subluxated vertebra is much less than the normal rotation. The illustrations in the bottom right hand corners of each photograph are of the right L3 facet trajectory.

When pelvic weight bearing and side-shift are transferred to the right the joint tightens so much that it affects the local blood supply. This is a lesion and is greatly compounded when the person attempts to further straighten or forward bend.

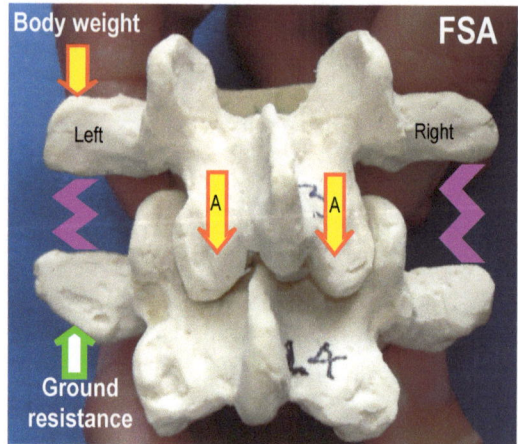

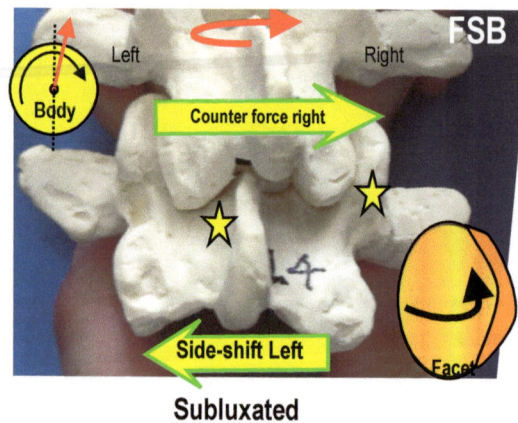

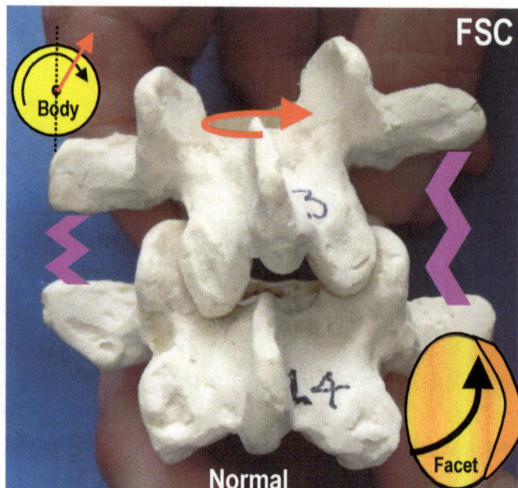

Normal

Line of Gravity Changes due to Lumbar Flexion Right Subluxations

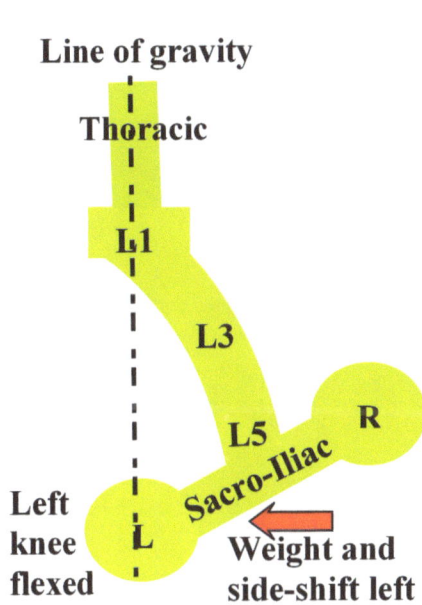

Line of gravity

Thoracic

L1

L3

L5

Sacro-Iliac

R

Left knee flexed

L

Weight and side-shift left

**Figure 3a
Normal**

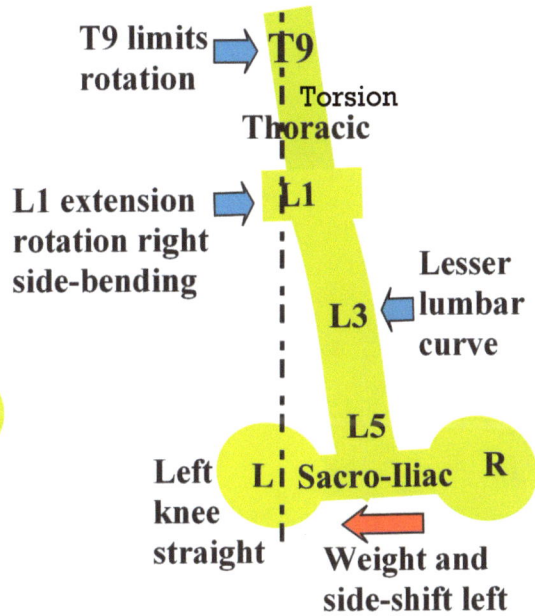

T9 limits rotation → T9

Torsion Thoracic

L1 extension rotation right side-bending → L1

Lesser lumbar curve ← L3

L5

Left knee straight

Li Sacro-Iliac R

Weight and side-shift left

**Figure 3b
Group subluxation**

Figures 3a and 3b above contrast the differences in the lumbar curve when the L3-L4 vertebrae becomes subluxated in flexion and a normal curve. The implication of the lesser side-bending curve is that the weight bearing line of gravity is not dissipated at L1 and is allowed to continue up the thoracic spine to approximately T9 or higher.

Why thoracic extension with rotation to the right is barred

The intension is to side-bend left and rotate the thoracic vertebrae to the right in backward bending in keeping with the lumbar.

T10 is used in our example. In the lumbar this is a flexion movement but in the thoracic it is an extension movement.

When pelvic weight bearing and side-shift are to the left, T11 side-shifts to the left. Counter resistance from above side-shifts T10 to the right across the facets of T11 and the vertebra rotates and side-bends left.

Remember, the intention was for T10 to rotate right.

This conflict of rotation creates an area of extreme torsion and is shown in **figure FSD.**

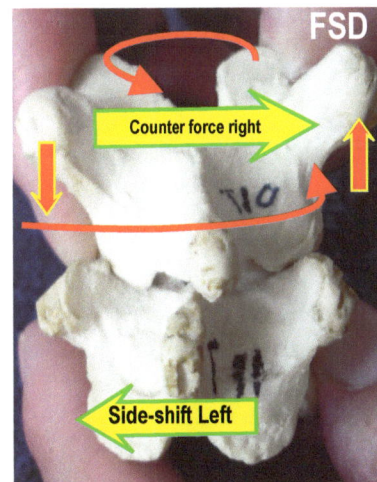

T10 Rotation and Side-bending to the left not right.

89

Typical L1-2
L3-L-R Recap of Flexion to the Right

The subluxation forces that are placed on the L4-L3 joint are also placed on L2-L1 joint and sacroiliac joint.

In preparation for how the L1-2 joints subluxate, this page is a quick recap on the normal physiological movement that takes place during flexion with rotation to the right.

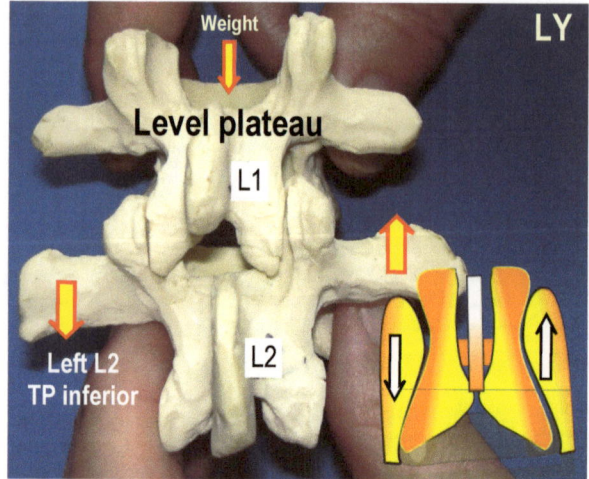

L2 side-bends left

L1-2 normal physiology recap

L1 acts as a counter lever in the vertical position during lumbar rotation and side-bending movements. When the left knee flexes, L2 follows the side-bending of the weight-bearing left pelvis. This aligns the right L2 facets to the middle of the right L1 facet, as shown in **figure LY.**

When the pelvis side-shifts to the left, L2 is pulled in the same direction and the two aligned facets engage to block the side-shift. This is shown in **figure LZ**.

If these movements are taken to their physiological limit, they do not lock; therefore, this is not how the L2-L1 joint becomes subluxated.

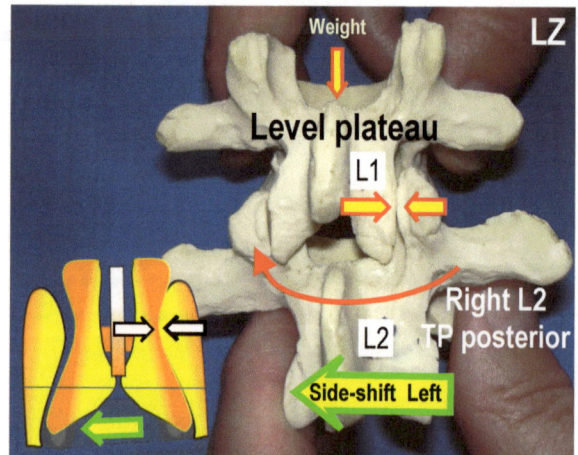

L2 rotates right whilst L1 blocks this movement to protect the thoracic vertebrae from rotating left.

L3-4 subluxation

The production and alignment of the L1-2 subluxation is influenced by the already subluxated L3-4 joint below. The subluxated L3-4 joint is for easy reference is illustrated in **figure FSBa**.

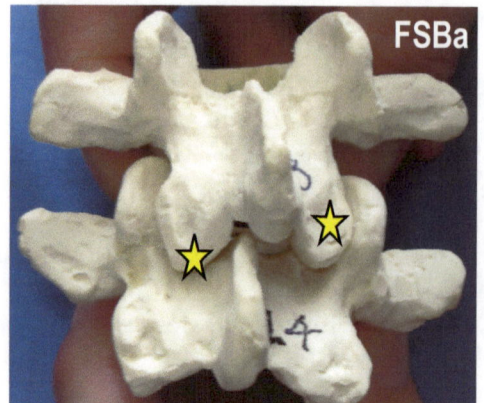

L2-L1
L3-L-R Flexion Subluxation to the Right

If the weight bearing left knee is not flexed and the lumbar is flexed in readiness to rotate right, the facets of L2 and L1 approximate in parallel. The inferior border of the L1 facets are brought into close proximity with the L2 lamina. Due to weight bearing on the left, the left facet of L2 is marginally side-bent left. This is an incorrect starting point and is shown in **figure FSF** and **FSFa**.

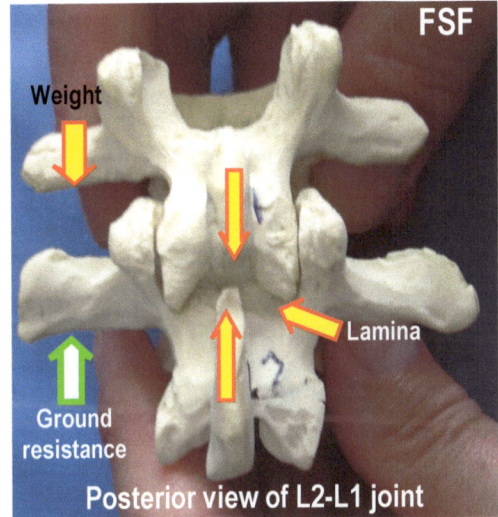

FSF

Weight

Ground resistance

Lamina

Posterior view of L2-L1 joint

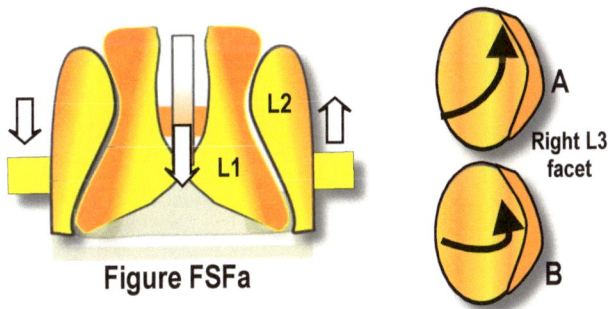

L2

L1

A

Right L3 facet

B

Figure FSFa

Figures FSG and **FSGa** show L2 following the pelvic side-shift left. A quick reminder of what happened at L3 below. The facet of L3 should have rotated in an arc, as shown in **'A'** above but instead subluxated and only marginally rotated and side-bent, as shown in **'B'** without arcing.

This has the knock-on effect of stopping the right facets of L1 from following the rotation arc of L3 and smoothly sliding up the right L2 facet. As L2 rotates right, the right facet of L1 becomes wedged against the L2 facet, as shown in **figure FSGb**. Because the right facet of L2 cannot move up the right facet of L1, L1 is forced to side-bend right.

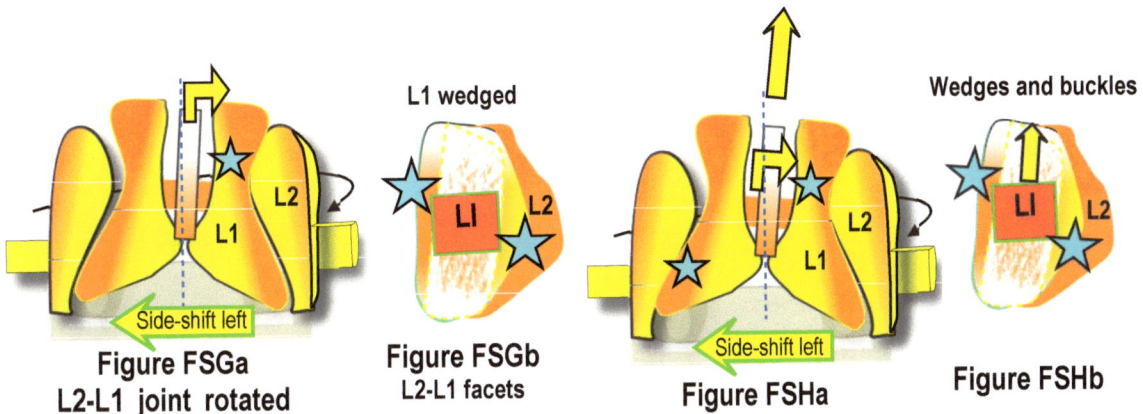

FSG

Side-shift left

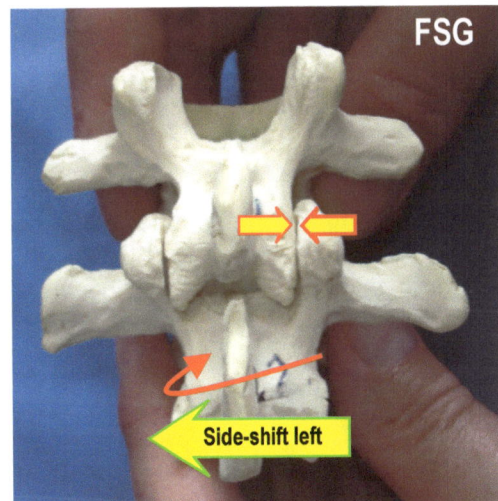

Side-shift left

Figure FSGa
L2-L1 joint rotated

L1 wedged

L1

L2

Figure FSGb
L2-L1 facets

Side-shift left

L2

L1

Figure FSHa

Wedges and buckles

L1

L2

Figure FSHb

L1-T12
L3-L-R Flexion Subluxation to the Right

Continuing on from the previous page, **figure FSGb** showed how the L1 facet got wedged just over halfway up the L2 facet and caused a minor subluxation. This subluxation is further compounded when the person leans forward without changing their direction of side-shift.

The thoracic column levers the facets of L1 superiorly as shown on the previous page in **figures FSHa** and **FSHb**. As the misaligned right facet of L1 gets dragged superiorly, the joint buckles. The force of the side-shift to the left rotates and side-bends the destabilized L1 vertebra to the right. A photograph of this final stage is shown in **figure FSH**.

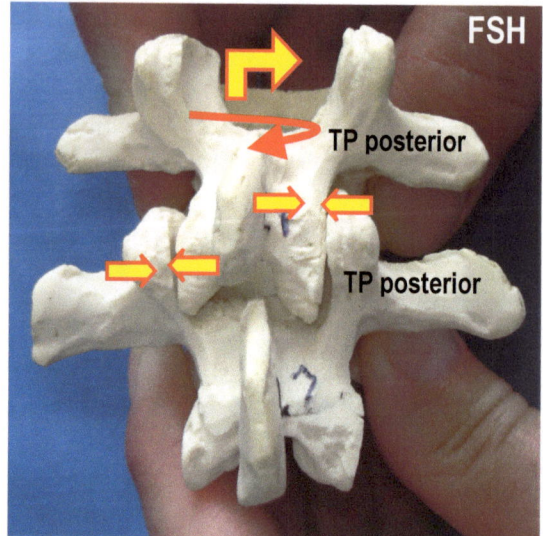

FSH

TP posterior

TP posterior

The L1-T12 joint

In normal physiology, lumbar flexion pelvic side-shift is blocked at L1, therefore T12 should have no way of rotating. However, **figure 3b** showed how the misaligned subluxated lumbar spine allowed the pelvic side-shift to pass to the left of L1.

Figure 3b also showed that the pelvic side-shift to the left does not come back into the mid-line until approximately T9 to T7 and therefore creates huge stability problems, along with extreme tightness.

For reference, **figures LCH** and **LCHa** show the L1-T12 joint in neutral.

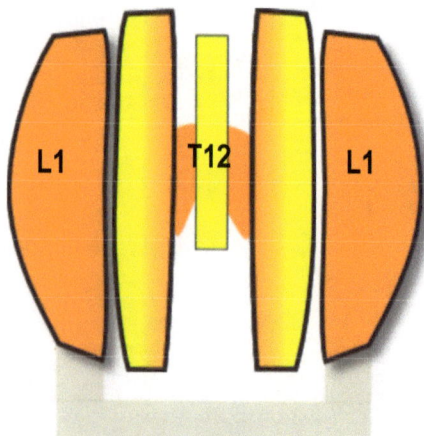

Figure LCHa
L1-T12 in neutral

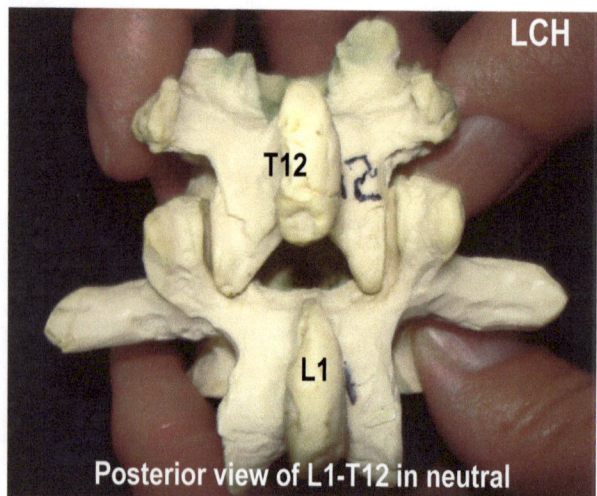

LCH

Posterior view of L1-T12 in neutral

L1-T12
L3-L-R Flexion Subluxation to the Right

Stage one

In thoracic extension (backward bending) T12 approximates with L1. **Figure FSR** illustrates the facet angles of L1. It can be seen that the rotation and side-bending to the right of the L1 facets is followed by the superior facets. The superior facets of L1 do not touch the T12 facets, as shown in **figure FSS**. However, this is an incorrect starting point for T12 to rotate right.

Stage two

Figure FST illustrates the next stage when pelvic side-shift forces L1 to the left. As L1 side-shifts to the left the inferior part of the right L1 facet engages against the inferior part of the right T12 facet. As side-shift continues, T12 buckles and rotates up the L1 facet, as shown in **figure FSU** and **FSV**.

Stage one

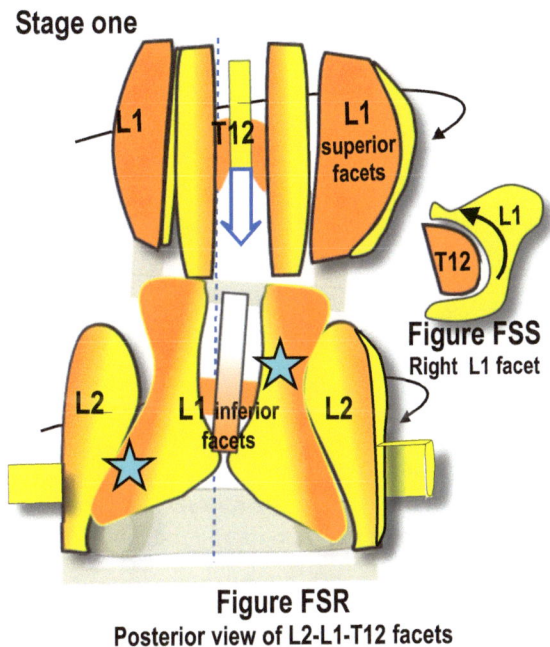

Figure FSS
Right L1 facet

Figure FSR
Posterior view of L2-L1-T12 facets

Stage three

Figure FSW illustrates the upward pull on the right side of the T12 facet when the person leans forward without change in side shift. The distorted T12 facet is dragged up the L1 right facet where it becomes firmly wedged. This is the final stage of the subluxation. **Figure FSX** illustrates T12 being forced to rotate right as the side-shift to the left buckles and side-bends T12 left. **Figure FSY** illustrates T12 subluxated approximately one third of the way up the L1 facet.

Stage two

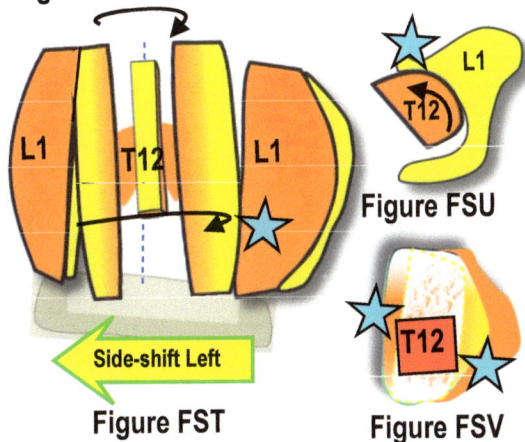

Figure FST

Figure FSU

Figure FSV

Side-shift Left

Stage three

Thoracic flexion
Pulls T12 upwards

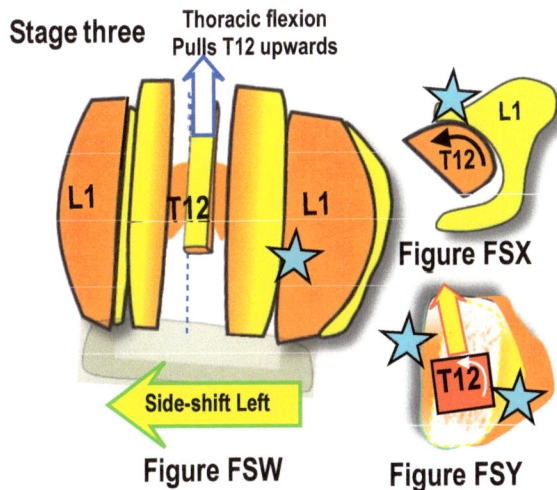

Figure FSW

Figure FSX

Figure FSY

Side-shift Left

Sacroiliac
L3-L-R Flexion Subluxation to the Right

Figure FSZ is a photograph of the final stage of the T12 subluxation. T12 is rotated and side-bent to the right in thoracic extension.

The right transverse processes of L1 and T12 are posterior and the spinous processes are approximated.

The sacroiliac joint flexion recap

Figure FSK is a brief recap of the normal physiological movement for rotation right in lumbar flexion.

When weight and pelvic side-shift are directed to the left and the left knee flexed the sacroiliac 'A' facets engage and align the acetabulum and head of the femur to angle anteriorly, medially and superiorly. This results in left knee flexion.

The flexed left knee has two advantages,

1. It side-bends the lumbar vertebrae, and
2. Rotates the pelvis and lumbar to the right.

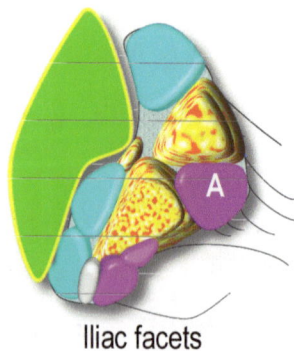

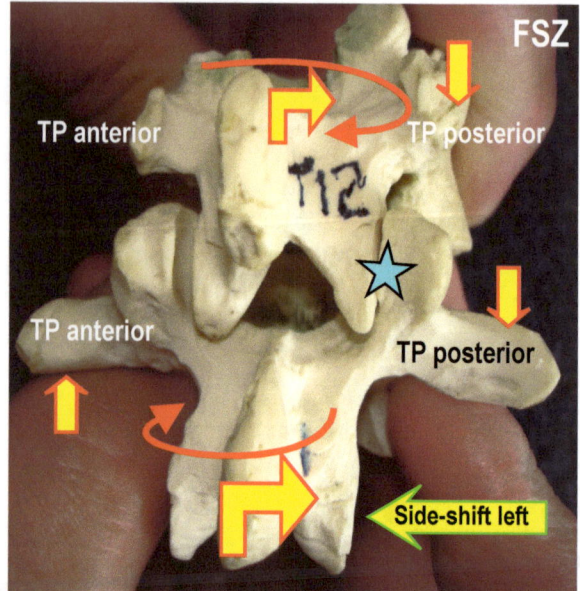

Posterior view: L1-T12 Flexion subluxation

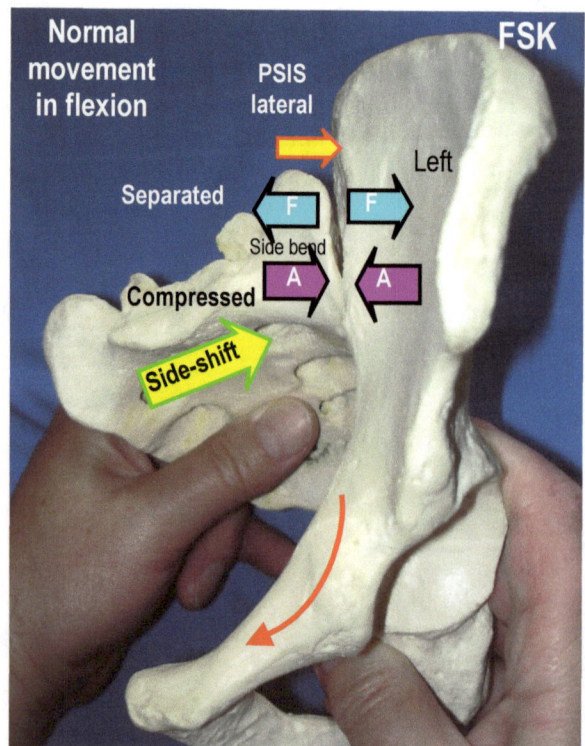

Anterior view of left sacroiliac joint

Iliac facets

Sacroiliac
L3-L-R Flexion Subluxation

The lumbar vertebrae are flexed (backward bent). Backward leaning also comes from the hips and knees.

A sacroiliac flexion subluxation will take place when a person is standing with both knees straight. With no left knee flexion the sacroiliac joints remain level so the left 'A' facets are unable to engage as they would normally do during their normal physiological flexion movement.

Instead of body weight being directed through the sacroiliac 'A' facets it incorrectly stays at the 'point of pivot'. This is acceptable when standing up straight and reservedly swaying the pelvis from side to side but not when backward bending is present. See **figure FSL**.

When backward bending, weight bearing and side-shift are directed at the left sacroiliac joint, with no facet orientation the joint becomes unstable with no facet directed rotation to the right.

If the person forces rotation right using the 'M' force muscles from above spinal rotation is forced on the unstable sacral facets and causes the sacral 'A' facet to slide over the iliac 'A' facet and overlap the joint border. See **figures FSM** and **FSMa**.

The perimeter overlap triggers the ligaments to clamp and stop any further dislocation and this locks the subluxation in. The PSIS is medial and inferior and the ASIS, superior and lateral. Effectively the left sacroiliac joints are locked tightly and constitute a **sacroiliac subluxation.**

With side-shift still to the left and the lumbar joints subluxated above, when the person straightens as they would to walk, they forcibly lever the left Ilium including the locked sacroiliac joint forward. This compounds the sacroiliac subluxation. **This is an Innominate sub-lesion.**

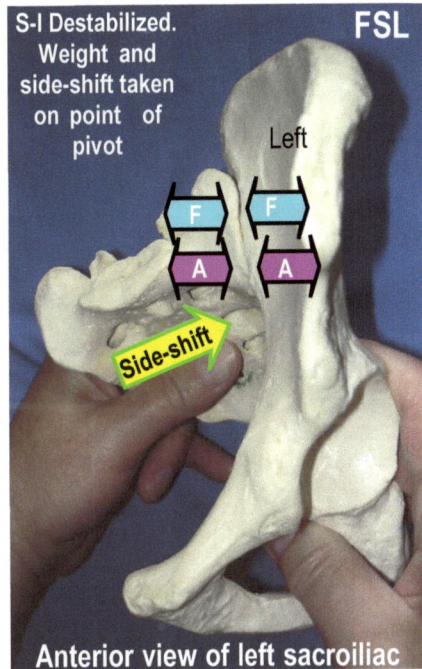

FSL
S-I Destabilized. Weight and side-shift taken on point of pivot
Left
F F
A A
Side-shift
Anterior view of left sacroiliac

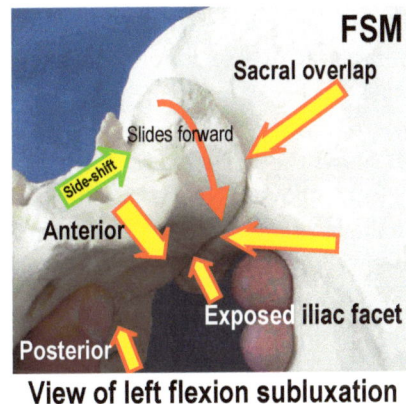

FSM
Sacral overlap
Slides forward
Side-shift
Anterior
Exposed iliac facet
Posterior
View of left flexion subluxation

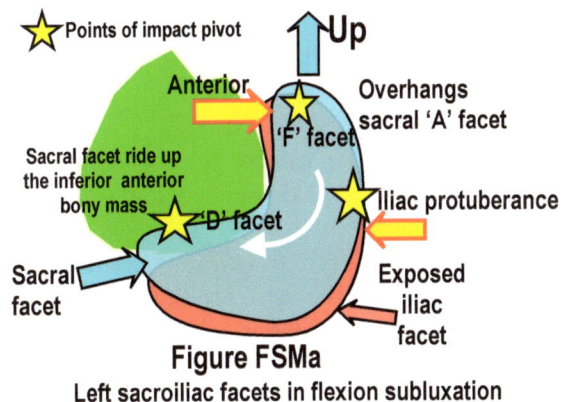

Points of impact pivot
Up
Anterior
Overhangs sacral 'A' facet
'F' facet
Sacral facet ride up the inferior anterior bony mass
'D' facet
Iliac protuberance
Sacral facet
Exposed iliac facet
Figure FSMa
Left sacroiliac facets in flexion subluxation

Sacroiliac
L3-L-R Flexion Subluxation

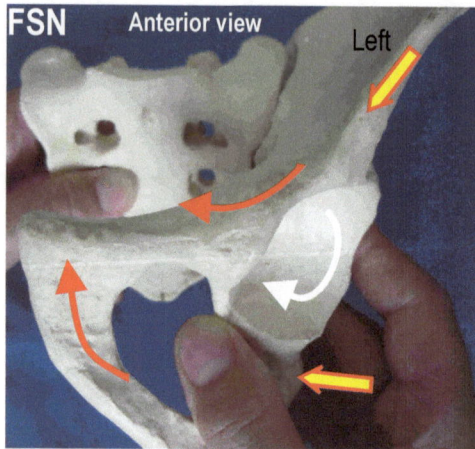

Normal physiological movement

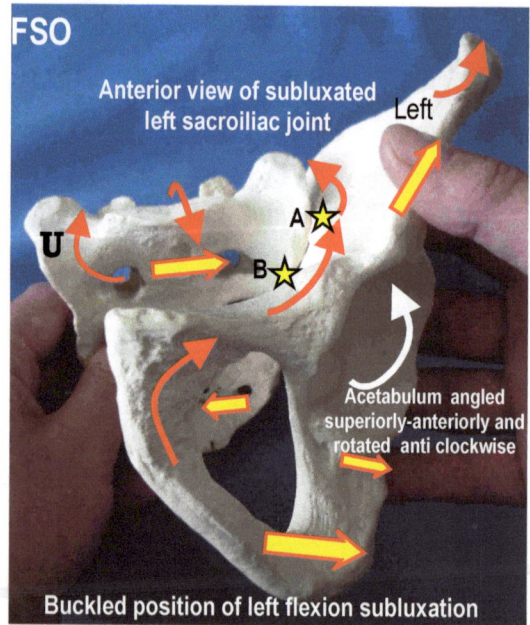

Buckled position of left flexion subluxation

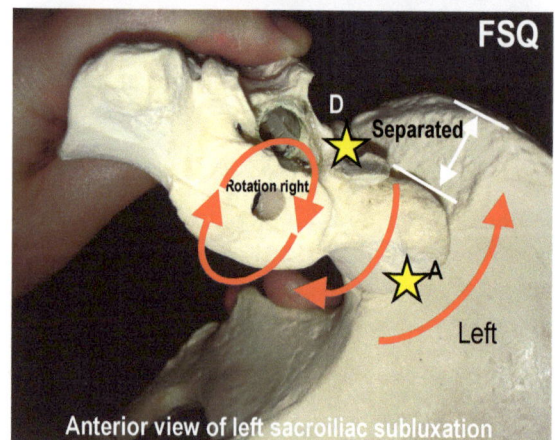

Anterior view of left sacroiliac subluxation

For comparison purposes, **figure FSN** shows the direction of forces during normal physiological flexion. **Figure FSO** shows the buckled position of the left Ilium and its affect on the angle of the acetabulum, pubic ramous and iliac crest in the flexion subluxation. The yellow stars show the points of impact. The upward arrow (U) shown in white on the right side of the sacral base denotes the minor upward tilt that takes place.

Figure FSQ shows the subluxated sacrum in relation to the Ilium from above. Note that the base of the sacrum on the left side is anterior in relation to the left Ilium and that the posterior superior iliac crest is medial.

Two stages take place simultaneously to create the flexion subluxation. To make it easier to understand, **figure FSQa** illustrates the two stages in block form:

Stage one, the inferior part of the Innominate is pushed outward to create side-bending to the left;

Stage two, the left Innominate remains posterior and buckles in relation to the sacrum. It is important to remember that it is the sacrum that moves on the weight bearing Ilium.

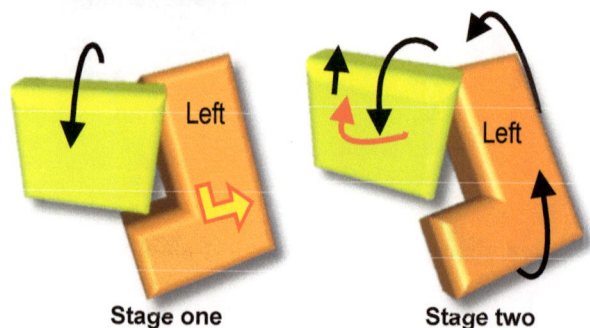

Figure FSQa
Block anterior views of the left sacroiliac subluxation in formation

Sacroiliac
L3-L-R Flexion Subluxation

The purpose of this page is to illustrate that in the L3-L-R flexion subluxation the sacrum slides anterio-inferiorly on the left. This incorrectly rotates the sacrum right in a distorted manner that both mis-aligns the Ilium and tilts its base forward.

Figure FSR is a photograph of the left side of the S/I flexion subluxation. The left side of the sacrum rotates right and slides anterio-inferiorly. This lifts the apex of the sacrum and dips the base.

In this position the right side of the sacrum due to the lack of knee flexion on the left is balanced on the 'point of pivot' and easily forced to rotate right and slide posterio- superiorly.

For better visualization **figure 9b** illustrates the angle of the subluxated sacrum .

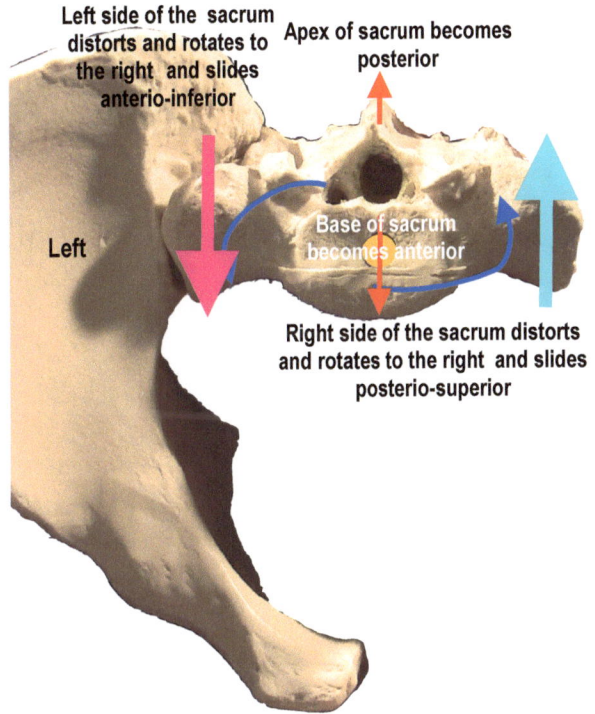

Figure 9bb and **9c** illustrate the difference in position between the normal alignment of the innominate and the flexion subluxated left Innominate.

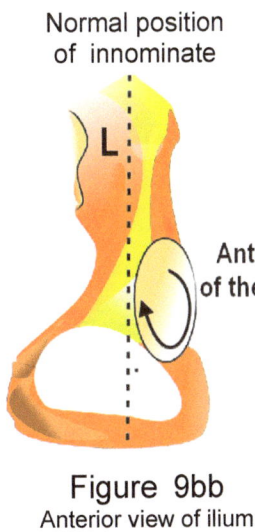

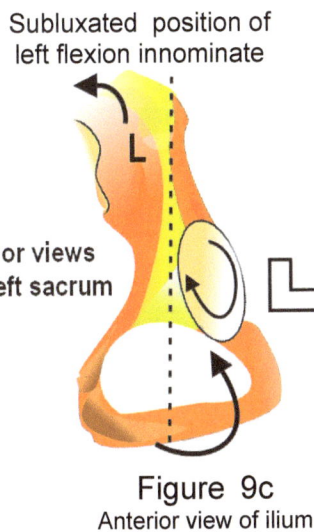

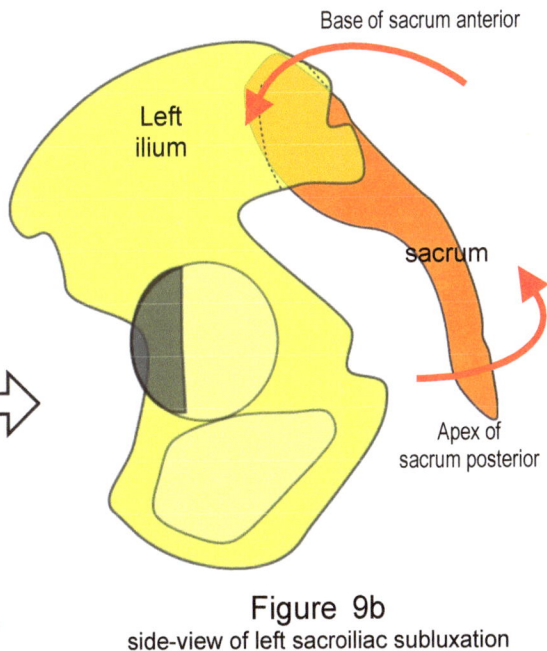

Left side of the sacrum distorts and rotates to the right and slides anterio-inferior

Apex of sacrum becomes posterior

Left

Base of sacrum becomes anterior

Right side of the sacrum distorts and rotates to the right and slides posterio-superior

Figure FSR
View from above of left flexion sacroiliac subluxation

Normal position of innominate

Subluxated position of left flexion innominate

L

L

Anterior views of the left sacrum

Figure 9bb
Anterior view of ilium

Figure 9c
Anterior view of ilium

Base of sacrum anterior

Left ilium

sacrum

Apex of sacrum posterior

Figure 9b
side-view of left sacroiliac subluxation

Consequences of a Left Flexion Subluxation on the Right Sacroiliac

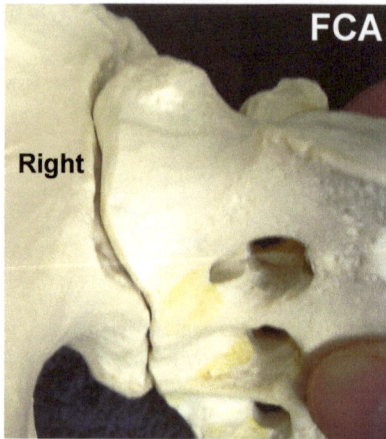

FCA

Right

Neutral starting position
Anterior view of right
sacroiliac joint

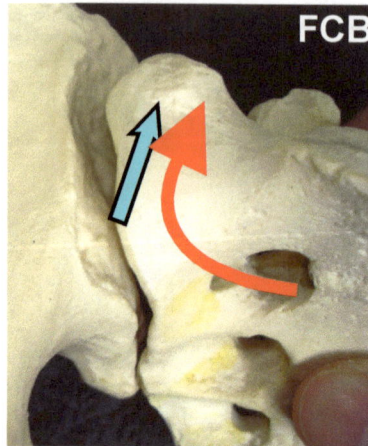

FCB

Sacrum side-bent left

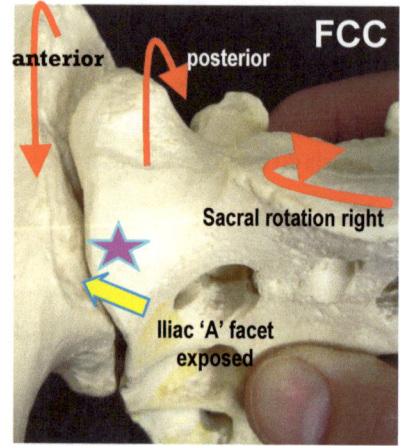

FCC

anterior   posterior

Sacral rotation right

Iliac 'A' facet
exposed

Sacral base dragged posteriorly

Without left knee flexion pelvic side-shift to the left becomes exaggerated. See chapter one. This causes the right side of the sacroiliac joint to be weak and vulnerable.

Like the left side, without left knee flexion to align the sacroiliac facets the right side of the sacroiliac joint takes its point of axes from the 'point of pivot'. The distorted sacral rotation to the right emanating from the left, slides the sacral 'F' facet superiorly over the iliac 'F' facets where it lodges over the superior border of the iliac 'F' facet and against the bony mass.

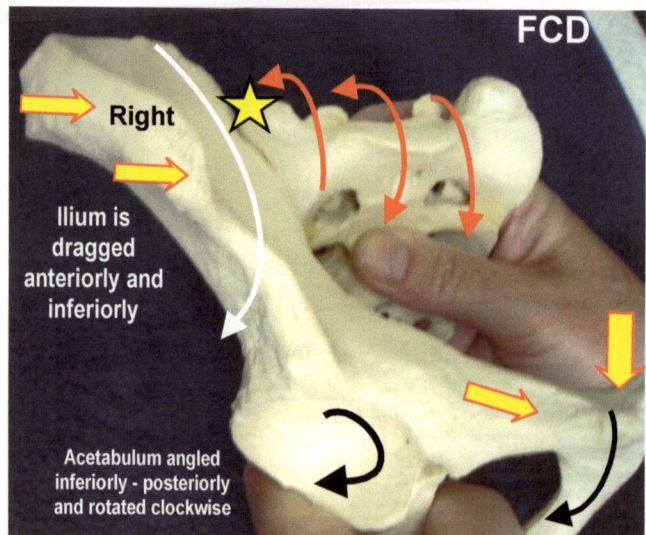

FCD

Right

Ilium is
dragged
anteriorly and
inferiorly

Acetabulum angled
inferiorly - posteriorly
and rotated clockwise

Figure FCA shows for reference the neutral position of a right sacroiliac joint.

Figure FCB shows the sacral rotation and slide superio-posterior against right iliac 'F' facet.

Figure FCC shows the Iliac'A' facets exposed and the positional relationship between the sacral and iliac facets. This is a sacroiliac subluxation.

Figure FCD shows the position of the sacrum is distorted and rotated posteriorly on the right in contrast to the anterior rotation on the left. The right acetabulum is inferior, medial and posterior. The anterior superior iliac spine is medial, anterior and inferior and the pubic tubercle is posterior, inferior and medial.

Illustrations
Right Iliac Flexion Subluxation

Figure 9J shows the position of the right sacral facet as it rides up and impacts against the right superior bony mass of the Ilium. Note that there are three points of impact pivot:

1. The anterior superior iliac bony mass
2. The mound between the 'A' iliac facet and the 'F' iliac facet.
3. The 'B' iliac facet.

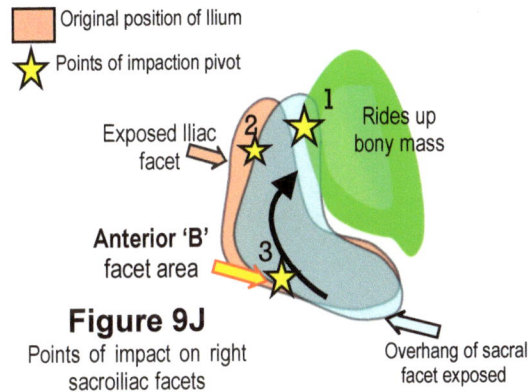

Figure 9L illustrates the position of the right Innominate immediately after the flexion subluxation has taken place on the left.

Figure 9M illustrates the position of the Ilium when the person leans backward in order to stand upright. The 'F' facet of the sacrum is levered posteriorly over the 'F' facet of the Ilium into the bony mass.

The Innominate is side-bent right and tipped anteriorly. This rotates the acetabulum posteriorly, medially and inferiorly and causes the weight of the person to channel through their right leg to their toes.

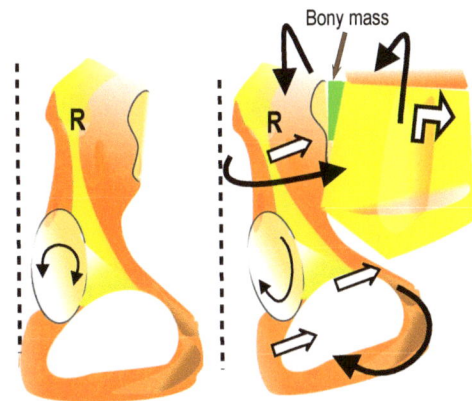

Figure 9K is an anterior view illustration of the type of distortion the subluxated sacroiliac joints inflict on the pelvis.

When weight and side-shift transfer to the right, the sacroiliac subluxations become blocked by the weight bearing and distorted right side of the pelvis. This tightens and distorts the pelvis further and with weight bearing locks-in the S/I subluxations.

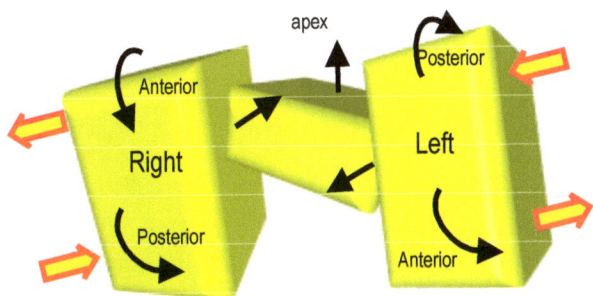

This is stage one of a pelvic lesion. Stage two comes when the person attempts to forward bend and this further tightens the pelvic lesion.

Original position of Ilium

Points of impaction pivot

Exposed Iliac facet

Anterior 'B' facet area

Rides up bony mass

Figure 9J
Points of impact on right sacroiliac facets

Overhang of sacral facet exposed

Bony mass

Figure 9L   **Figure 9M**
Anterior views, showing the effect the left
Sacroiliac flexion subluxated pattern has on the right side.

apex

Anterior

Posterior

Right

Left

Posterior

Anterior

Figure 9K
Anterior view of Sacroiliac joint group
L3-L-R subluxation

Lumbar Flexion Subluxation Pattern

All of the transverse processes are posterior on the right

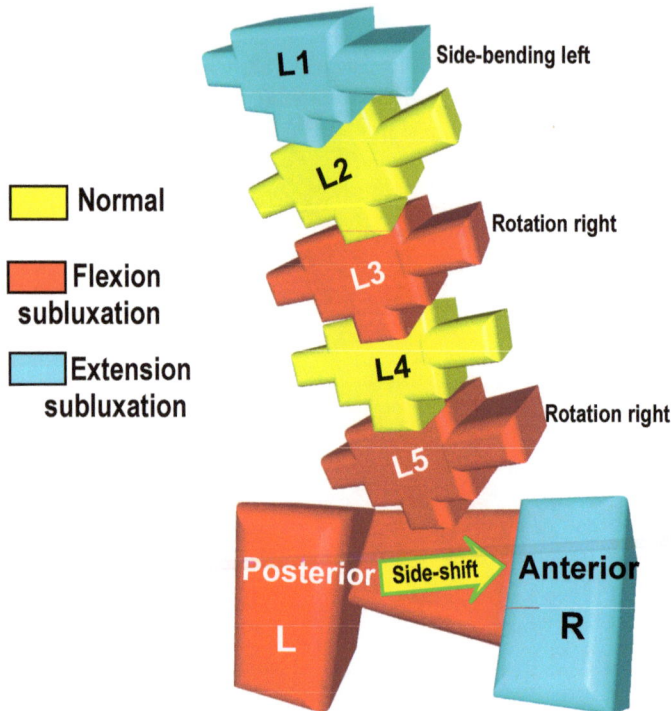

L1 — Side-bending left

□ **Normal**

■ **Flexion subluxation**

□ **Extension subluxation**

L2

L3 — Rotation right

L4

L5 — Rotation right

Posterior → Side-shift → **Anterior**

L   **R**

Figure 6
Posterior view of lumbar and sacroiliac joints

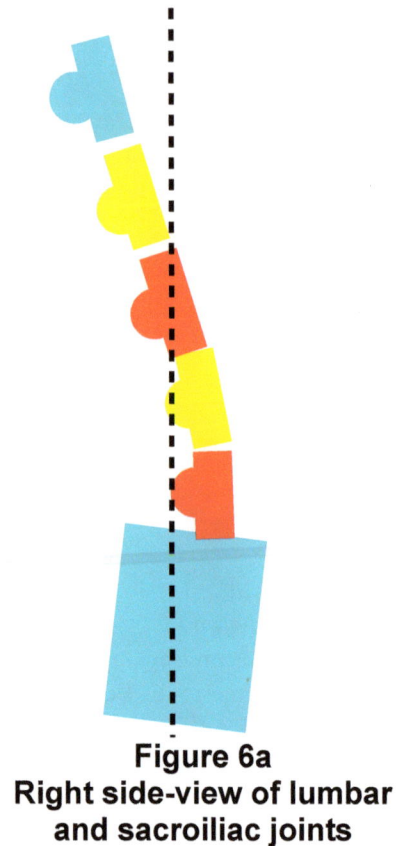

Figure 6a
Right side-view of lumbar and sacroiliac joints

With the subluxation elements of the lumbar and sacroiliac joints put together, **figure 6** shows the theoretical lumbar vertebrae flexion subluxation pattern. The flexion subluxations are in red.

Although L1 is backward bent, because the subluxation locked with side-bending and rotation to the right, (the same side) it is technically an extension subluxation.

Figure 6a provides a right side-view of the sacroiliac and lumbar joints. L1 is shown in backward bending.

Finally, the side-bending left and the rotation right of the pelvis rotates L4 to the right against L3. In doing this the right superior facet of L4 becomes further compacted against the subluxated inferior right L3 facet. This double locks in the L3 subluxation. For the same reason the L5 subluxation also becomes double locked.

The further the base of the sacrum moves anteriorly the greater the torsion on L4. This can make visual and palpable differentiation of L4-L3 very confusing, as it feels and looks as if L4-3 has side-bent right.

Left-Right Pelvic Flexion Lesion
Part One

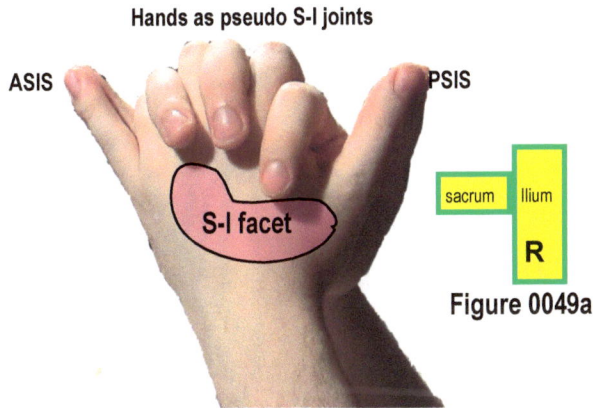

Hands as pseudo S-I joints

ASIS PSIS

S-I facet

sacrum | Ilium

R

Figure 0049a

Figure 0049
The Hands as an S-I Joint and pelvis

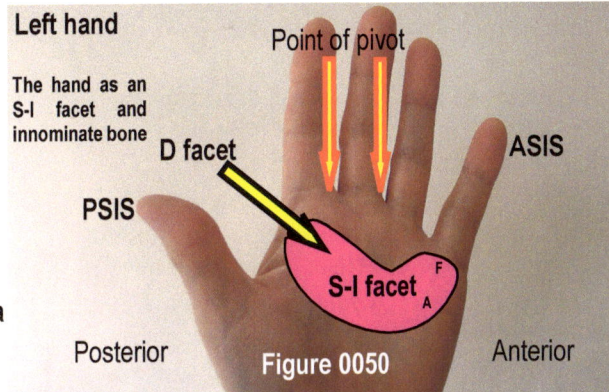

Left hand

The hand as an S-I facet and innominate bone

Point of pivot

D facet

ASIS

PSIS

S-I facet

Posterior   **Figure 0050**   Anterior

The pelvic lesion locks-in the sacroiliac subluxations and forces them to become sacroiliac lesions. At the same time the lesioned pelvic forces compound the lesions in the spine and rib cage.

A Pelvic lesion is reinforced each and every time a leg becomes weight bearing. Particularly the right leg It is difficult to show how a pelvic lesion is inflicted with actual bones therefore, I have illustrated how the pelvis becomes lesioned with a practical example.

Do this self test

In these hand examples your elbows act as your knees/legs and the right hand the combination of the side of the Ilium and sacrum, see **figure 49A**.

Start by putting your hands together as per **figure 0049** and imagine the S-I facets are positioned in the palms of your hands as per **figure 0050**.

Place your hands together in an upright position as per **figures 0051, 0051A and 00050B**.

Keep your elbows level. Now draw your hands towards you body to simulate pelvic flexion (backward bending) as per **figures 0052, 0052A and 0052B**.

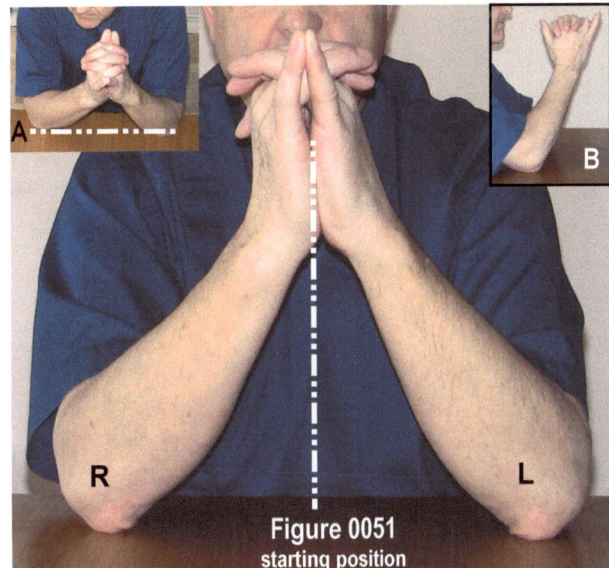

R   L

Figure 0051
starting position

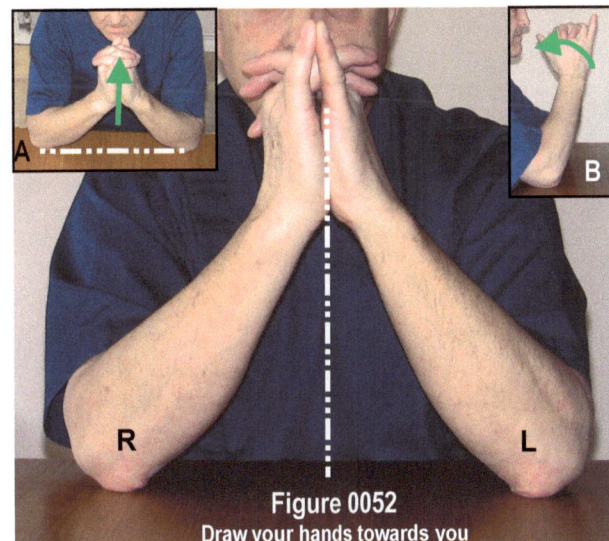

R   L

Figure 0052
Draw your hands towards you

101

Left-Right Pelvic Flexion Lesion
Part Two

Next place your weight on your left elbow.

Look at **figures 0053** and **0053C** and draw your right elbow towards the left elbow to simulate pelvic side-shift to the left. At the same time rotate your hands right to simulate rotation to the right from the spine. Your right elbow will move to the left and towards your body. This is the position the subluxated left S/I facets would angle the pelvis. See **figure 0053B**. (Side-bent right and rotated right).

Refer to **figure 0053D** below and squeeze your index and middle fingers together to simulate the 'point of pivot' shown in **figure 0053B**. The 'point of pivot' is the area where the facets are in subluxation. I.e. 'D' facets.

In **figure 0053A** note that the position of the little finger on the right hand which represents the ASIS is anterio-superior. And that the left thumb, which represents the PSIS, is posterio-inferior.

Next, transfer your weight to your right elbow. This will fractionally lift your left elbow off the table. Move your left elbow towards your right to simulate pelvic side-shift right, as per **figures 0054** and **0054A**. With the 'D' facet as the point of pivot (see **figure 0055/1)** your left elbow will move away from your body and rotate your hands further to the right. This locking simulates the knock-on position of the pelvis when the right S/I facets become subluxated.

Position recap
• Both of your arms and hands should now be to the left of the mid line.
• Your hands should be side-bent to the right and rotated to the right.
• Your right elbow (leg) posterior and medial and your left elbow (leg) anterior to your right elbow and slightly medial.
• This represents the position of the pelvis in the bi-lateral flexion S/I subluxation.

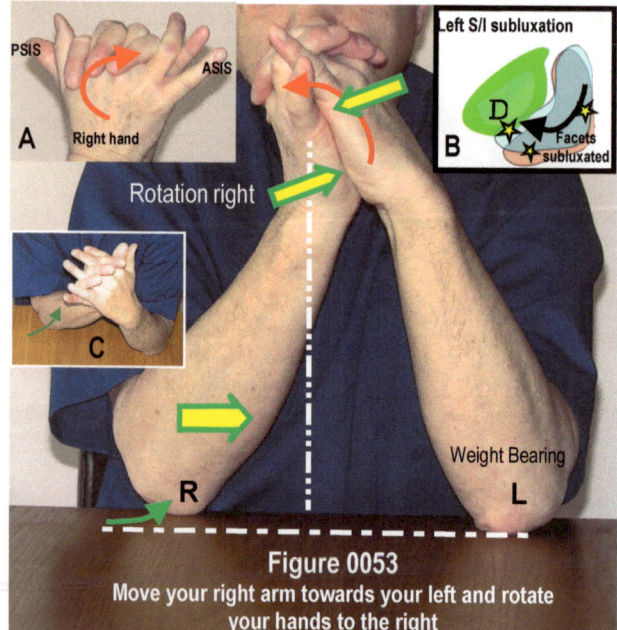

Figure 0053
Move your right arm towards your left and rotate your hands to the right

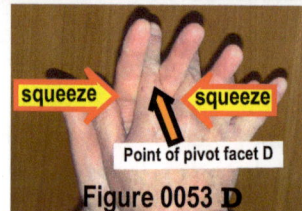

Figure 0053 D

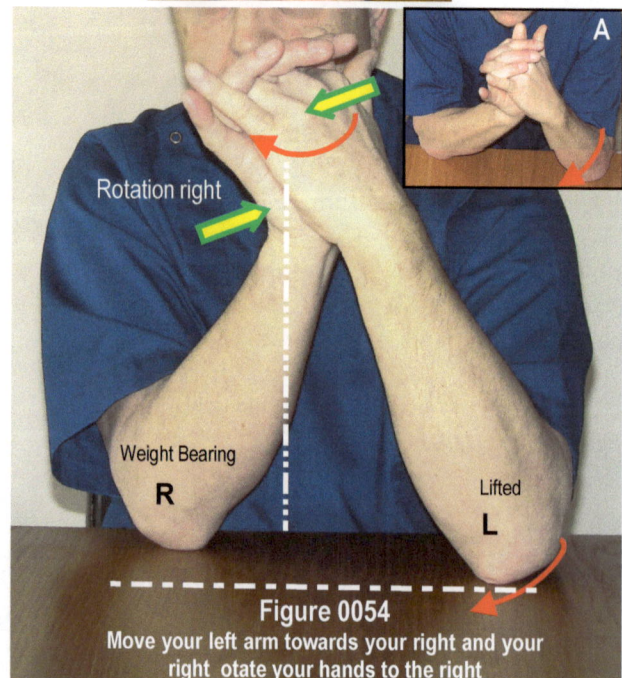

Figure 0054
Move your left arm towards your right and your right otate your hands to the right

Left-Right Pelvic Flexion Lesion
Part Three

Iliosacral lesions are created in the pelvis when a person then walks forward.

Figure 0055 illustrates the 'point of pivot', situated at the subluxated 'D' facets on the left. This is a fixed point that is locked in by the S/I subluxations.

Refer to **figures 0056, 0056A, 0056B** and **0055/2**. Body weight is directed back to the left elbow (leg) and the person strides forward with their right elbow (leg). To do this they side-shift their pelvis to the left. Because the point of pivot is at the posterior, the anterior parts of your hands become rotated to the left.

Your right elbow will be anterior in relation to your left and closer to the mid line. This forces the heel of your left hand behind the heel of your right hand (the point of pivot) and effectively rotates your hands (pelvis) to the left.

Next refer to **figures 0057, 0057A, 0056B** and **0055/3**. Body weight is directed back to the right elbow (leg) with side-shift of your hands (pelvis) to the right the person strides forward with their left elbow (leg). With the rotational force directly posterior and to the right of the 'point of pivot' your hands (pelvis) rotate further to the left.

Your left elbow (leg) will be anterior and rotated outwards in relation to your right. Your right will also be turned outward but not as much as the left. The angle of the hands (pelvis) which are locked in side-bending to the right will cause your right elbow (leg) to be physiologically shorter whenever weight is placed on the right elbow (leg).

This is a 'complicated lesion' as it set out with pelvic rotation to the right but then ended up with forced rotation to the left. This lesion is reinforced and amplified every time weight is placed on the legs.

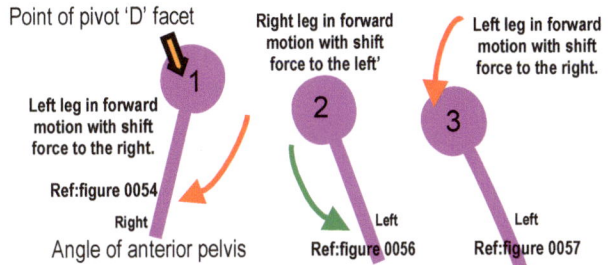

Point of pivot 'D' facet

Left leg in forward motion with shift force to the right.
Ref:figure 0054
Right
Angle of anterior pelvis

Right leg in forward motion with shift force to the left'
Left
Ref:figure 0056

Left leg in forward motion with shift force to the right.
Left
Ref:figure 0057

Figure 0055 aerial view
shows how S/I facets are forced to rotate left

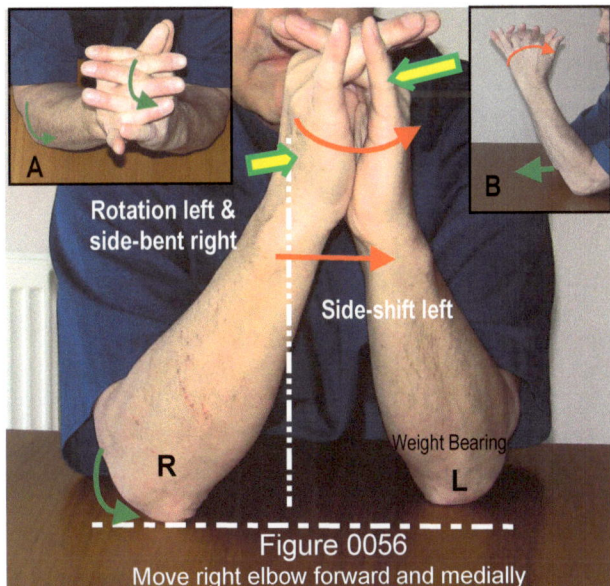

Rotation left & side-bent right
Side-shift left
Weight Bearing
R
L

Figure 0056
Move right elbow forward and medially

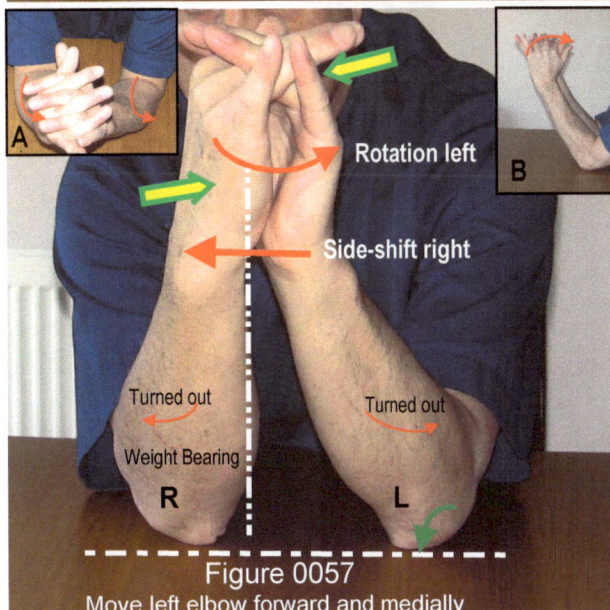

Rotation left
Side-shift right
Turned out
Turned out
Weight Bearing
R
L

Figure 0057
Move left elbow forward and medially

L3-Left-Right Lumbar-Pelvic Flexion Lesion Pattern

The reactive force that travels up the legs compounds the pelvic lesion on weight bearing. The L5-sacral joints which started out being subluxated with rotation to the right are levered to rotate in lesion to the left. This makes the left transverse process of L5 posterior. This is a very tight lesion and capable of causing much pain.

Because of the pelvic and lumbar rotation to the left the whole spine becomes generally rotated to the left.

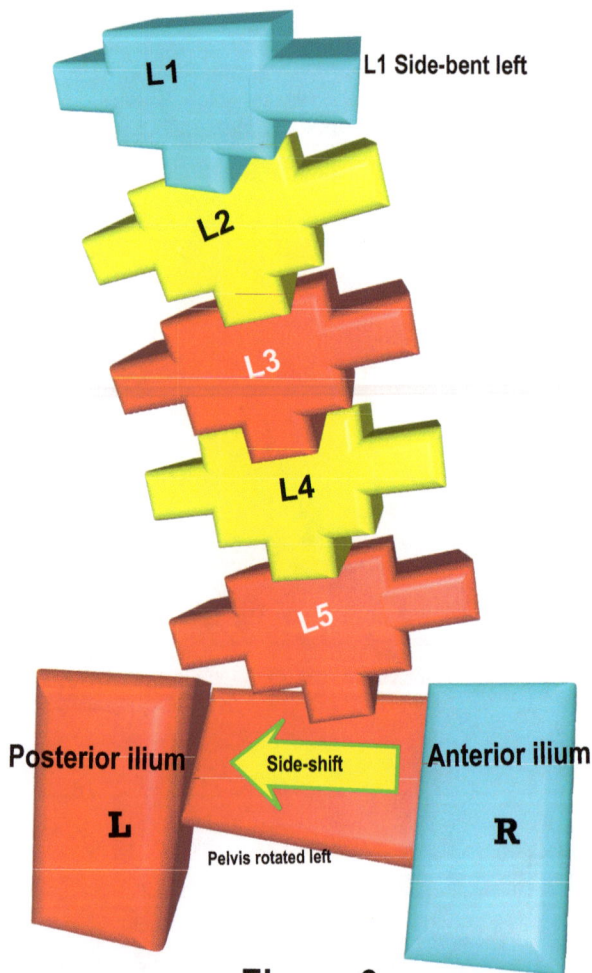

Figure 6c
Posterior view of lumbar and sacroiliac joints

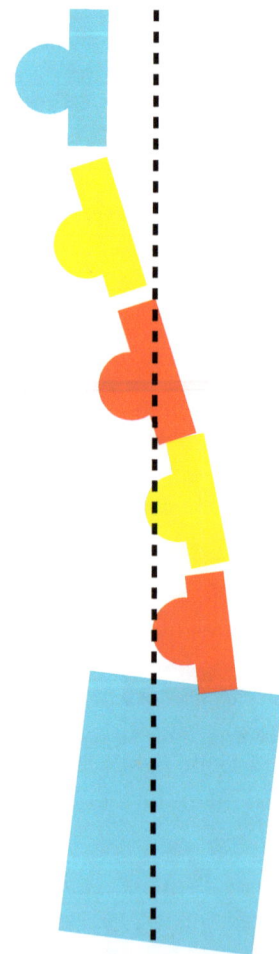

Figure 6d
Right side-view of lumbar and sacroiliac joints

Normal   Flexion lesion   Extension lesion

Chapter Eight

L3-Right-Right
Extension Lesions of the Lower Back

Extension subluxations in the lumbar vertebrae are caused in lumbar extension (forward bending) in the absence of left knee flexion. This creates a misaligned starting position for normal lumbar side-bending to follow. When weight bearing and side-shift are transferred to the right, the initial rotation right and correct trajectory of the lumbar and sacroiliac facets are askew.

When forced side-bending is applied from above using the 'M' force, the joint subluxates. This subluxation is compounded when weight and side-shift are transferred to the left leg and lumbar flexion is attempted. It then becomes a lesion.

Figure 2 is an illustration of the hypothetical forces placed on the lumbar and sacroiliac joints in extension (forward leaning), with rotation to the right.

It can be seen that L3 takes the maximum bending and stress and that the secondary areas of stress are taken at L2-L1 and L5 and the right sacroiliac joint.

L3-L4 is therefore the area of prime torsion.

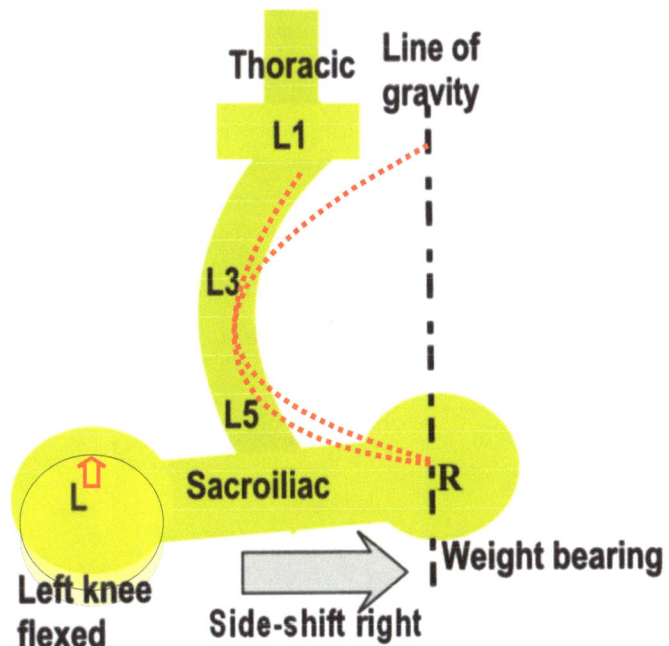

Thoracic Line of gravity

L1

L3

L5

Sacroiliac R

Weight bearing

L
Left knee flexed

Side-shift right

Figure 2

105

The Principles of a Lumbar Extension Lesion
Part One

Extension subluxation

The principle of how an extension subluxation is created is illustrated here together with the two additional forces that convert a subluxation into an osteopathic lesion.

You may find it useful to refresh your memory of normal physiological lumbar extension rotation before completing this test. See pages 21 and 22.

Do this self test

By doing these hand movements yourself you will gain an understanding of how lesions are created and the kind of tightness and pain they are capable of inflicting.

Lumbar extension lesion with rotation to the right

Figure 0045 is an illustration of the starting point. Make sure your hands are clasped tightly together. Your palms and the heels of hands should also be pressed into one another.

Joints have very little slack. In these illustrations think of your elbows as knees, the base of your hands as the pelvis and your interlaced fingers as the L3-4 joint.

To create a subluxation your knees would not be flexed, so make sure your elbows are level and on a flat surface and in line with each other. See **figure 0045A**.

Place your body weight on your right elbow and try not to allow too much play in your wrists.

To simulate lumbar extension (forward bending) push your hands away from your body as shown in **figures 0046 and 0046A**. This provides us with pseudo lumbar extension.

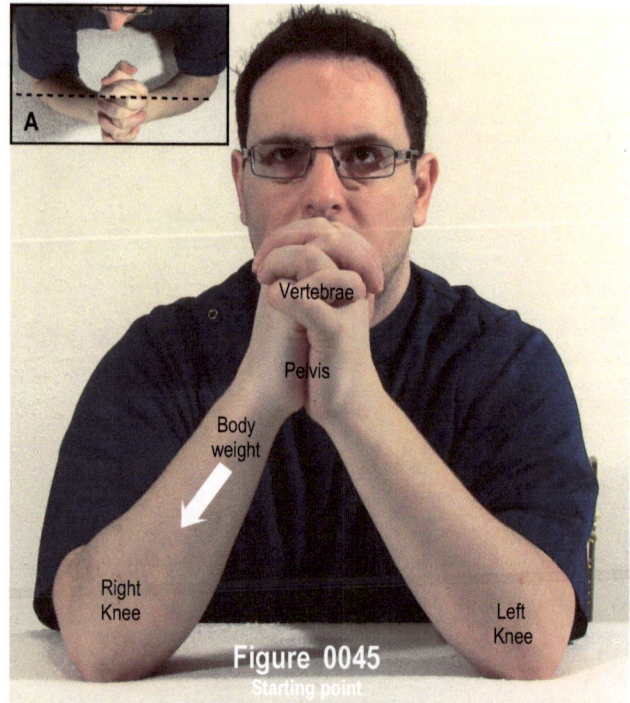

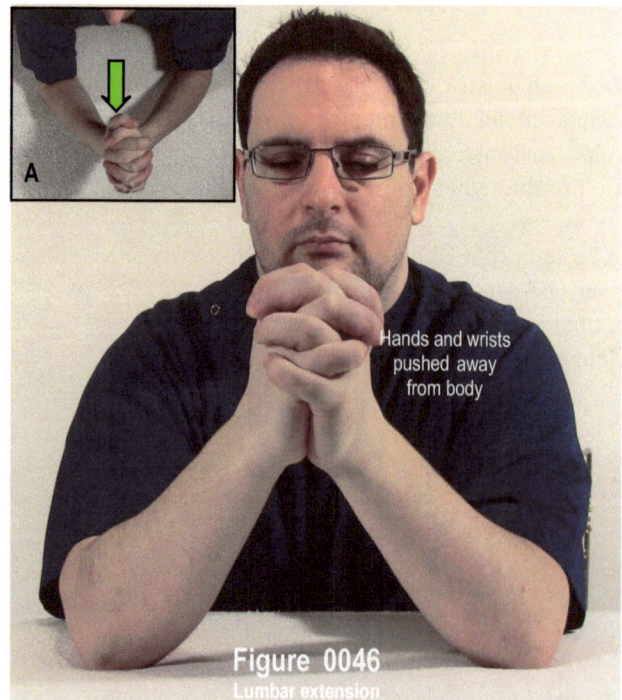

A

Vertebrae

Pelvis

Body weight

Right Knee

Left Knee

Figure 0045
Starting point

A

Hands and wrists pushed away from body

Figure 0046
Lumbar extension

The Principles of a Lumbar Extension Lesion
Part Two

Pelvic side-bending and rotation are restricted by the non flexed knees, therefore, there is no general precursor pelvic rotation or side-bending. This forces the lumbar joint articulations to start from a misaligned position.

Side-shift your left elbow towards your right to simulate pelvic side-shift right as shown in **figure 0047A**. No rotation or side-bending take place.

To rotate both hands to the right, the action has to be forced from above using the 'M' force. But when you attempt to rotate your hands to the right the action is blocked. This is because with your hands away from your body (extended) your hands side-bend to the right.

Now draw your hands towards your body to simulate a person attempting to straighten into spine neutral. You never quite make it and the tightness in your fingers becomes uncomfortable. See **figure 0047B**. This is a lumbar extension subluxation to the right.

Extension lesion to the right

See **figure 0048**. To compound the subluxation side-shift your right elbow towards your left to simulate pelvic side-shift to the left. Notice that your fingers now rotate right a little and tighten more acutely on each other and result in an increase in discomfort or pain.

See **figure 0048D**. Now attempt to draw your hands towards your body to simulate a person attempting to stand upright and feel your fingers bite into each other to the point of turning your knuckles white. Note that the closer you draw your hands to your body the tighter your hands become.

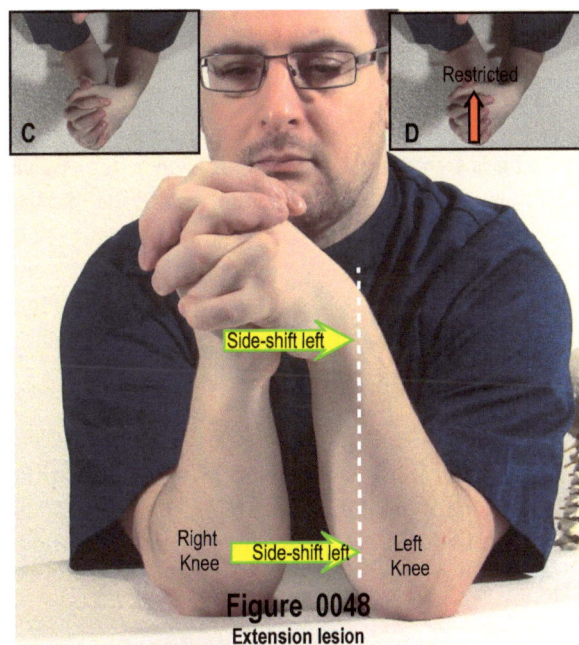

Figure 0047
Extension Subluxation

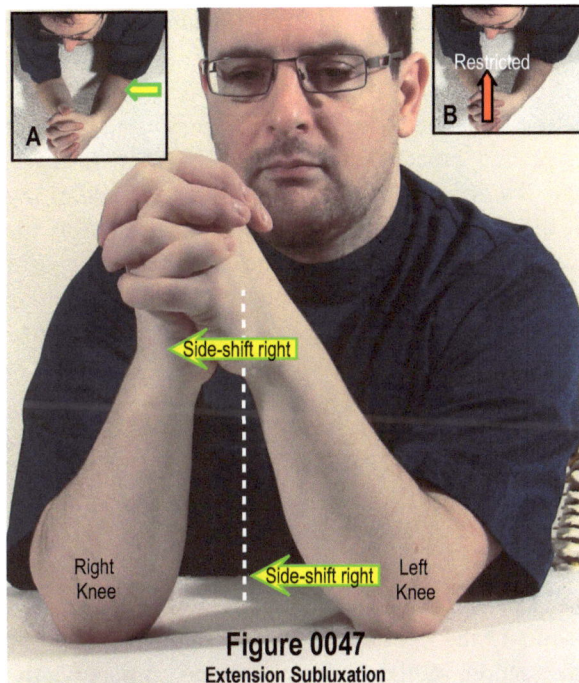

Figure 0048
Extension lesion

Look at the overall position of your hands. Your elbows are basically level, the left elbow only slightly anterior. In normal physiology lumbar extension with rotation to the right is created by rotation and side-bending to the same side. In the lesion, side-bending with rotation to the same side, the opposite way round. Worse is to come when the pelvis buckles to the right.

L4-L3
Extension Lesion to the Right

Initially a person leans forward and the lumbar vertebrae are are placed in a state extension, as shown in **figure ESA**.

When the left knee is not flexed for reasons of lack of space or bad practice the right S/I 'F' facet does not engage. If weight is then placed on the right side of the body, the pelvis does not rise and cannot rotate to the right. Without the pelvic rise and rotation to the right L4-L3 is unable to align into the correct starting position for local 'M' force side-bending to follow.

Without pelvic 'G' force rotation and correct side bending to the right, rotation at L3-4 to the right has to be forced using the 'M' force. This is shown in **figure ESA**

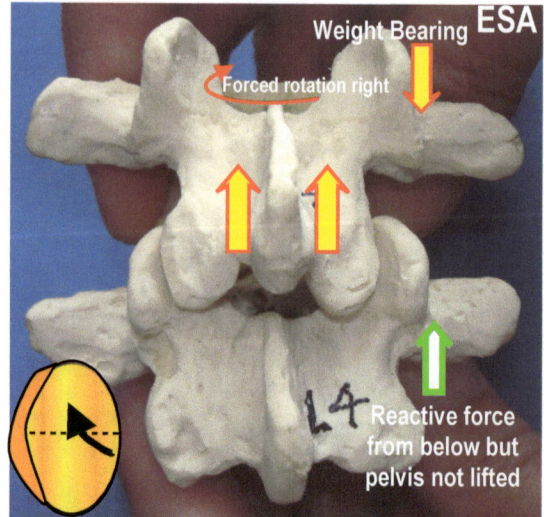

Figure ESB shows what happens when the pelvis side-shifts to the right and the 'G' force drags L4 in the same direction. With counter-resistance from above the L3 facets are forced to articulate across the facets of L4 on an incorrect trajectory that forces the left L3 facet to impact into the side of the left L4 facet.

This binding is tightened into a subluxation when pelvic side-shift is maintained on the right and the person backward bends (lumbar flexion), as shown in **figure ESC**. The vertebral column acts as a long lever and forces the left facet of L3 inferiorly and laterally on the left L4 facet and this increases the impaction. The more the person straightens the tighter the subluxation becomes.

The illustrations in the bottom left side corners of the photographs are of the left L3 facet trajectory. The 'body' in the top left hand corner shows the degree of rotation.

When pelvic weight bearing and side-shift are transferred to the left the joint tightens to the point where it can affect the local blood supply. This is a lesion and is greatly compounded when the person attempts to further straighten or backward bend.

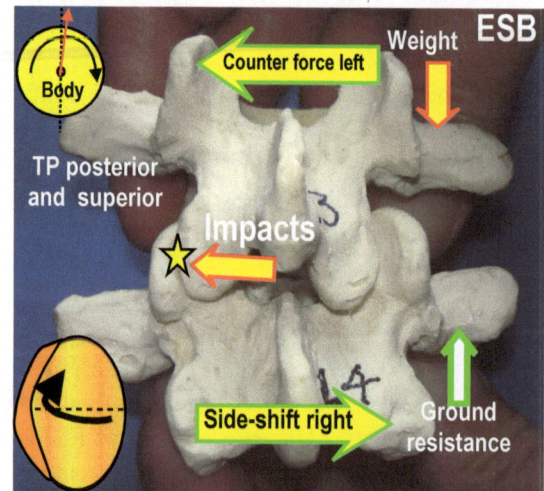

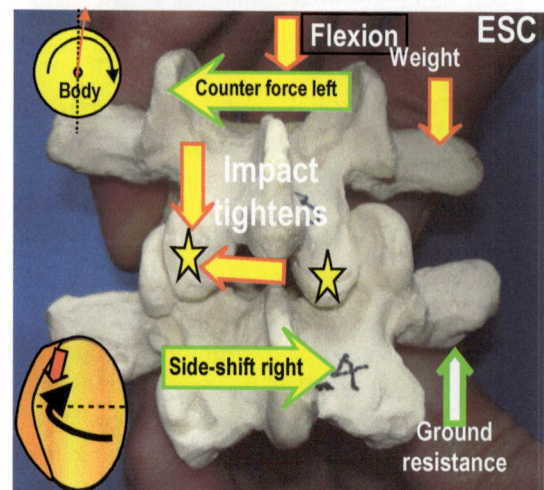

L4-L3 Subluxation Vs Normal Rotation

A practical example of this type of subluxation occurs when a standing person keeps their legs straight and bends forward and rotates to the right. If the person then straightens whilst continuing to rotate to the right the spinal joints will subluxate.

Commonly this type of action can be traced to people who dig or shovel incorrectly or lift when rotated in a tight space.

Figure ESD is an exaggeration of the normal extension rotation to the right movement and is shown for comparison against the subluxated version shown in **figure ESC.**

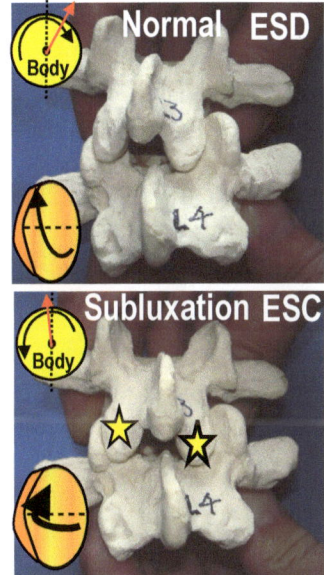

The forces that are placed on L4-L3 are also placed on L2-L1 and the sacroiliac joint. So let's look at the L2-L1 joint next. To briefly recap on the normal physiological movement of the L2-L1 joint, L1 acts as a counter lever in the vertical position during lumbar rotation movements. When the left knee flexes, L2 follows the pelvic side-bending. However, the weight bearing down the right side of the body meets the upward ground resistance at the pelvis and counters this side-bending to a point. L1-L2 rotate right along with the pelvis and the combination of this movement positions the left L2 facet just below the upper part of the left L1 facet, as shown in **figure ESD**.

When the pelvis side-shifts to the right, it fully levels the pelvis and side-shifts L2 in the same direction. This causes L2 to side-bend right and engage against the level left L1 facet. This is shown in **figure ESDa**. If these movements are taken to their physiological limit, they do not lock; therefore this is not how the L2-L1 joint becomes subluxated in extension to the right.

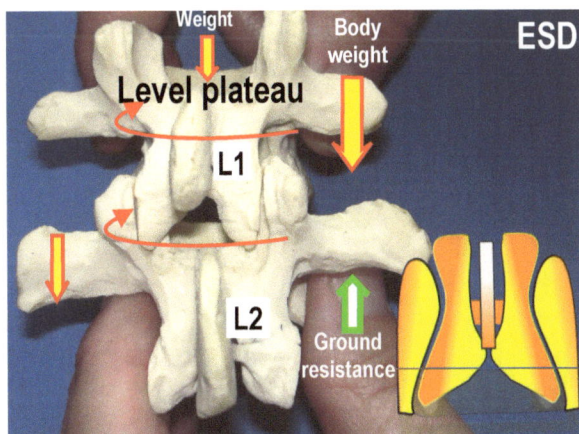

General rotation right

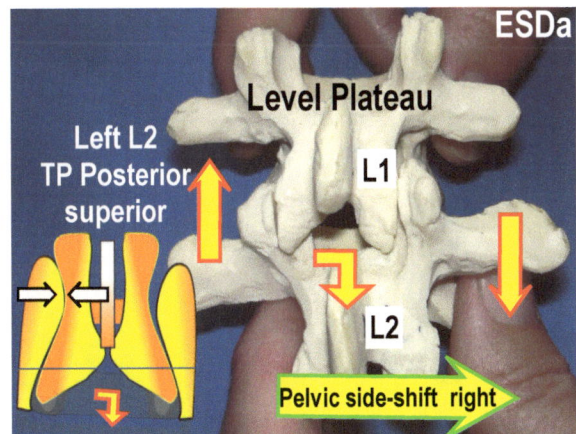

L2 side-bends right and L1 remains level

L2-L1
Extension Subluxation to the Right

If the left knee is not flexed and the body weight is taken on the right leg, no lumbar side-bending to the left or pelvic rotation to the right can take place. Due to the weight bearing on the right, the left facets of L2 become marginally side-bent right. This is an incorrect starting point and is shown **figures ESE** and **ESEa**. See **figures LBB** and **LBBa** on page 51 for comparison.

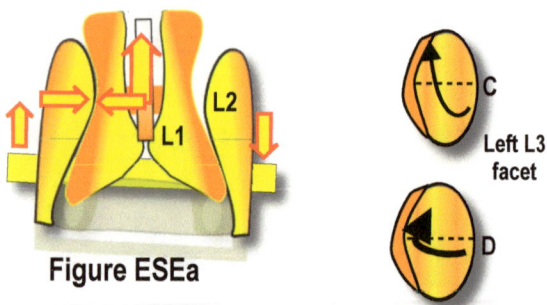

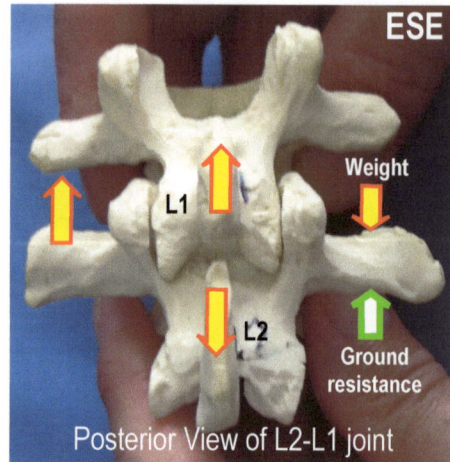

Posterior View of L2-L1 joint

ESE

Weight

Ground resistance

Figure ESEa

Left L3 facet

C

D

Figure ESG and **ESGa** show L2 following the pelvic side-shift right. A reminder of what happened at L3 below. The left facet of L3 should have side-bent in an arc, as shown in 'C' above but it subluxated and side-bent as shown 'D' *without arcing.* This has the knock-on effect of stopping the facets of L1 from following the side-bending arc of L3 and sliding smoothly up the L2 facet.

As L2 side-bends right the left facet of L1 becomes wedged against the L2 facet as shown in **figure ESGb**. Because the left facet of L2 cannot move up the left facet of L1, L1 is forced to side-bend left as shown in **figure ESGa.**

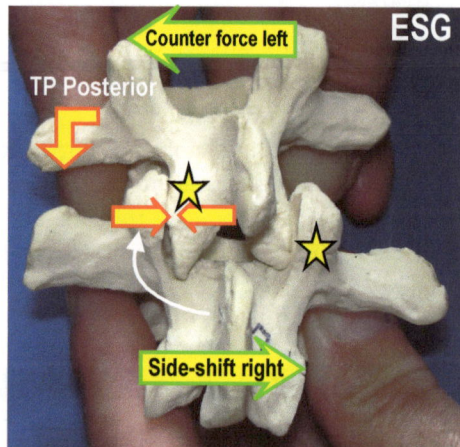

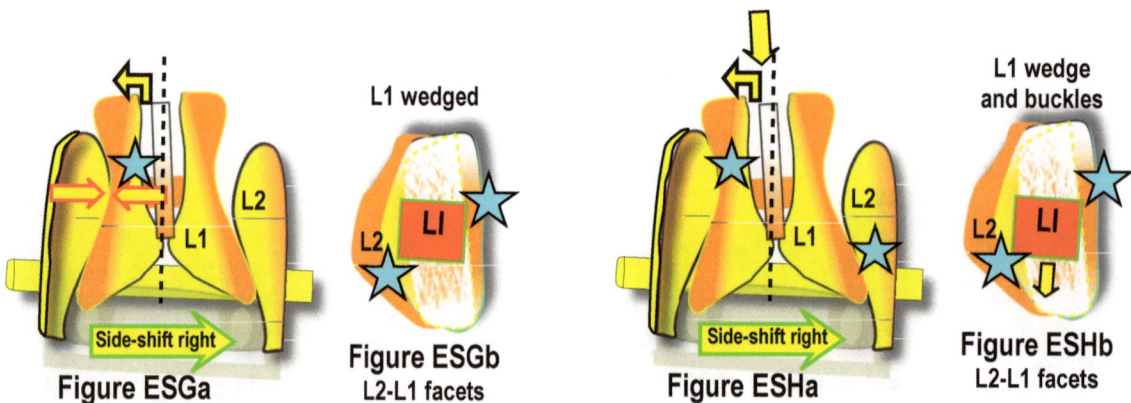

ESG

Counter force left

TP Posterior

Side-shift right

Side-shift right

Figure ESGa

L1 wedged

Figure ESGb
L2-L1 facets

Side-shift right

Figure ESHa

L1 wedge and buckles

Figure ESHb
L2-L1 facets

L2-L1
Extension Subluxation to the Right

To continue on from the previous page, **figure ESGb** showed how the L1 facet got wedged just over halfway up the left L2 facet and caused a minor subluxation. This subluxation is further compounded when the person leans backwards without changing the direction of side-shift.

The thoracic column levers the facets of L1 inferiorly as shown on the previous page in **figures ESHa** and **ESHb.** As the misaligned left facet of L1 gets dragged inferiorly, the joint buckles.

The force caused by the side-shift to the right, side-bends the destabilized L1 vertebra to the left. A photograph of the final stage of this subluxation is shown in **figure ESH**.

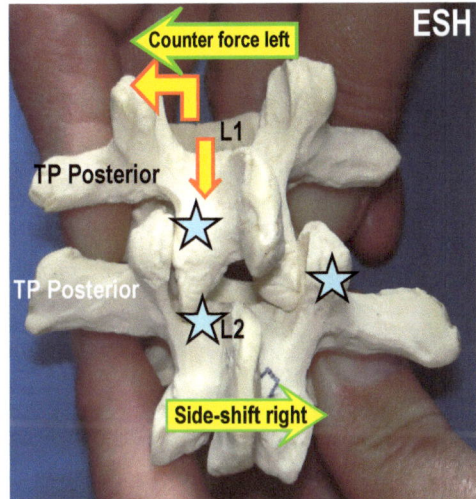

The L1-T12 joint
In normal physiological lumbar extension, side-shift passes to the right of L1. This provides T12 along with all the thoracic vertebrae above with the ability to rotate. This side-shift is not blocked in the subluxated lumbar vertebrae.

For reference, **figures LCH** and **LCHa** show the L1-T12 joint in neutral.

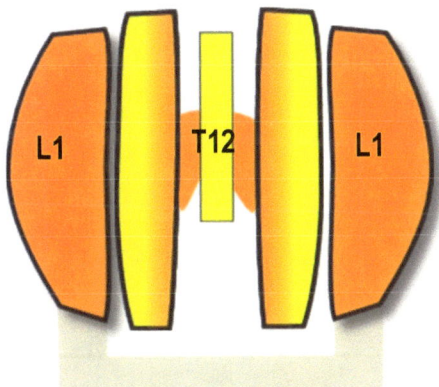

Figure LCHa
L1-T12 in neutral

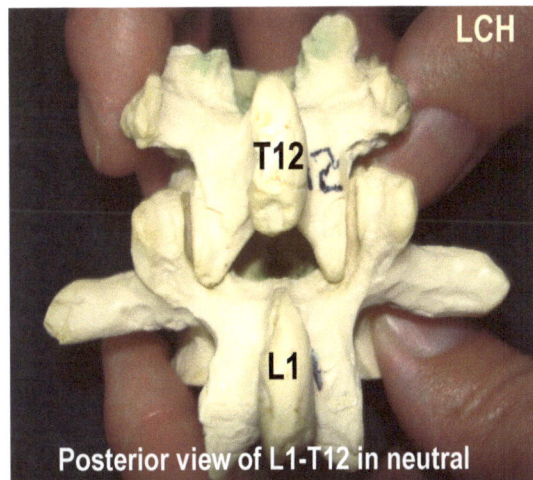

Posterior view of L1-T12 in neutral

L1-T12

Extension Subluxation to the Right

Stage one

In thoracic flexion, (forward bending) T12 separates with L1. **Figure ESF** illustrates the subluxated angles of the L1 facets. It can be seen that the rotation and side-bending to the left by the inferior L1 facets is reflected in the superior L1 facets. The superior facets of L1 do not touch the T12 facets, as shown in **figure ESFa.** However, this is an incorrect starting point for T12 to rotate left.

Stage two

Figure EFSb illustrates the next stage when pelvic side-shift forces L1 to the right. As L1 side-shifts to the right the inferior part of the left L1 facet engages against the inferior part of the left T12 facet. As side-shift continues, T12 buckles and rotates up the L1 facet, as shown in **figures EFSc** and **EFSd.**

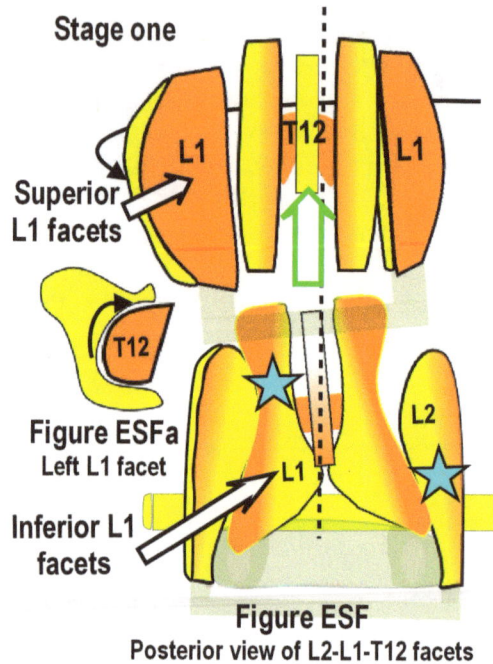

Figure ESFa
Left L1 facet

Figure ESF
Posterior view of L2-L1-T12 facets

Stage three

Figure ESFe illustrates the downward thrust on the left side of the T12 facet when the person leans backwards without change in side shift. The distorted T12 facet is dragged down the L1 right facet where it becomes more firmly wedged.

This is the final stage of the subluxation. **Figure ESFf** illustrates T12 being forced to rotate left as the side-shift right buckles and side-bends T12 left. **Figure FSY** illustrates T12 subluxated one third of the way up the L1 facet.

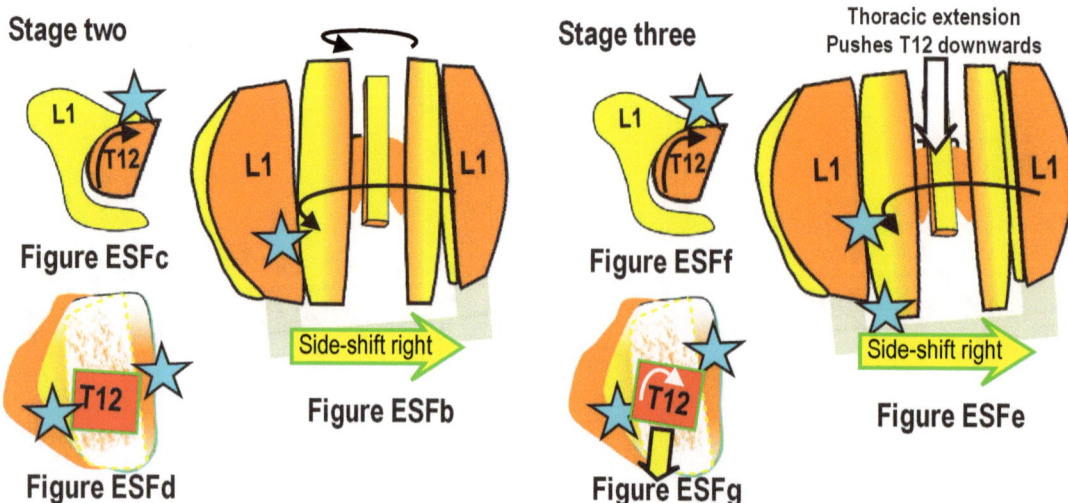

Figure ESFc

Figure ESFd

Figure ESFb

Side-shift right

Figure ESFf

Figure ESFg

Figure ESFe

Side-shift right

Thoracic extension
Pushes T12 downwards

Sacroiliac
Extension Subluxation to the Right

Figure ESJ is a photograph of the final stage of the T12 subluxation. T12 is rotated and side-bent to the left in thoracic flexion.

The left transverse processes of L1 and T12 are posterior and the spinous processes are separated.

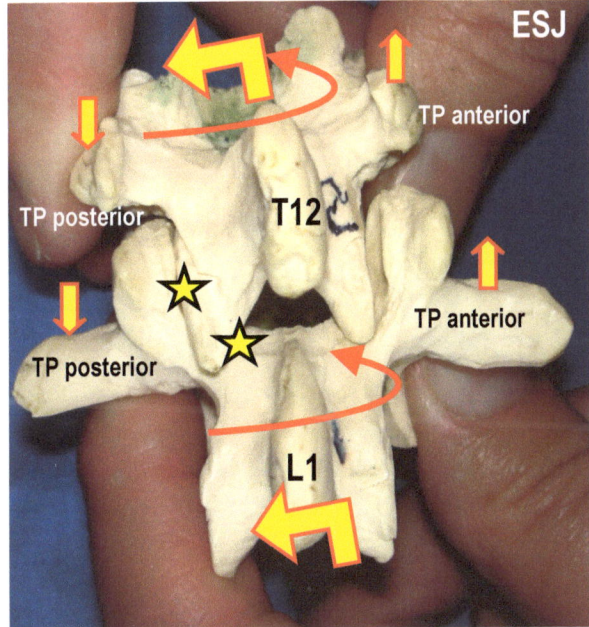

The sacroiliac join extension recap

Figure ESK illustrates the normal physiological movement of the sacroiliac joint when a person rotates to the right in extension.

When weight and pelvic side-shift are directed to the right, the sacroiliac 'F' facets engage and align the acetabulum and head of the femur to angle posteriorly, laterally and inferiorly. This results in a weight bearing straight right leg.

On the opposite side the left knee is mildly flexed by the engagement of the 'A' facets and provides a general 'G' force rotation of the pelvis and lumbar to the right.

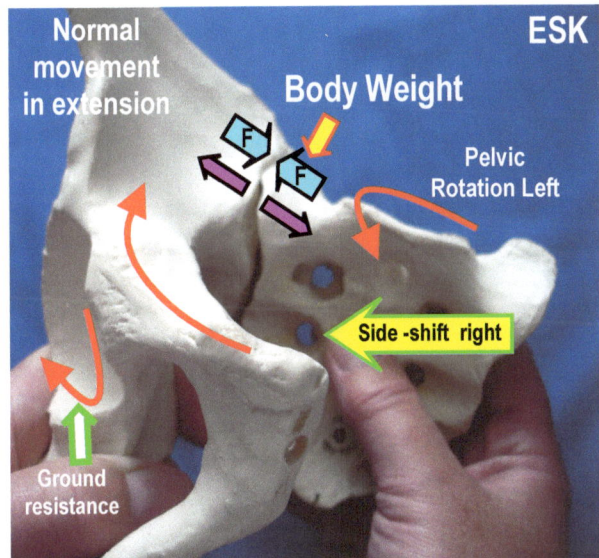

Posterior view:
Extension subluxation at L1-T12

Anterior view of right sacroiliac joint

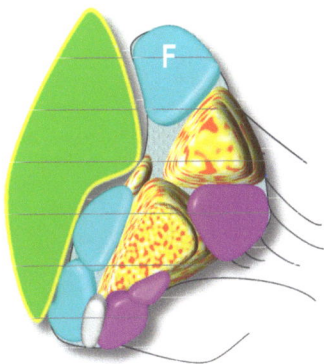

Sacroiliac
Extension Sub-Lesion to the Right

The lumbar vertebrae are extended (forward bent). Forward bending also comes from the hips and knees.

A sacroiliac extension subluxation will take place when a person is standing with both knees straight. With no left knee flexion the sacroiliac joints remain level so the right 'F' facets are unable to engage as they would during their normal physiological movement.

Instead of body weight being directed through the sacroiliac 'F' facets, it incorrectly passes through the 'point of pivot'. This is acceptable when standing up straight and reservedly swaying the pelvis from side to side but not when forward bending is present. See **figure ESM.**

When forward bending and weight bearing is directed at the right sacroiliac joint, with no facet orientation the joint becomes unstable with no rotation to the right.

If the person forces rotation right using the 'M' force muscles from above, instead of the S/I 'F' facet engagement, contact is kept with the 'point of pivot'. With forced rotation to the right the sacral 'F' facets are forced to slide over the iliac 'F' facets and overlap the joints posterior facet border. See **figures ESN** and **ESNa**. This triggers the ligaments to clamp and stop any further dislocation and locks the subluxation in. The PSIS is lateral and superior and the ASIS, inferior and medial. Effectively the right side sacroiliac joints are locked tightly together in this position. **This is a sacroiliac subluxation.**

With side-shift still to the right and the lumbar joints subluxated above, when the person straightens as they would need to do to walk, they forcibly lever the left Ilium including the locked sacroiliac joint backward. This compounds the sacroiliac subluxation. **This is an Innominate sub-lesion.**

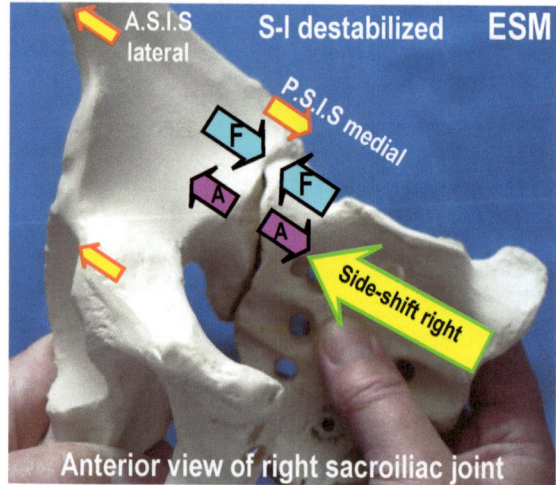

A.S.I.S lateral — S-I destabilized — ESM
P.S.I.S medial
F
A
F
A
Side-shift right
Anterior view of right sacroiliac joint

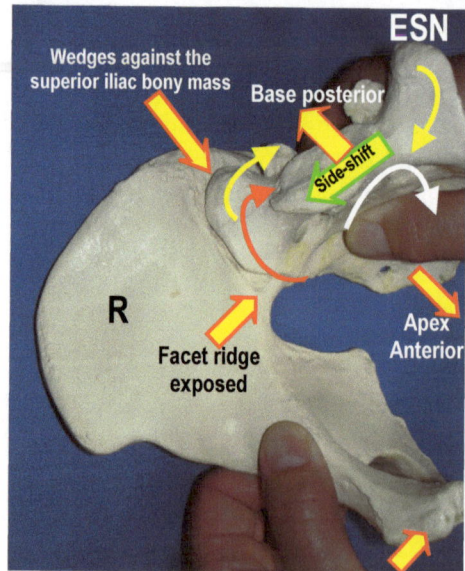

ESN
Wedges against the superior iliac bony mass
Base posterior
Side-shift
R
Facet ridge exposed
Apex Anterior

Points of impact pivot

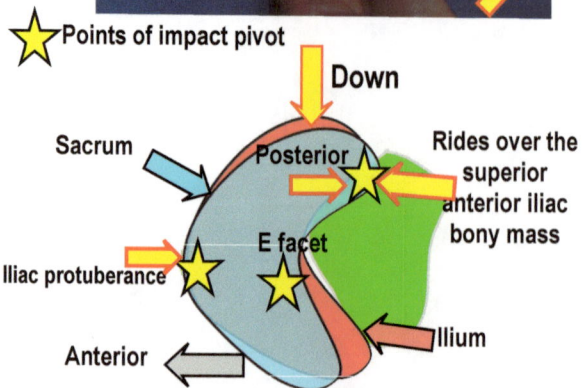

Down
Sacrum
Posterior
Rides over the superior anterior iliac bony mass
Iliac protuberance
E facet
Ilium
Anterior

Figure ESNa
Right sacroiliac facets in extension subluxation

Sacroiliac
Extension Subluxation to the Right

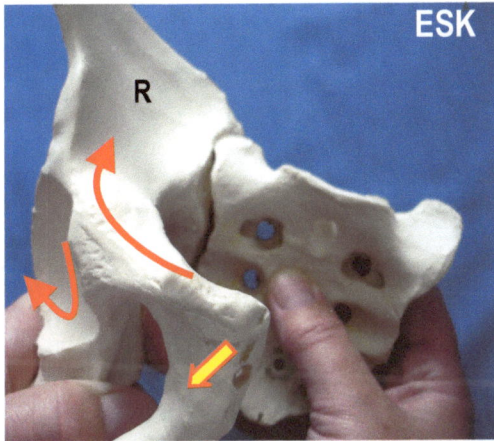

Normal physiological movement

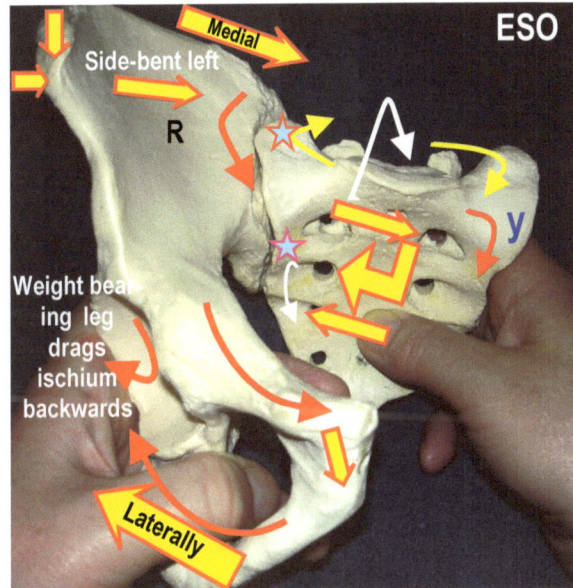

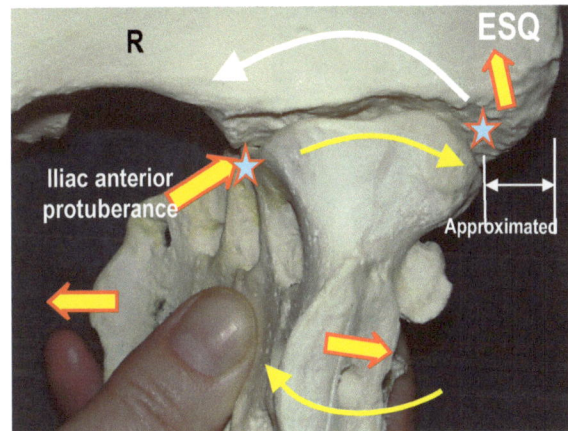

For comparison purposes, **figure ESK** shows the direction of pelvic forces during normal physiological extension with rotation to the right.

Figure ESO shows the buckled position of the right Ilium and its affect on the angle of the acetabulum, pubic ramous and iliac crest in the extension subluxation. The blue stars show the points of impact. The downward arrow (y) shown in blue on the left side of the sacral base denotes the minor inferior tilt that takes place.

Figure ESQ shows the subluxated sacrum in relation to the Ilium from above. The base of the sacrum on the right side is posterior in relation to the right Ilium and the posterior superior Iliac crest lateral.

Two stages take place simultaneously to create the extension subluxation. To make it easier to understand **figure ESQa** illustrates the two stages in blocks:

Stage one, the base of the sacrum subluxates posteriorly and causes the right Innominate to rotate to the left, and;

Stage two, the sacrum rides up the right anterior Iliac protuberance and side-bends the inferior part of the Ilium, left. The sacrum subluxates against the weight bearing Ilium.

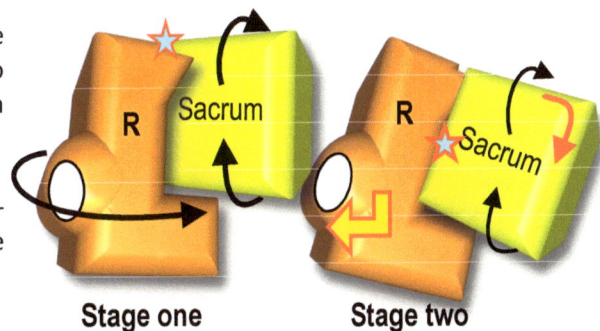

Figure ESQa
Anterior view of right sacroiliac extension subluxation

Extension Subluxation Pattern
from Right to Left Ilium

To recap with left knee flexion the right S/I facets should have engaged the 'F' facets and the left the 'A' facets. However, with no left knee flexion both sides of the S/I joint were forced to start from their points of pivot.

Wrong footed and unstable, the right side of the sacrum was forced to rotate posteriorly over and past the 'F' facets where it collides with the bony mass.

Conversely the left side of the sacrum is over rotated anteriorly where it passes over the iliac A' facet and to overlap its perimeter.

Figure 9 BA illustrates the general position of the subluxated sacroiliac joint.

Figure CESB is view from above of the left S/I joint and shows the relative positions of the sacrum and Ilium.

Figures CESBC and **9BA** illustrate the buckling displacement of the left acetabulum in the subluxated left sacroiliac joint.

In summary the distorted pelvis as a whole is side-bent right and rotated left.

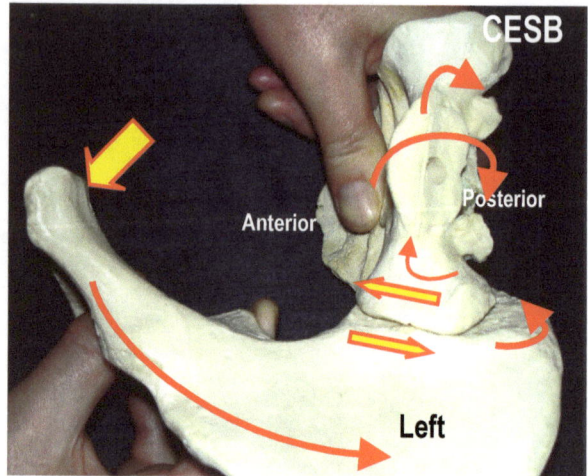
CESB
Anterior
Posterior
Left

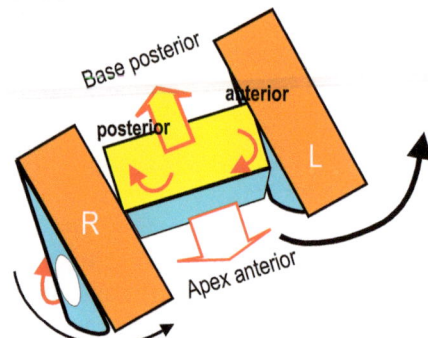
Base posterior
anterior
posterior
Apex anterior
R
L

Figure 9 BA
Aerial view of
sacroiliac joint

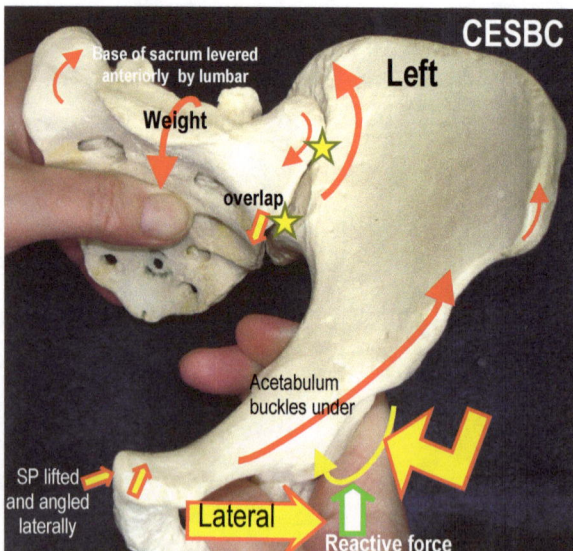
CESBC
Base of sacrum levered anteriorly by lumbar
Left
Weight
overlap
Acetabulum buckles under
SP lifted and angled laterally
Lateral
Reactive force

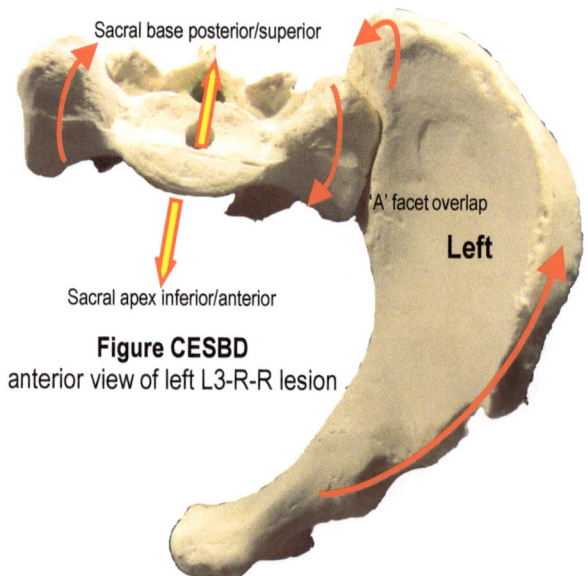
Sacral base posterior/superior
'A' facet overlap
Left
Sacral apex inferior/anterior

Figure CESBD
anterior view of left L3-R-R lesion

Points of Facet Impact
Left Ilium

It should be remembered that because the side-shift was originally taken on the weight bearing right, the sacroiliac ligaments and muscles on the left automatically slackened. Thus the left sacroiliac joint had no resistance to the forced sacral rotation to the right from above.

Figure 9E shows the points where the sacral facets impact against the iliac facets.

Point 1) is at the anterior perimeter of the iliac 'A' facet at the meeting with the superior iliac protuberance.

Point 2) is at the inferior posterior border of the iliac 'D' facet, where it meets the foothills of the inferior anterior iliac bony mass.

Points 3) form the anterior border of the iliac facets.

When weight and side-shift transfer to the left sacroiliac joint, the subluxations become wedged in. The left leg is lifted and angled anteriorly by the buckled acetabulum. The consequence of this is that the left leg has further to reach the ground. In normal physiology when weight bearing and side-shift pass through the acetabulum the reactive upward force directs the posterior superior S/I facets to engage. However, because the subluxated 'A' facets are locked in engagement the Ilium is forced to buckle and lift the Ilium from underneath in a posterior trajectory.

The apex of the sacrum is thus forced to rotate medially and superiorly and push the right Ilium laterally, superiorly and anteriorly. This is shown in block form in **figures P1** and **P2** and technically a **pelvic lesion** and the factor the locks in the S/I subluxations.

The anterior base of the sacrum, particularly on the left, causes the spine to be twisted right and angled anteriorly and is the cause of the L3-R-R forward bent posture.

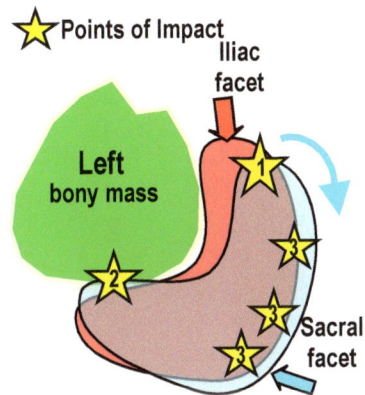

Points of Impact
Iliac facet
Left bony mass
Sacral facet

Figure 9E

S/I L3-R-R final subluxation stage

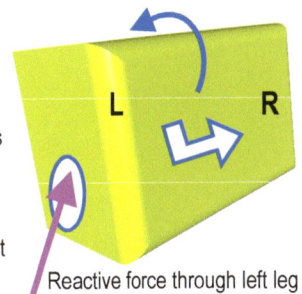

The subluxated left S/I causes acetabulum to move laterally and superiorly. This changes the wight distribution relationship between inwardly inclined acetabulum and S/I facet

P1

L   R

Reactive force through left leg

Side view of left innominate with subluxated S/I joint in block form.

Pelvic L3-R-R lesion

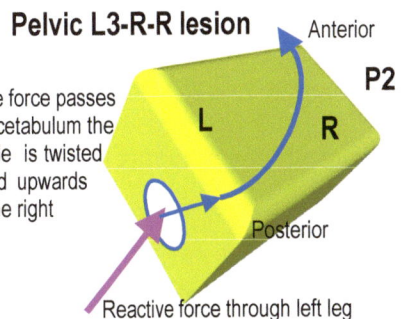

When the reactive force passes through the left acetabulum the pelvis as a whole is twisted posteriorly and upwards towards the right

Anterior
P2
L   R
Posterior

Reactive force through left leg

Side view of L3-R-R pelvic lesion in block form.

Extension pelvic Lesion in Block Form When Side-Shift to the Left to Level

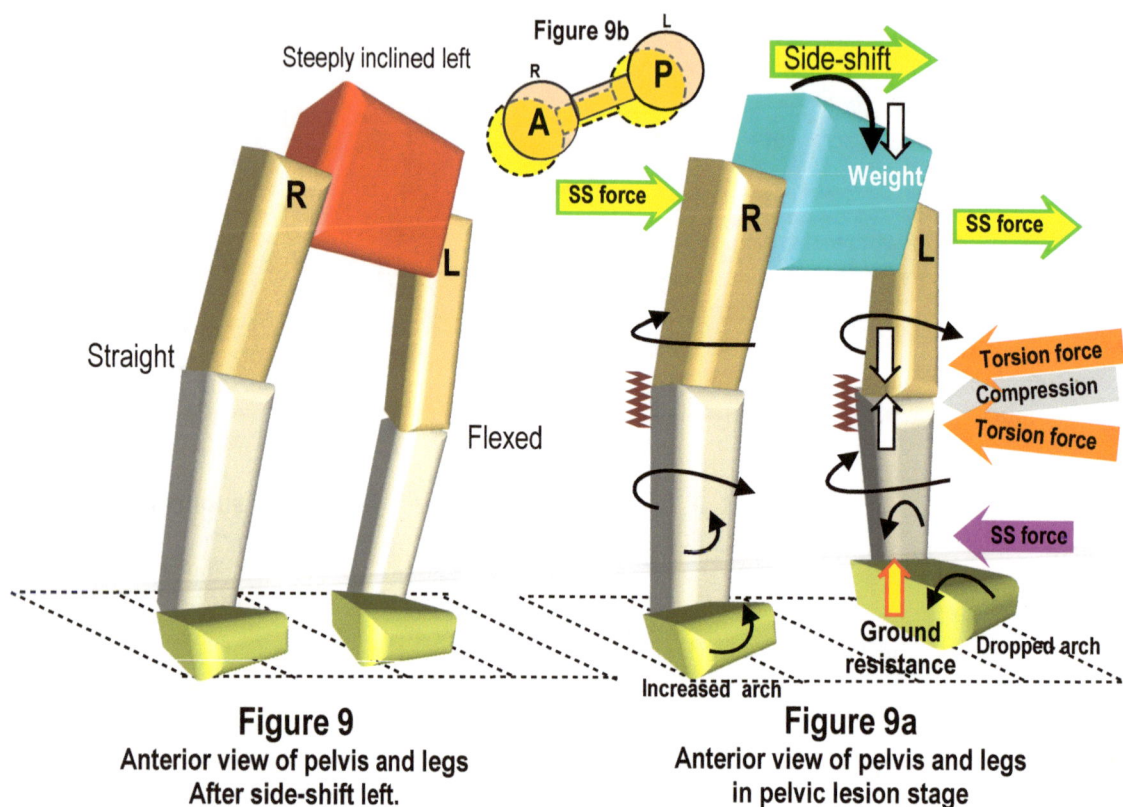

Steeply inclined left

Figure 9b

Side-shift

Weight

SS force

R

L

SS force

Straight

Flexed

Torsion force

Compression

Torsion force

SS force

Ground resistance

Dropped arch

Increased arch

Figure 9
Anterior view of pelvis and legs
After side-shift left.

Figure 9a
Anterior view of pelvis and legs
in pelvic lesion stage

Figure 9 illustrates in block format the angles of the pelvis, legs and feet just from the left sacroiliac subluxation stage. At this stage weight bearing has just changed from the right foot to the left. Note that the left foot is anterior to the right. The pelvis as a whole is side-bent left and rotated left.

Figures 9a illustrates in block format the conflicting angles of the pelvis, legs and feet after the body has tried to level the sacral base by side-shifting the weight distribution to the left. In completing this manoeuvre the left side of the pelvis and feet are positioned further posteriorly which exaggerates the torsion placed on the pelvis. **Figure 9b** demonstrates how the side-shift to the left emphasises the posterior position of the left buttock.

Figure 9a also shows the adverse forces placed on the feet, knees and hips. The right foot is turned inward causing ground resistance to return up the posterior lateral side of the foot and leg, whilst the more weight bearing left foot has the ground force resistance travelling up the medial anterior foot. This resistance puts a myriad of strains and counter-strains on the instep of the left foot, ankle knee, and hip, sacroiliac and above.

Finally notice that because the pelvis is twisted anteriorly the right foot is now anterior.

Changes after Side-Shift Left

Figure 10 shows the pelvis and lumbar when the initial lower back subluxation pattern developed as weight bearing and ground resistance were applied. The overall lumbar concavity is on the right. The extension subluxations are shown in blue.

Figure 10a shows the complications that develop in the lower back when pelvic side-shift transfers to the left. Note that the shape of the lumbar curve is reduced as conflicting weight bearing and ground resistance meet. The flexion subluxation is shown in red.

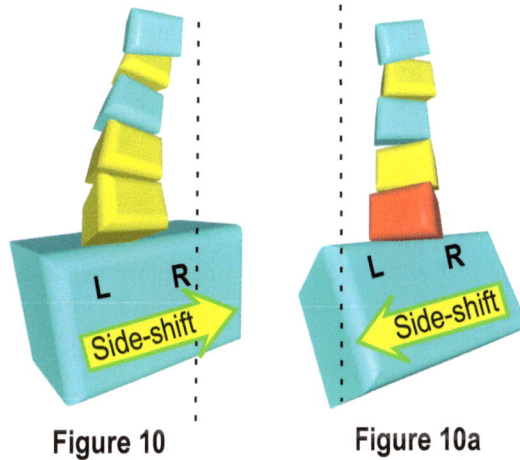

Figure 10

Figure 10a

Ground Force

Figure 10b, shows how the side-shift to the left attempts to level the sacral base. As the left leg becomes the dominant weight bearing leg, ground resistance returning up the left leg is referred up the left hand side of the spine where it crosses over to the right side at approximately T3. The upward misalignment of the sacrum on the left together with the side-shift to the left as shown in **figure 3D**, creates a new set of movements and subluxations up the spine that are locked in by the subluxated left sacroiliac joint. This makes for very interesting lesion permutations.

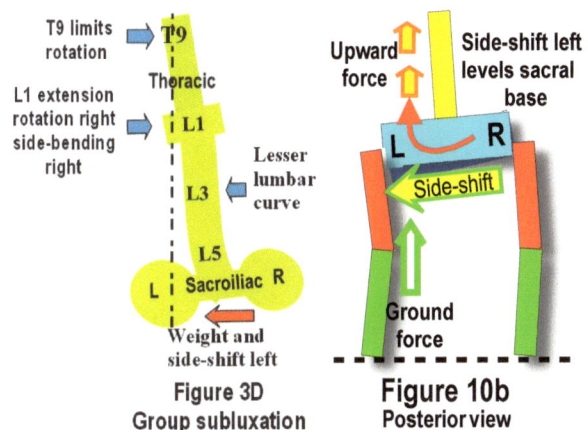

Figure 3D
Group subluxation

Figure 10b
Posterior view

Extension Feet

The positions of the feet shown in **figure 11** are of a person with an extension subluxation pattern. The right foot is anterior with an increased arch. Note that the weight bearing part of the right foot is towards the posterior lateral part of the foot. The left foot has a dropped arch due to the weight distribution on the medial anterior part of the foot. The toes of the left foot are angled laterally.

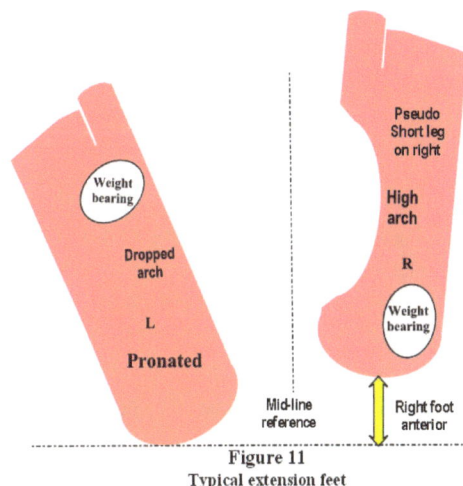

Figure 11
Typical extension feet

119

Left Leg Drag

Figure 11A illustrates the forward leaning posture of the L3-R-R person. If they stood or walked around like this they could have balance problems.

Figure 11B shows the compensations the body makes to keep the body upright. In particular note how far the knees have to flex to keep the lumbar more vertical. Also note that the midline has moved further anteriorly. This is the posture Lisa has had to adopt to stand upright in **figure 11C.**

Figure 11C is a side-view of Lisa standing. Note how the line of gravity passes through the area of her cervico-dorsal junction and causes her shoulders to become rounded. Also note that her forward-bent posture causes the angle of her neck to be pushed forward.

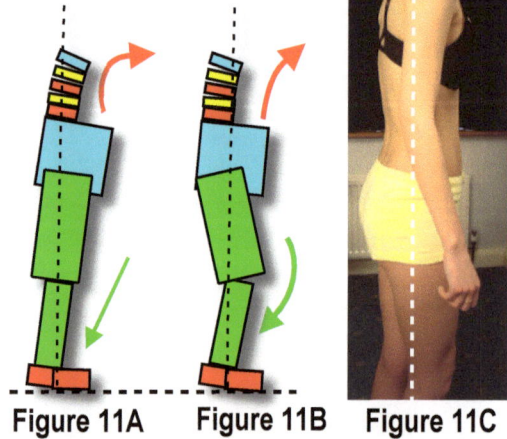

Figure 11A   Figure 11B   Figure 11C

Knee drop test

The standing feet are placed side by side and flat on the floor. Observe the sacrum and ask the person to keep their left leg straight and flex their right knee keeping their heel firmly on the floor. This directs all movement to the pelvis. The person should be able to do this with no detectable pain or restriction on the sacroiliac joint as the knee is being flexed in the direction of the left subluxation.

When the person is asked to flex their left knee as shown in **figure CESBF** under the same circumstances the person will most often experience difficulty flexing the knee fully and feel pain just above the posterior base of their right sacrum. This is because the sacrum on the right side cannot rotate posteriorly as it is blocked by the bony mass, as shown in **figure ESQa.**

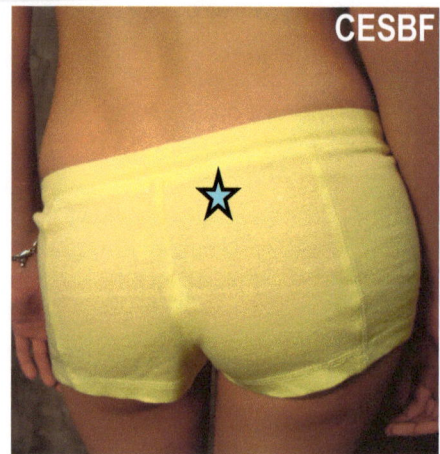

CESBF

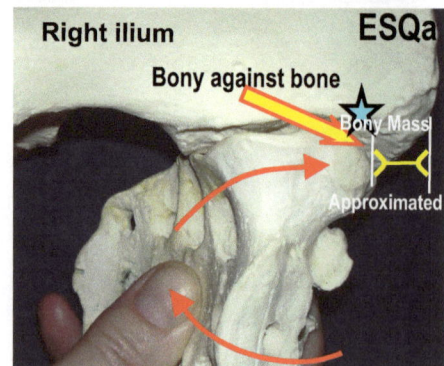

Right ilium   ESQa
Bony against bone
Bony Mass
Approximated

120

Theoretical Lumbar Extension Subluxations

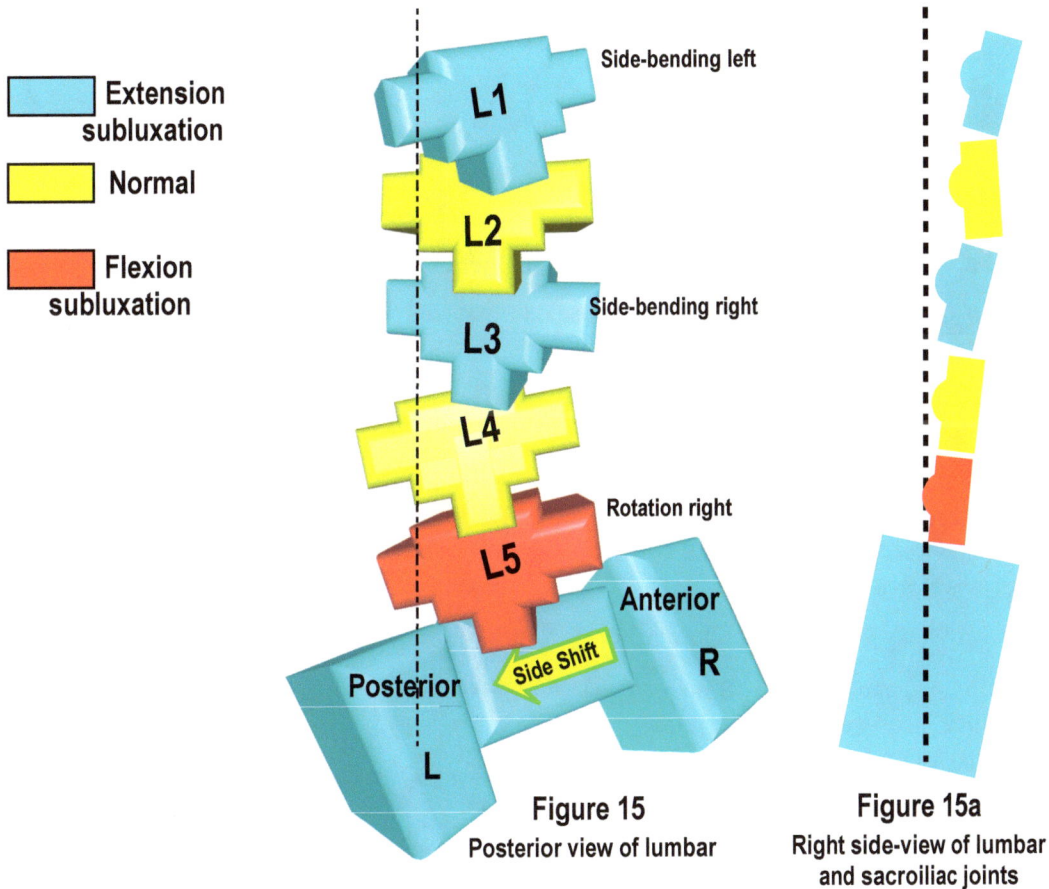

Extension subluxation

Normal

Flexion subluxation

Side-bending left

L1

L2

Side-bending right

L3

L4

Rotation right

L5

Anterior

R

Side Shift

Posterior

L

Figure 15
Posterior view of lumbar

Figure 15a
Right side-view of lumbar and sacroiliac joints

Figure 15 shows the theoretical lumbar vertebral extension subluxation pattern when all elements of the lumbar and sacroiliac joints are put together. When L5 subluxates, it can become compacted and unbalanced.

Figure 15a is a side-view taken from the right side. As can be seen, there is a loss of lumbar flexion and that the pelvis and lumbar are both leaning forward. L1 is forward bent and rotated and side-bent left.

Finally, because the pelvis has become rotated and side-bent left, L4 is forced to rotate left against L3. In doing this the left superior L4 facet is forced to compact still further against the subluxated left L3 facet. This double locks in the L3 subluxation. Conversely, for the same reason the L5 subluxation is prized open, which makes the joint unstable.

Right-Right Pelvic Extension Lesion Part One

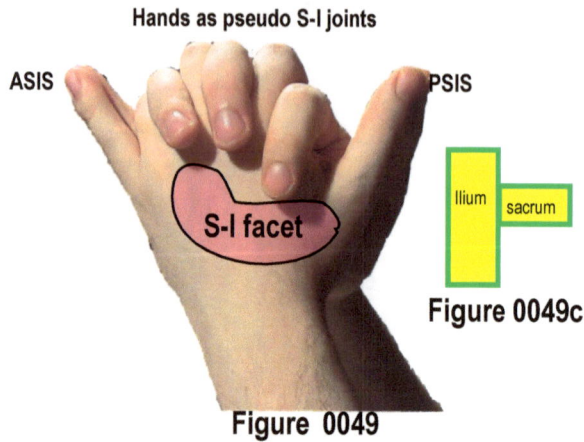

Hands as pseudo S-I joints

ASIS PSIS

S-I facet

Figure 0049

Ilium sacrum

Figure 0049c

Right hand

Point of pivot

ASIS

F facet

Anterior S-I facet Posterior

PSIS

Figure 0058
The hand as an S-I facet and innominate bone

Pelvic lesions lock-in the sacroiliac subluxations and turn them into contorted sacroiliac lesions whilst compounding the lesions already in the spine and rib cage.

Pelvic lesions are reinforced each and every time a leg becomes weight bearing. Again, as with the flexion pelvic lesion this lesion is difficult to show with actual bones. Therefore, I have illustrated how the pelvis becomes lesioned by practical example using your own hands.

Do this self test

In these hand examples your elbows act as your knees/legs and each hand the combination of the side of the Ilium and sacrum, see **figure 49c**.

Start by placing your hands together as per **figure 0049** and imagine the S-I facets are positioned in the palms of your hands as per **figure 0058**.

Place your hands together in an upright position as per **figures 0059, 0059A** and **00059B**.

Keep your elbows level. Now push your hands away from you body to simulate pelvic extension (forward bending) as per **figures 0060, 0060A and 0060B.**

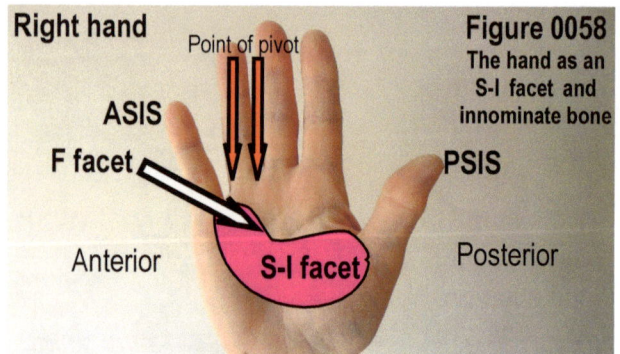

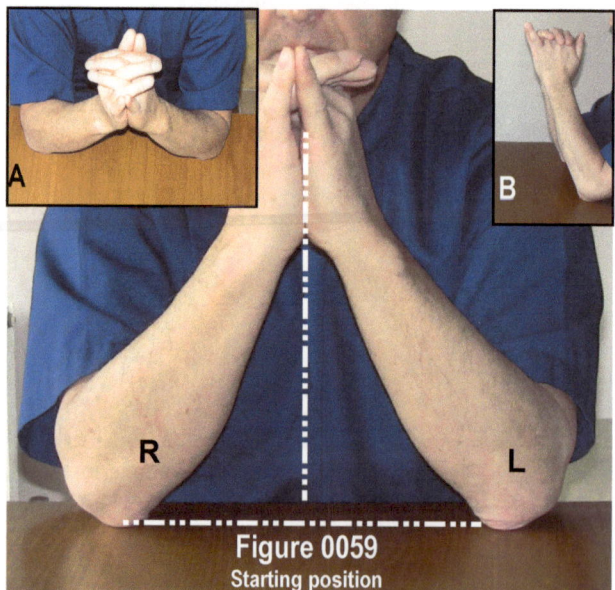

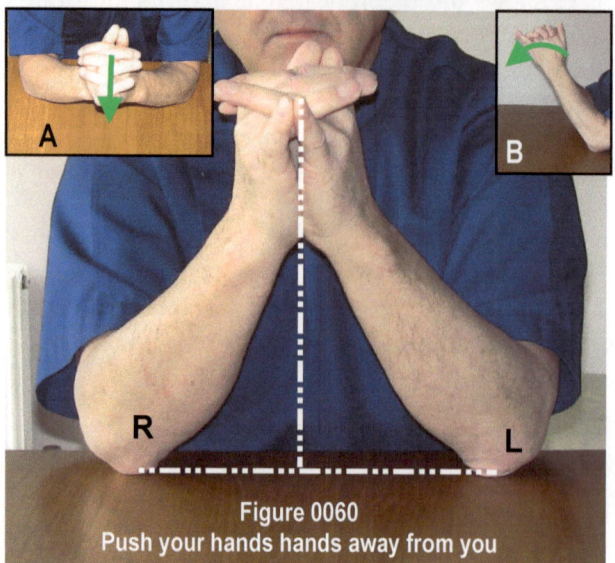

R L

Figure 0059
Starting position

R L

Figure 0060
Push your hands hands away from you

Right-Right Pelvic Extension Lesion Part Two

Look at **figures 0061** and **0061C** and place your weight on your right elbow and push your left elbow towards your right to simulate pelvic side shift to the left. At the same time rotate your hands right to simulate forced rotation to the right from the spine. Your left elbow will move to the right and away from your body. This is the position the subluxated S/I facets would angle the pelvis. See **figure 0061B**. (Side-bent right and rotated right).

Refer to **figure 0061D** and squeeze your little, ring and middle fingers together to simulate the 'point of pivot' shown in **figure 0061B**. The 'point of pivot' is the area where the facets are in subluxation. Ie 'F' facets.

In **figure 0061A** note the position of the little finger on the right hand which represents the ASIS is anterio-superior. And that the left thumb, which represents the PSIS, is posterio-inferior.

Next, transfer your weight to your left elbow which will fractionally lift your right elbow off the table. Move your right elbow towards your left to simulate pelvic side-shift right, as per **figures 0062** and **0062A**. With the 'F' facet as the point of pivot your elbow will move away from your body and rotate your hands further to the right. This locking simulates the the knock-on position of the pelvis when the right S/I facets become subluxated.

Position recap

• Both of your arms and hands should now be to the right of the mid line.
• Your hands should be side-bent to the left and rotated to the right.
• Your right elbow (leg) posterior and lateral and your left elbow (leg) anterior to your right elbow and slightly medial.
• This represents the position of the pelvis in the

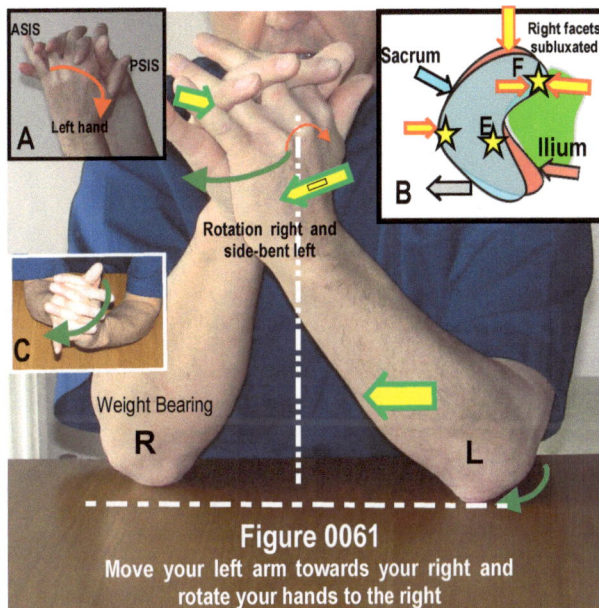

Figure 0061
Move your left arm towards your right and rotate your hands to the right

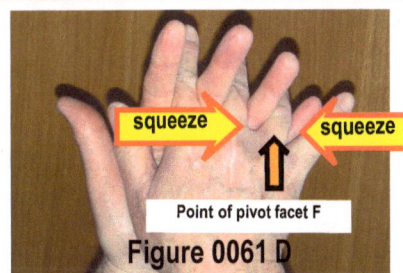

Figure 0061 D

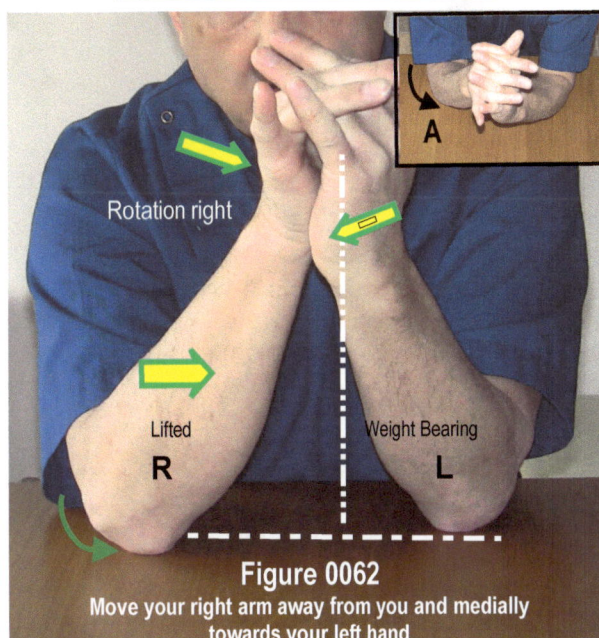

Figure 0062
Move your right arm away from you and medially towards your left hand

123

Right-Right Pelvic Extension Lesion
Part Three

Iliosacral lesions are created in the pelvis when a person then walks forward.

To recap **figure 0061D** illustrated the 'point of pivot', situated at the subluxated 'F' facets on the right. This is a fixed point that is locked in by the S/I subluxations.

Refer to **figures 0063, 0056A**. Body weight is directed back to the right elbow (leg) and the person strides forward with their left elbow (leg). To do this they must side-shift their pelvis to the right. Because the point of pivot is at the anterior, the posterior parts of your hands become rotated to the right and your left elbow will be anterior in relation to your right and closer to the mid line.

Next refer to **figures 0064, 0064A** and direct your body weight back to the left elbow (leg) and side-shift of your hands (pelvis) to the left and move your right elbow(leg) away from you to simulate when the person strides forward. With the rotational force directed at the anterior part of your hands the 'point of pivot' your hands (pelvis) will move away from you and inferiorly and rotate further to the right.

Your right elbow will be anterior and angled inwards in relation to your left which will be angled outward.

When you place your weight on both elbows you will notice that your left elbow (leg) lifts because the hands (pelvis) are side-bent left which makes the left elbow (leg) physiologically shorter. Or if you balance the weight, it forces your hands (pelvis) to side-shift further to the right.

This is a pelvic extension lesion.

Like the flexion lesion this lesion is reinforced every time a person puts weight on their feet, and walks forward.

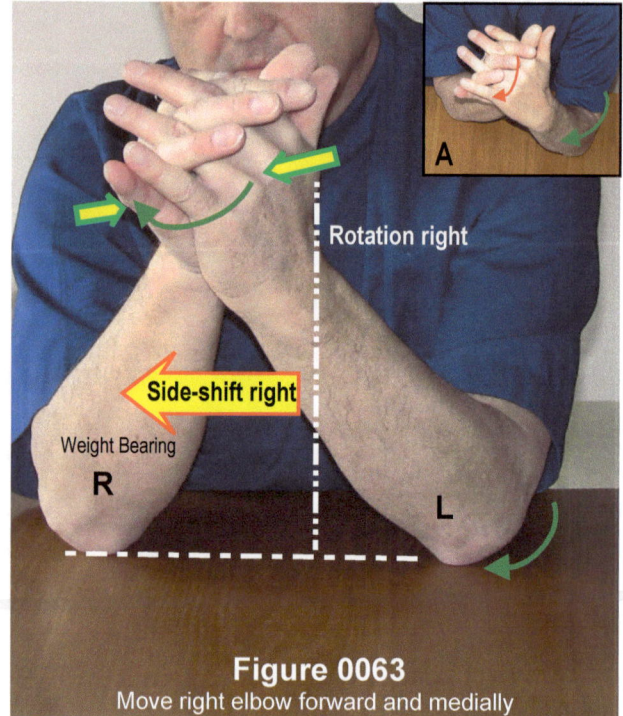

Rotation right

Side-shift right

Weight Bearing

R

L

A

Figure 0063
Move right elbow forward and medially

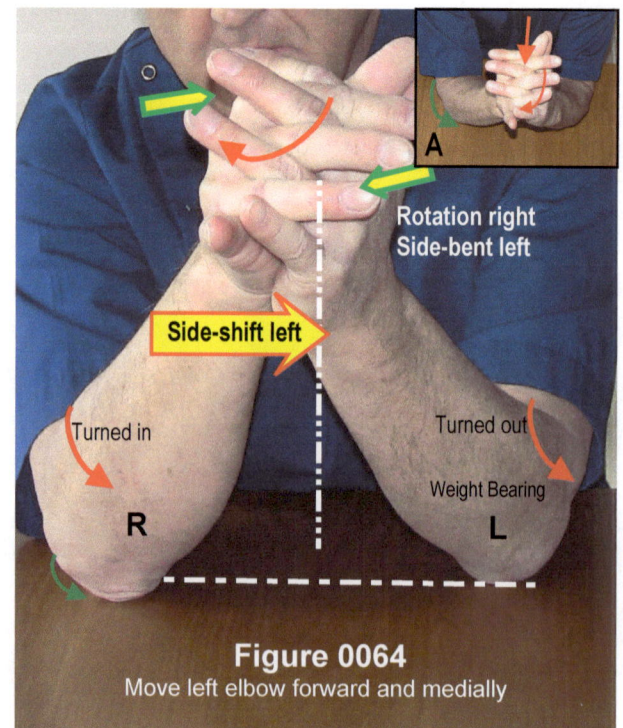

Rotation right
Side-bent left

Side-shift left

Turned in

Turned out

Weight Bearing

R

L

A

Figure 0064
Move left elbow forward and medially

Theoretical Lumbar Pelvic L3-R-R Lesion

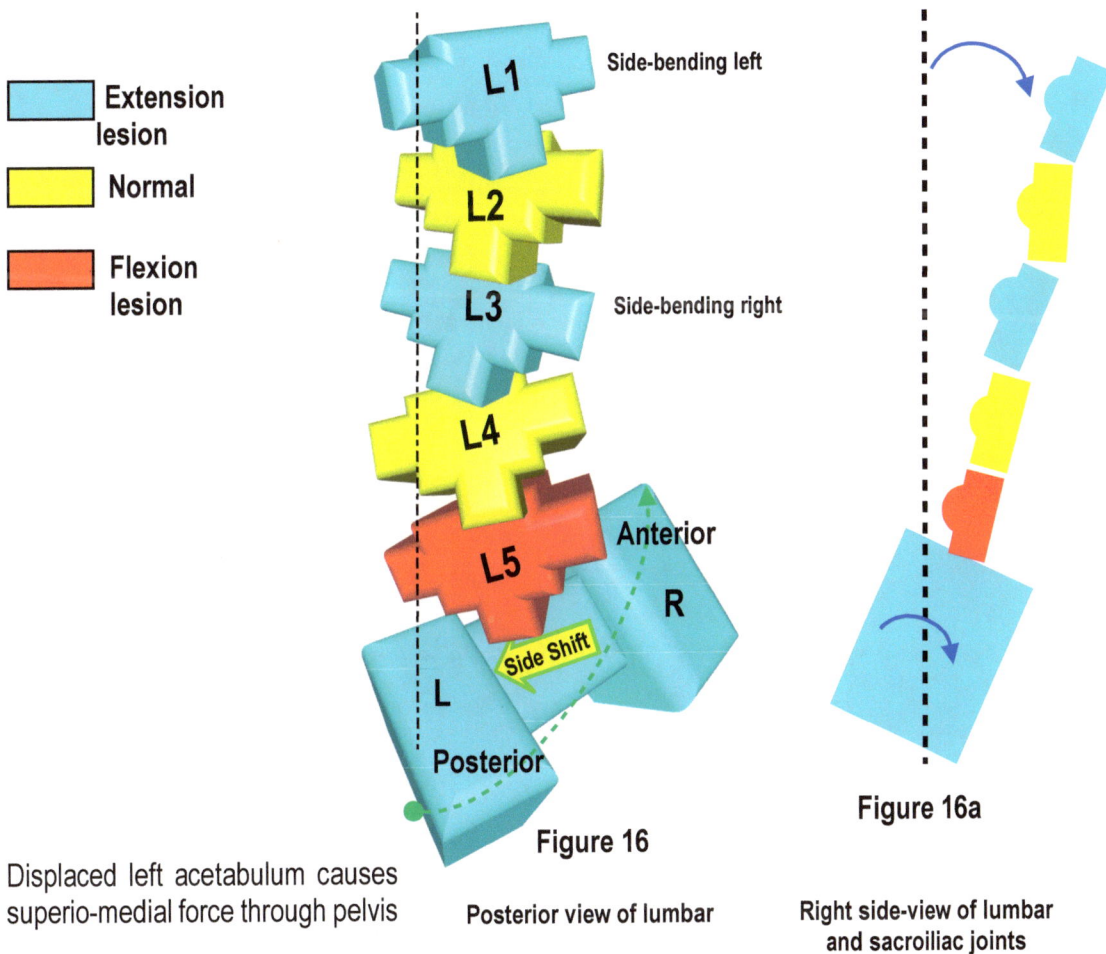

Extension lesion

Normal

Flexion lesion

L1 — Side-bending left

L2

L3 — Side-bending right

L4

L5

Anterior

R

Side Shift

L

Posterior

Figure 16

Posterior view of lumbar

Figure 16a

Right side-view of lumbar and sacroiliac joints

Displaced left acetabulum causes superio-medial force through pelvis

Figures 15 and 15a show the theoretical effects of the pelvic lesion complication. Note the lumbar is forced to incline anteriorly on the right.

With the displaced left acetabulum, reactive ground force passes up the left leg and twists the inferior half of the left Ilium medially and superiorly thus forcing the right Ilium to move anteriorly and superiorly every time the left leg becomes weight bearing. This locks in the pelvic lesion and reinforces all the spinal lesions above.

Comparison Lesion Patterns in Pelvic and Lumbar L3-R-R and L3-L-R

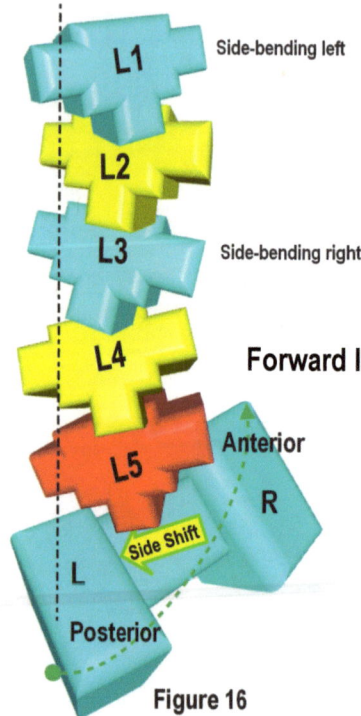

Side-bending left — L1

L2

Side-bending right — L3

L4

Forward leaning

L5 Anterior

R

Side Shift

L

Posterior

Figure 16

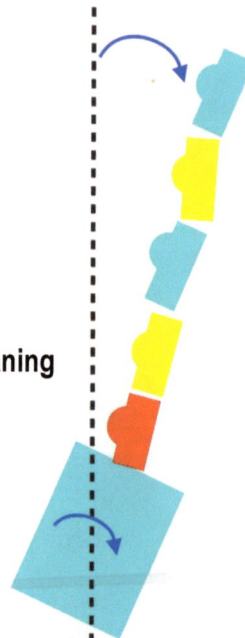

Figure 16a

L3-right-right pelvis and lumbar pattern

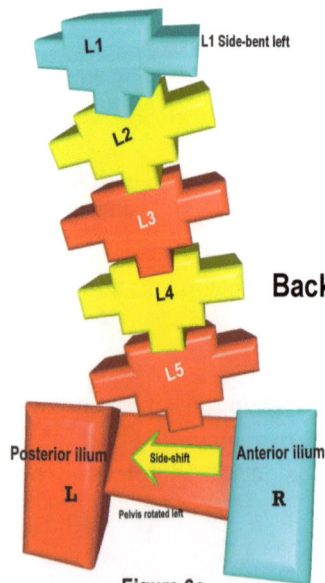

L1 L1 Side-bent left

L2

L3

L4 **Backward leaning**

L5

Posterior ilium Side-shift Anterior ilium

L R

Pelvis rotated left

Figure 6c
Posterior view of lumbar
and sacroiliac joints

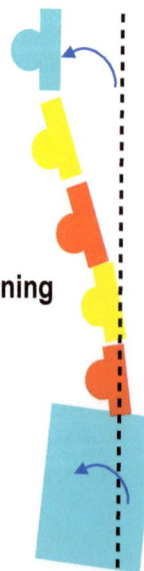

Figure 6d
Right side-view of lumbar
and sacroiliac joints

L3-left-right pelvis and lumbar pattern

126

Chapter Nine

Lesions of the Thoracic Joints

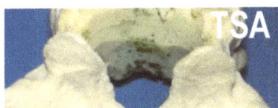
TSA

When you look at the almost flat surfaces of the anterior facets of T7 it is difficult to see how T6 can become subluxated, but it does.

Figure TSD shows T6 taken to its extreme limit. This is not how the joint subluxates.

Figure 1 shows the 'G' force side-shift passing to the right of the thoracic column in normal thoracic flexion (forward bending)

Figure 2 shows the 'G' force blocked at L1 to prevent it from passing to the left of the thoracic column in thoracic extension (backward bending).

Figure 4 shows L1 side-bent left and the additional driving 'G' force side-shift caused by the pelvic/lumbar L3-R-R subluxation pattern below. The extra 'G' force will overdrive the side-ways movement.

Figure 5 shows L1 side-bent right and the 'G' driving force side-shift incorrectly passing to the left caused by the pelvic/lumbar L3-L-R subluxation pattern below.

Figure 3D shows the driving 'G' force side-shift incorrectly passing to the left of L1 in the L3-L-R subluxation pattern.

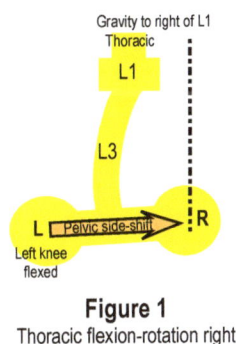

Figure 1
Thoracic flexion-rotation right

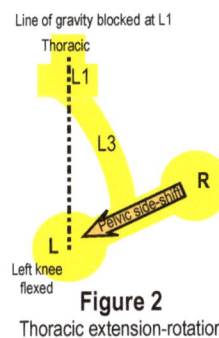

Figure 2
Thoracic extension-rotation

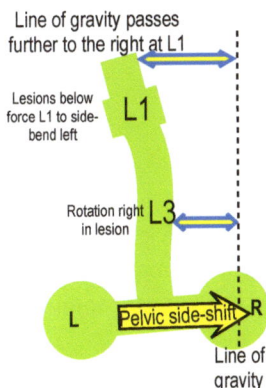

Figure 4
Thoracic flexion-rotation right
Lesioned in L3-R-R pattern

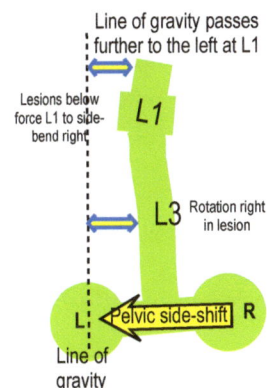

Figure 5
Thoracic extension - rotation right
Lesioned in L3-L-R pattern

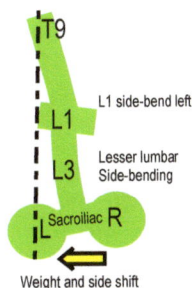

Figure 3D
Group lesion

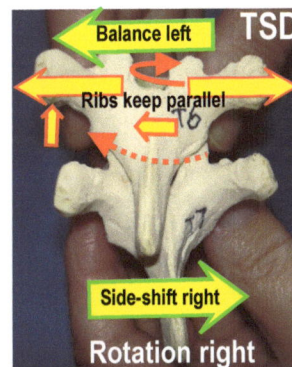
Balance left   TSD
Ribs keep parallel
Side-shift right
Rotation right

Theory Points of Stress
Rotation Right in Thoracic Flexion

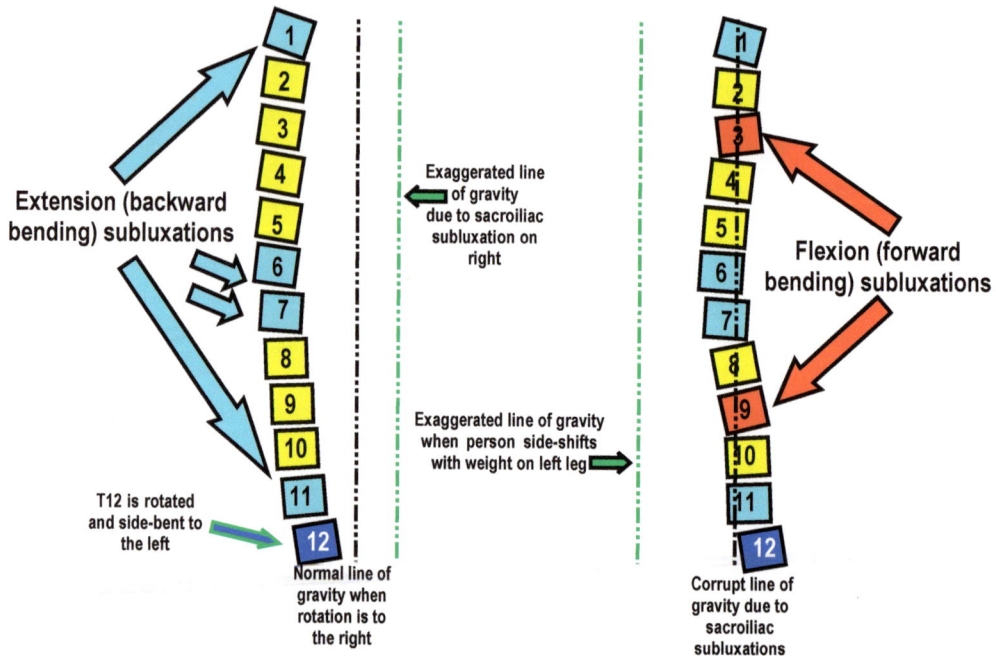

Extension (backward bending) subluxations

Exaggerated line of gravity due to sacroiliac subluxation on right

Exaggerated line of gravity when person side-shifts with weight on left leg

Flexion (forward bending) subluxations

T12 is rotated and side-bent to the left

Normal line of gravity when rotation is to the right

Corrupt line of gravity due to sacroiliac subluxations

Figure 16A
Shows the pelvic side-shift and weight bearing and their effect of their thoracic spine in thoracic flexion.

Figure 16B
Shows the pelvic side-shift and weight bearing and their effect of their thoracic spine in thoracic extension.

Figure 16A is an illustration of the points of maximum stress when a person bends forward and rotates right in the L3-R-R subluxation pattern. *Corrupt pelvic 'G' force weight bearing and side-shift are to the right.* Because T12 becomes locked as a part of the lumbar vertebrae subluxations it is not considered here as part of the thoracic flexion pattern. Therefore the lowest mobile thoracic vertebra is T11.

By simple division, the maximum bending and stress is taken at the mid-point between T11 and T1, which is T6/T7, and the secondary areas of maximum stress are taken at the two ends, T1 and T11. These vertebrae will therefore be the most likely sites for thoracic flexion subluxations to lesions.

See **figure 16B**. By simple division when the person straightens, the mid-point between the subluxated T1 and T6 is T3 and the mid-point between T7 and T11 is T9. When the corrupted 'G' force side-shift and weight bearing transfer to the left, the line of gravity passes through the thoracic spine at approximately T9.

However, when the person stands upright perched on their left leg to balance the level of their pelvis as L3-R-R people do, the line of gravity passes much further to the left. This is shown by the dotted red line. This then makes T9 and T3 the most likely sites of maximum stress. These vertebrae will therefore be the most likely sites for thoracic extension subluxations to lesions.

T6
Flexion Subluxation to the Right

Reference figure 16A page 128

The thoracic flexion subluxation begins when the person leans forward taking their weight on their right leg with their left knee straight. This stretches the thoracic joints apart. Note, the 'G' force will be further to the right than normal due to the pelvic and lumbar subluxations below. Also bear in mind at the starting point, the thoracic column is already leaning to the left, courtesy of L1.

Using T6/7 as an example, T7 follows the exaggerated 'G' force and side-shifts to the right. Whilst T6 follows the 'M' force from above and side-shifts to the left to create the typical step side-bending.

Because the 'G' force side-shift is over-exaggerated when the person straightens and maintains weight and pelvic side-shift to the right, the inferior edge of the left T6 facet impacts against the left pedicle of the T7 transverse process. The more the person attempts to straighten, the tighter the compaction. This is shown in **figure TSE.**

In an attempt to remain parallel, the ribs on both sides lock-in the compaction still further. The subluxation is locked in place by the subluxations below. Relative to the spinous process of T7, T6 is separated and to the left and relative to the left transverse process of T7, T6 is anterior and separated. The left T7 rib is separated from the left rib of T6 and the right is approximated. The left T6 facet is compacted and the right facet is destabilized.

Figure TSEa illustrates the effect the subluxated vertebra has on the ribs. The left rib is pushed laterally and inferiorly on the costo-transverse facet of T6 and causes the rib to subluxate in inspiration. Whilst on the right, the rib is pulled medially and superiorly which causes it to subluxate in expiration. **Figures TSEb** and **TSEc** are side views of the costo-transverse facets and illustrate how the ribs become subluxated in the angles of inspiration on the right and expiration on the left.

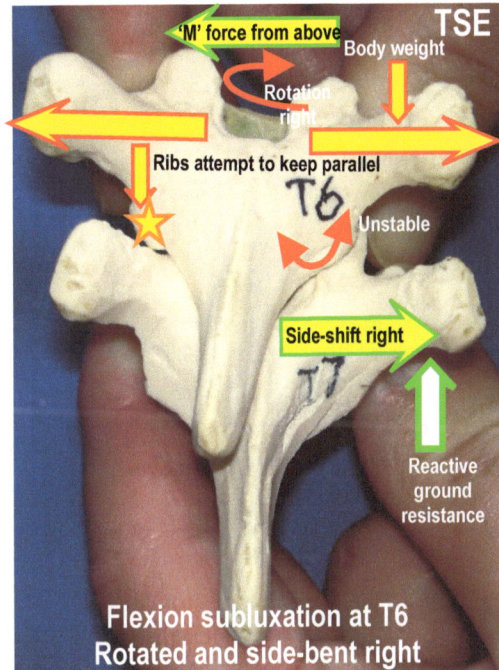

Flexion subluxation at T6
Rotated and side-bent right

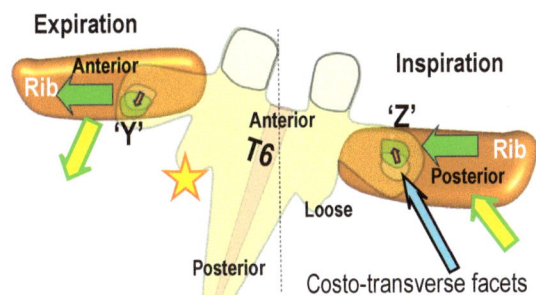

Figure TSEa
Simplified posterior view of rib flexion subluxation
Connection of ribs to vertebral body left off for clarity

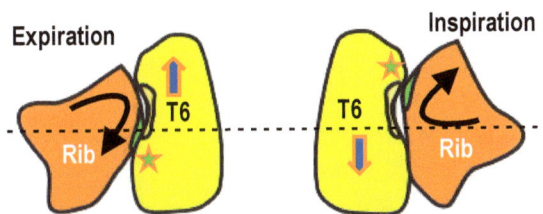

Figure TSEb	**Figure TSEc**
Left side-view of point 'Y'	Right side-view of point 'Z'

T3
Extension 'Complicated' Lesion to the Left

Reference figure 16B page 128.

Standing on their left leg and upright the thoracic spine is put into extension with reinforced side-shift and weight bearing to the left. Bear in mind in normal physiology thoracic extension (backward bending) rotation is prohibited.

Figure TSH illustrates what happens when the pelvic exaggerated 'G' force weight bearing and side-shift transfer to the left. T4 follows the exaggerated 'G' force and side-shifts to far too the left, at the same time the 'M' force counter-resistance from above causes the T3 facets to side-shift to the right across the convex facets of T4. This causes T3 rotation to the left.

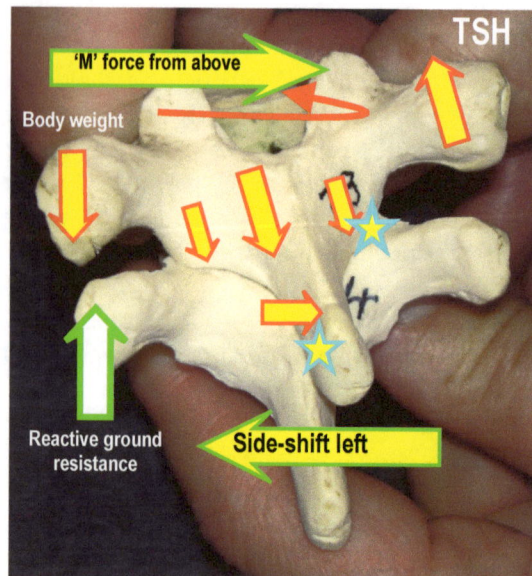

When the person forces their back to straighten the right facet of T3 is forced inferiorly where it impacts and rides up the right T4 lamina.

The ribs on either side fight to remain parallel and lock-in the subluxation further, particularly on the right. The T3 spinous processes are approximated and to the right of the T4 spinous process. The right transverse process of T3 is anterior and separated in relation to the right transverse process of T4. The right T4 rib is separated from the right rib of T3 and the left side is approximated. T9 will subluxate in the same way T3 does.

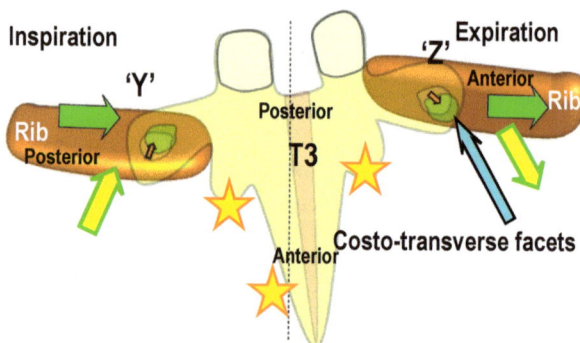

In this subluxation the ribs, illustrated in **figures TSHa, TSHb** and **TSHc** become locked in expiration on the right and inspiration on the left.

Technically a lesion locked with rotation and side-bending to the same side would constitute a thoracic flexion lesion. However because it is locked in thoracic extension it comes under the category of what the old Osteopaths called a complicated lesion. This reverse rotation locks-in all the thoracic vertebral subluxations and converts them into lesions.

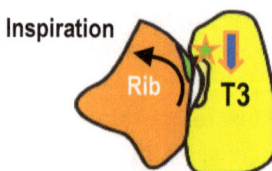

Figure TSHa
Simplified posterior view of rib extension subluxation
Connection of ribs to vertebral body left off for clarity

Figure TSHb
Left side-view of point 'Y'

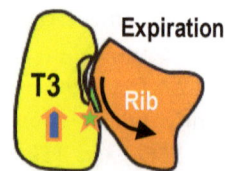

Figure TSHc
Right side-view of point 'Z'

L3-Right-Right Thoracic Spine in 3D and Scapulae Displacement

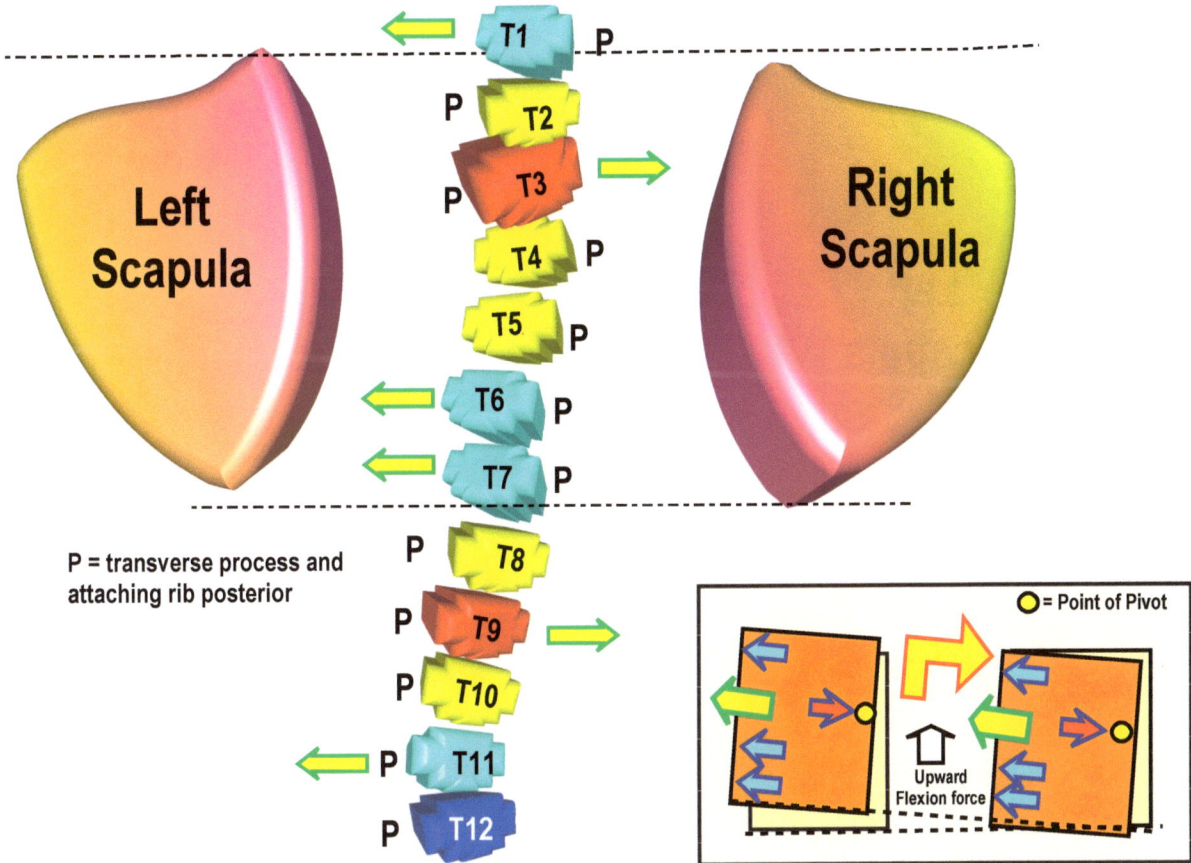

Left Scapula

Right Scapula

T1 P
P T2
P T3
T4 P
T5 P
T6 P
T7 P

P = transverse process and attaching rib posterior

P T8
P T9
P T10
P T11
P T12

Figure 17
Posterior view spine in 3D

○ = Point of Pivot

Upward Flexion force

Figure 17A
Box view of scapulae displacement

Figure 17 is a continuation of the previous pages and shows the rotation and side-bending in more detail along with the effect this pattern has on the scapula bones.

The scapulae follow the angles and side-shift of the spine, as simplified and demonstrated in **figure 17A**. The points of pivot although not shown in the illustration (for the sake of simplicity), attempt to de-side-bend the scapulae. Note that the subluxation pattern draws both shoulders superiorly, particularly on the left.

Note also that T11 follows the exaggerated rotation left of T12 even though it is rotated right.

The free vertebrae between the subluxated vertebrae are pulled in all directions and locked in a state of torsion.

L3-Right-Right Thoracic Theory Outcome

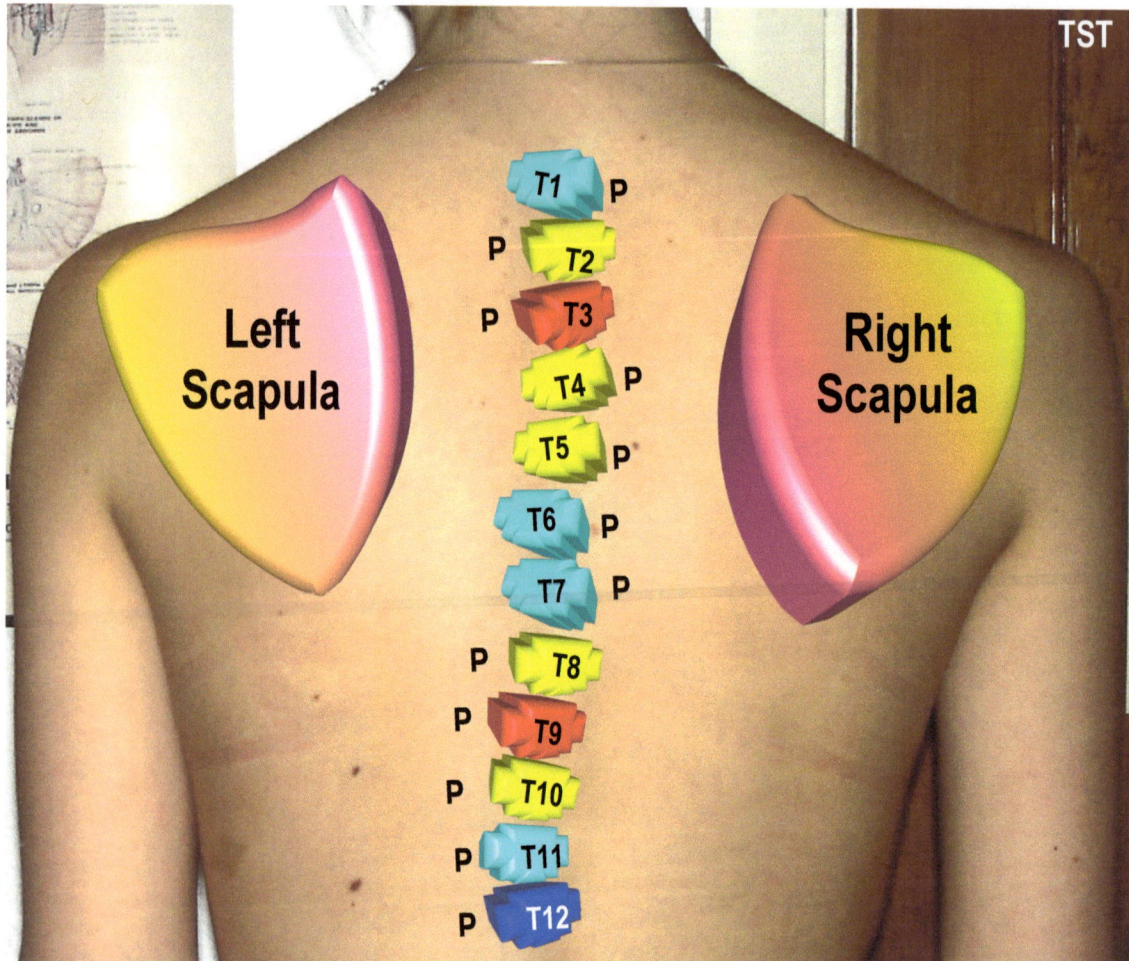

The above picture **figure TST** shows **figure 17**, transposed onto a picture of Lisa's back. It is not to scale.

The medial sides the scapulae follow the curves and shapes of the vertebrae and ribs. For example if you look at the right side of T6/7. The right transverse process is posterior which forces the attached rib posterior, therefore the medial inferior tip of the right scapula has no option other than to follow.

The angle of the right scapula has ramifications for the efficiency and integrity of the right gleno-humeral joint and bursa. The angle of the left scapula creates a torsion of opposite forces between the anterior transverse process of T1 and the posterior angle of the superior angle of the scapula.

Thoracic Posture
L3-Right-Right Subluxation Pattern

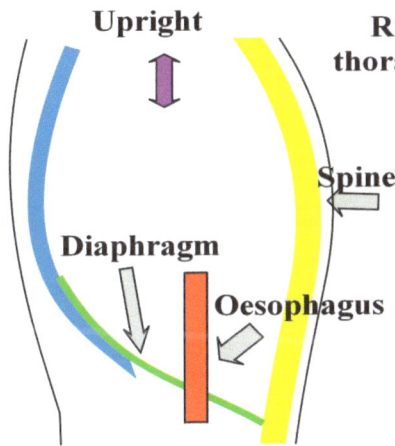

Figure 18
Normal shape of thoracic and rib cage

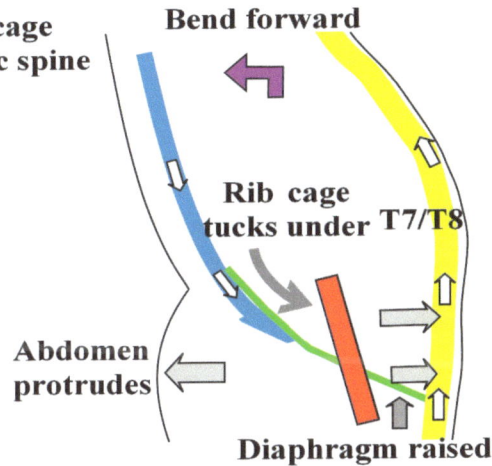

Figure 18a
Thoracic with flexion subluxations

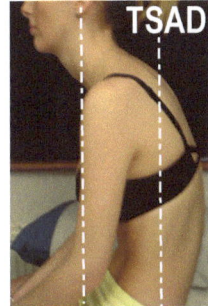

Figure TSAD is a picture of Lisa sitting in a slouched position, which is a common position for people sitting and eating in front of the television or sitting in front of a computer VDU.

Figure 18 shows a side-view of the position of a non subluxated spine. Note the Oesophagus is naturally positioned. It is illustrated to represent the soft tissue and vessels passing through the diaphragm.

The person who slouches forward increases the rounded shape of their shoulders and jutting jaw. The position also bulges their abdomen. Unlike the person free from the thoracic flexion lesion pattern who can straighten, the person with the lesion flexion pattern is constantly locked in a forward bent position. Therefore, the person feels more comfortable to slouch than sit up straight, which reinforces and adds to the problem.

If the person attempts to sit up straight it comes at the expense of exaggerating their thoracic extension subluxations, which can be very uncomfortable and therefore in a short time they will resume slouching forward again. No amount of pulling your shoulders back is going to correct this.

The diaphragm is dragged superiorly by the misaligned vertebrae and is therefore likely to affect the Oesophagus in some way as it passes through.

Theory
Rotation Right in Thoracic Extension

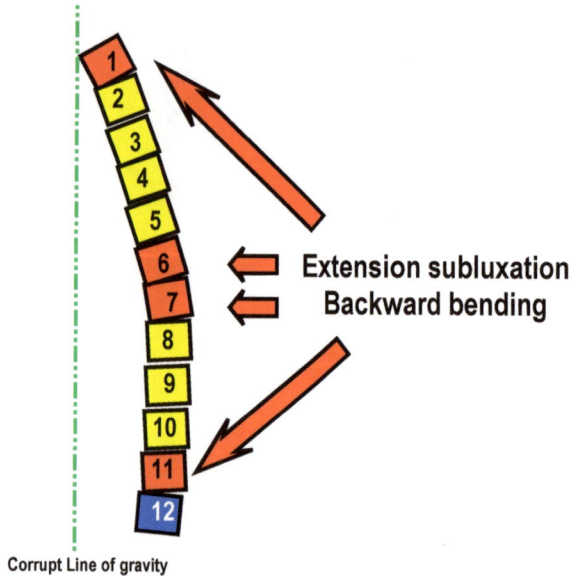

**Extension subluxation
Backward bending**

**Flexion subluxations
forward bending**

Corrupt Line of gravity

Corrupt Line of gravity

Figure 16C
Shows the pelvic side-shift and
weight bearing to the left and their
effect of their thoracic spine in
thoracic extension.

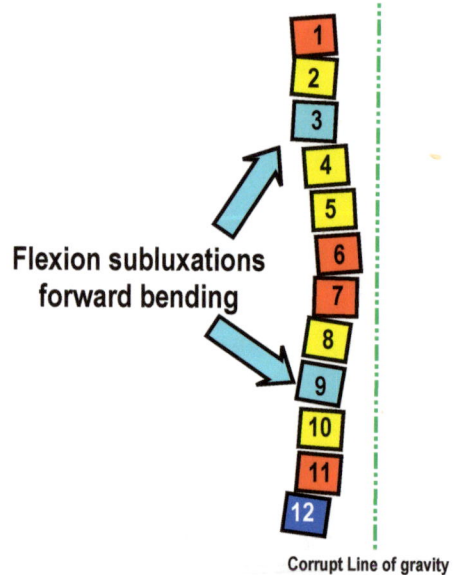

Figure 16D
Shows the pelvic side-shift and
weight bearing to the right and
their effect of their thoracic spine
in thoracic flexion.

Figure 16C is an illustration of the points of maximum stress when a person backward bends and rotates right. *Pelvic 'G' force weight and side-shift is subluxated to the left.* Because T12 became locked as part of the lumbar vertebrae subluxations it is not considered here as part of the thoracic extension pattern. Therefore the lowest free thoracic vertebra is T11.

By simple division, the maximum rotation, bending and stress is taken at the mid-point between T1 and T11, which is T6/T7, and the secondary areas of maximum stress are taken at the two ends, T1 and T11. Rotation with backward bending is not physiologically possible in the thoracic spine. Therefore, when rotation to the right in backward bending is forced, these four vertebrae will be the most likely sites for thoracic extension (impaction) lesions.

Bear in mind that the intention was to rotate right along with the pelvis and lumbar but these vertebrae would be levered into lesion with side-bending and rotation to the left in thoracic extension and not flexion. Again this is what the old Osteopaths called a 'complicated lesion'.

See figure 16D. By simple division when the person straightens, the mid-point between the subluxated T1 and T6 is T3 and the mid-point between T7 and T11 is T9. When the corrupted 'G' force side-shift and weight bearing transfer to the right, these will be the most likely sites for thoracic hyper-flexion lesions.

T6
Extension 'Complicated' Lesion to the Left

This type of subluxation is caused when a person wants to backward bend and rotate their right arm behind them. The thoracic spine is physiologically incompatible with this movement and if forced, thoracic extension subluxations will follow.

To begin with, the person leans backwards as shown in **figure TSJ.** This closely approximates the inferior tips of the T6 facets with the lamina of T7. Pelvic weight bearing is taken on the left leg and ground resistance rises up the left side of the spine. This approximates the left hand facet of T6 with the lamina of the left T7 facet still further.

When the subluxated pelvic 'G' force side-shifts to the left, as shown in **figure TSK,** T7 is forced to the left. In turn the resistant 'M' force from above side-shifts the facets of T6 to the right. This causes T6 to rotate to the left, which is the opposite direction the person wants to rotate.

The right facets of T6 impact against the lamina of T7. If the person then reaches out behind them and rotates right, for example to take hold of a car seat belt, the inferior tips of the T6 facets become levered to the left, where they impact further into the lamina of T7.

The ribs on either side fight to remain parallel and lock in the subluxation further, particularly on the right. The subluxation is so compacted that even as the person moves forward into the neutral position the right hand facets of T6 remain locked, bone against bone. These factors together typify this type of thoracic extension subluxation.

Posterior view of extension subluxation at T6

The T6 spinous process is approximated and to the right of the T7 spinous process. The right transverse process of T6 is anterior and separated in relation to the right transverse process of T7. The right hand T7 rib is separated from the right rib of T6 and the left side is approximated. T11, T7 and T1 will subluxate in exactly the same way as T3.

In this subluxation the ribs subluxate in the same torsions as those shown in **figures TSHa, TSHb** and **TSHc** There is no spare movement. On the right, the rib is locked in expiration and on the left, inspiration.

Technically this locking constitutes a thoracic flexion lesion.

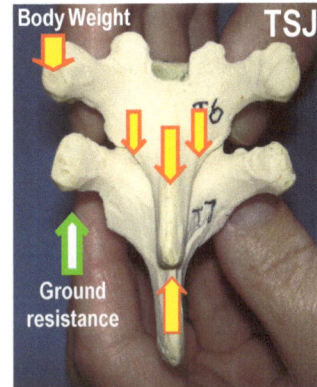

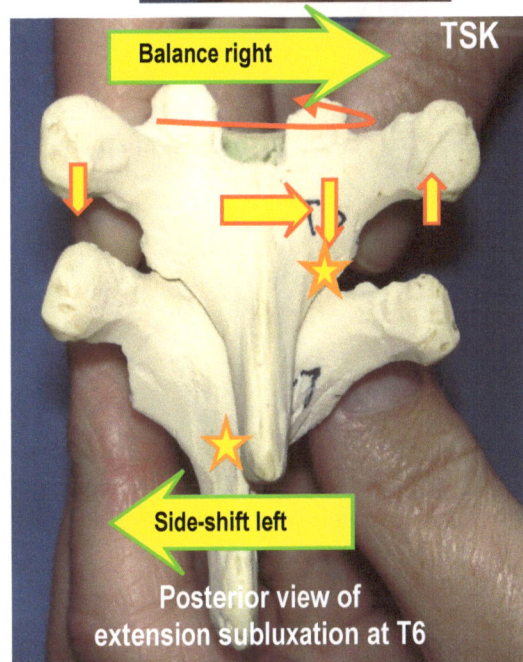

T3
Flexion Lesion to the Right

The thoracic backward-bending extension subluxations at T11 - T7 - T6 - T1 are locked in rigidly by bone against bone and the subluxated sacroiliac side-shift to the left.

To begin with, the person leans forward. This separates the inferior tips of the T3 facets from the lamina of T4. Pelvic 'G' force weight bearing and side-shift are then transferred to the right.

See **figure TSN.** T4 side-shifts along with the pelvic 'G' force to the right. At the same time the resistant 'M' force from above causes the T3 facets to side-shift left across the T4 facets, where they overlap the lateral lamina of T4.

When the person straightens into an upright position the inferior part of the left T3 facet impacts into the left T4 lamina. This causes the joint to buckle and side-bend right. The more the person straightens the more the joint buckles.

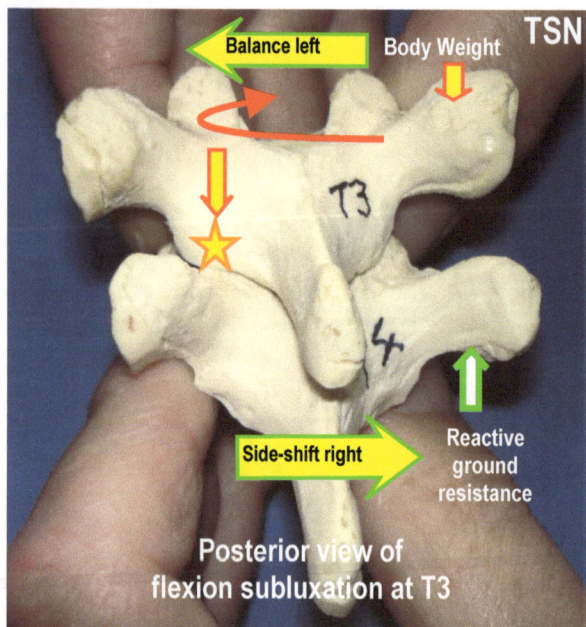
Posterior view of flexion subluxation at T3

In attempting to remain parallel, the ribs on both sides lock in the compaction still further. The subluxation is locked in place by the rigid subluxations below. Relative to the spinous process of T3, T4 is separated and to the right. And relative to the right transverse process of T3, T4 is anterior and separated. The right T4 rib is separated form the left rib of T3 and the left is approximated. The left T3 facet is compacted and the right facet is destabilized.

The ribs on either side fight to remain parallel and lock in the subluxation. In relation to the spinous process of T4, T3 is separated and to the left. And in relation to the left transverse process of T4, T3 is anterior and separated. The left T4 rib is separated from the left rib of T3 and the right is approximated. T9 will subluxate in exactly the same way as T3.

In this subluxation pattern the rib subluxations create the same torsions shown in **figures TSEa, TSEb** and **TSEc.**

On the right, the ribs becomes locked in inspiration and on the left, expiration.

The reverse rotation locks-in all the thoracic vertebral subluxations and makes them all lesions.

L3-Left-Right Thoracic in 3D and Scapulae Displacement

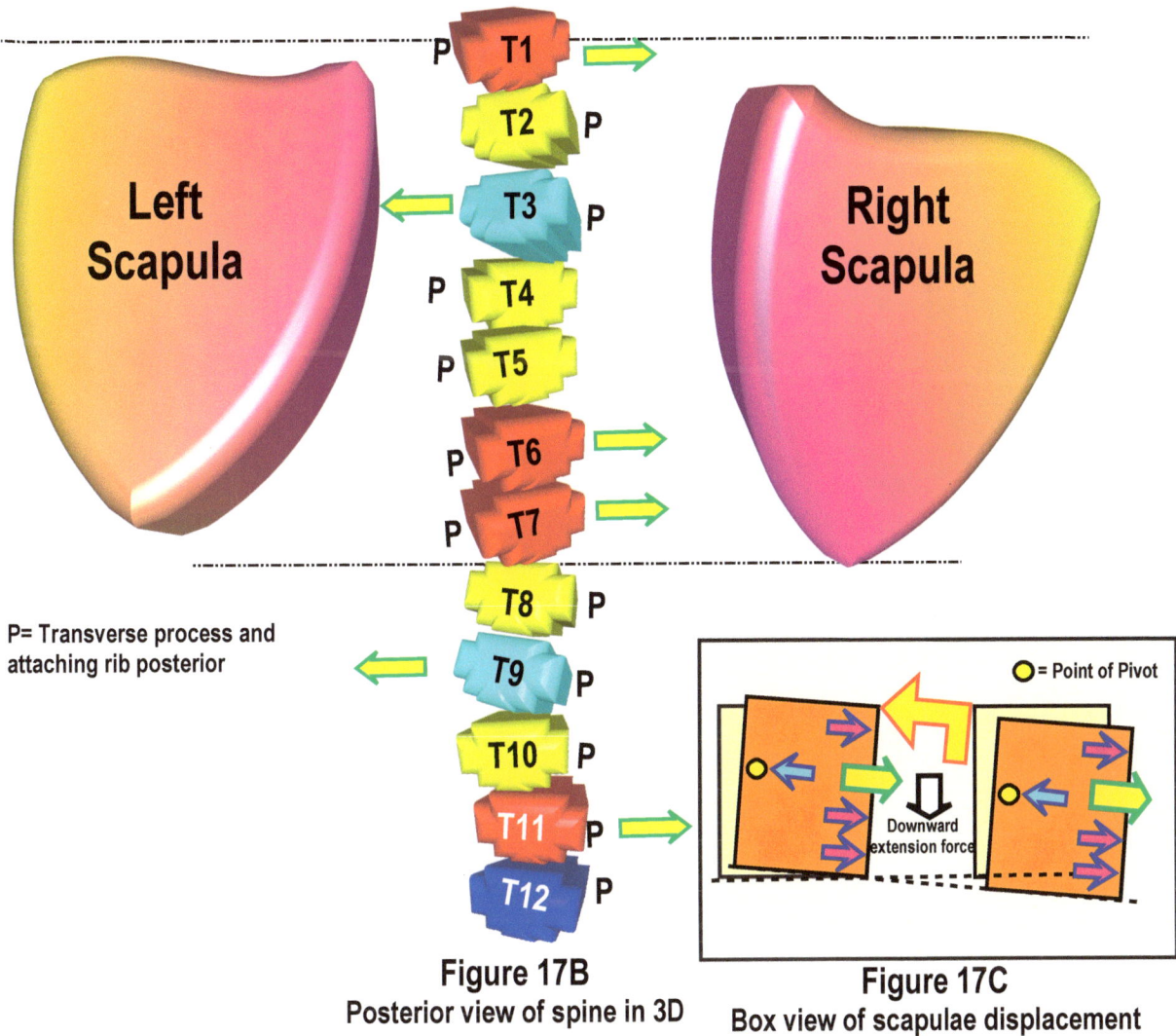

Left Scapula

Right Scapula

P T1

T2 P

T3 P

P T4

P T5

P T6

P T7

T8 P

T9 P

T10 P

T11 P

T12 P

P= Transverse process and attaching rib posterior

Figure 17B
Posterior view of spine in 3D

= Point of Pivot

Downward extension force

Figure 17C
Box view of scapulae displacement

Figure 17B is a continuation of the previous pages and shows the rotation and side-bending in more detail along with the effect this pattern has on the scapula bones.

The scapulae follow the angles and side-shift of the spine, as simplified and demonstrated in **figure 17C.** The points of pivot although not shown in the illustration (for the sake of simplicity), attempt to de-side-bend the scapulae. Note that the subluxation pattern draws both shoulders inferiorly, particularly on the right.

T11 follows the exaggerated rotation right of T12, though it is comparatively rotated left.

The free vertebrae between the subluxated vertebrae are pulled in all directions and locked in a state of torsion.

L3-Left-Right Thoracic Theory Outcome

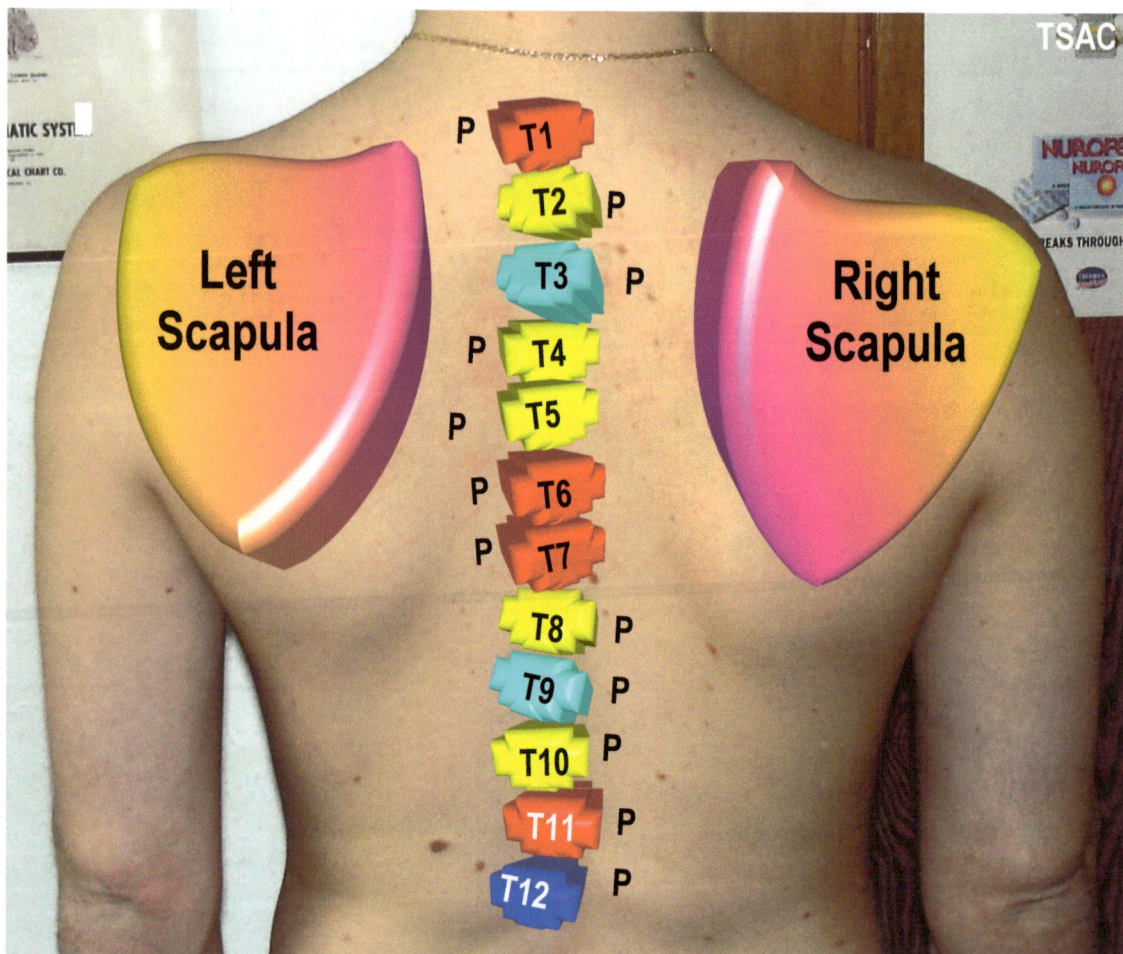

The above picture **figure TSAC** shows **figure 17B** transposed onto a photograph of Matthew's back. It is not to scale.

The medial sides of the scapulae follow the curves and shapes of the vertebrae and ribs. For example if you look at the left side of T6/7, the transverse process is posterior which forces the attached rib posterior therefore, the medial inferior tip of the left scapula has no option other than to follow.

Chapter Ten

Lesions of the Cervical Joints

Overview

With the exception of the C2/1 joint, there are two vulnerable areas within every cervical joint where lesions can occur. These areas are shown exaggerated in **figures CSA** and **CSB** below.

Figure CSA is a posterior view of a typical C3 cervical subluxation when rotation is locked to the left. The left facet of C3 is side-bent and rotated past its physiological limit and overlaps the inferior border of the left C4 facet. This brings the bony medial border of the C3 facet into direct contact with the medial bony surface of the lamina of C4. On its own, this is a minor subluxation.

Figure CSB is a side view taken from the left of the subluxated left C3 facet. The left superior perimeter of the C4 facet is wedged under the anterior tubercle of C3. This locks the joint and prevents C3 from de-rotation to the right.

The two areas interact and lock against each other and constitute a cervical lesion with rotation left.

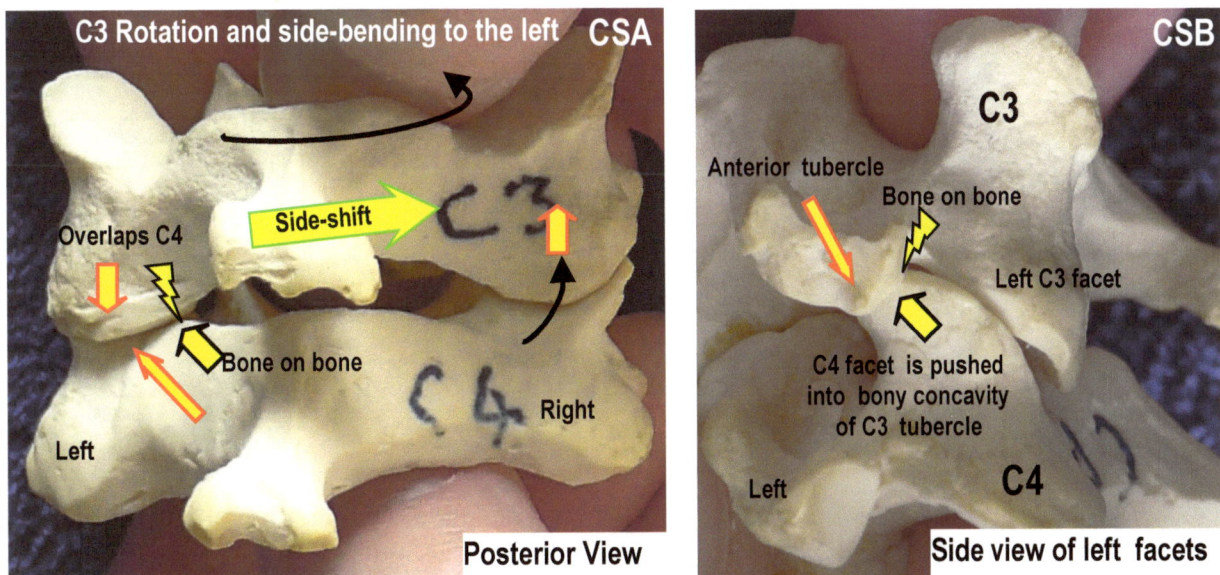

CSA — C3 Rotation and side-bending to the left

Overlaps C4 · Side-shift · C3 · Bone on bone · Left · Right · C4

Posterior View

CSB — C3

Anterior tubercle · Bone on bone · Left C3 facet · C4 facet is pushed into bony concavity of C3 tubercle · Left · C4

Side view of left facets

139

How the Cervical Joints Lock and Cause Extension and Flexion Lesions

Figure CSAa is a side-view of the left facets of C3-C4 in lesion. When the left C3 facet overhangs the inferior border of the left C4 facet and becomes lodged against the lamina, the superior tip of the C4 facet is pushed under the posterior recess of the left C3 anterior tubercle. A certain amount of facet buckle then takes place.

Figure CSAb shows a side-view of the left C3 tubercle. The posterior surface of the tubercle is slightly concave both vertically and horizontally and is illustrated in **figure CSAc**.

Figure CSAc illustrates the superior tip of the left C4 facet when it is forced against the left tubercle of C3. Bone is ground and wedged against bone and prevents C3 from de-rotation to the right.

Figure CSAd is an anterior left lateral view of the C3-C4 lesion with rotation to the left locked-in. Due to the proximity of the vertebral body's on the left side, side-shift to the right is restricted and prevents right facet dislocation.

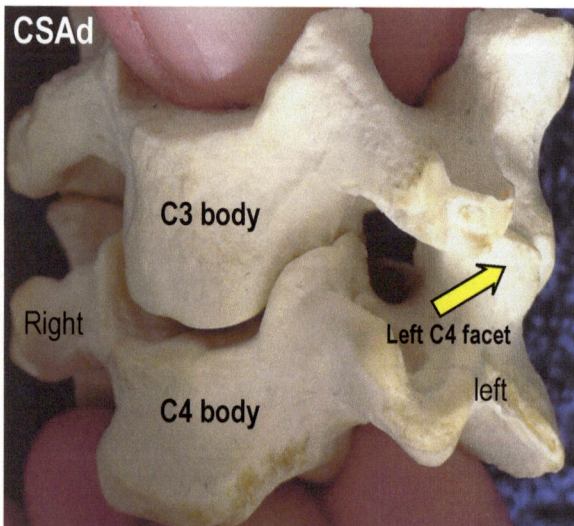

Anatomy of a lesion on the left cervical lesion

Cave like recess of the anterior C3 tubercle

Body

SP

C3

Bony area

C4 facet slips under recess of C3 tubercle

C4   left

CSAa

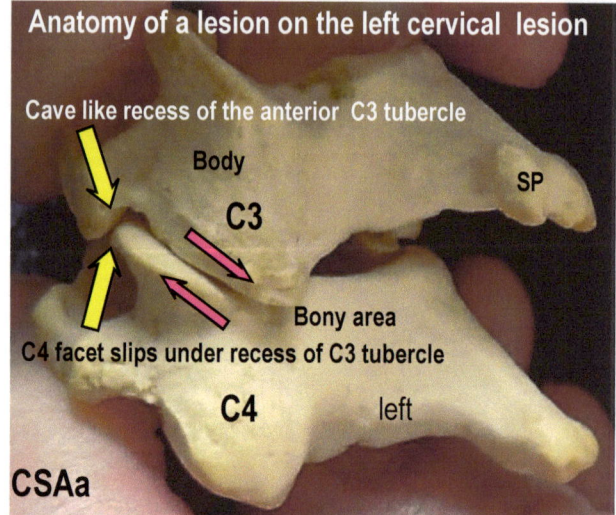

CSAb   Inferior view of the left half of C3

Anterior C3 tubercle

C3 facet

left

SP

C3 body

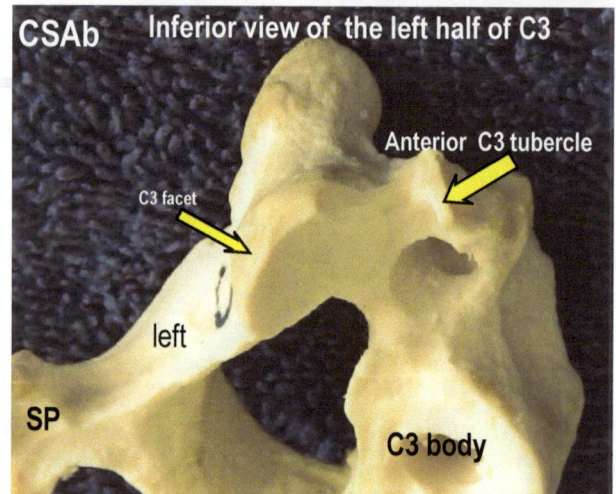

CSAd

C3 body

Right

Left C4 facet

left

C4 body

Anterior left lateral view showing relative positions of the C4 and C3 body's in a typical rotation to the left lesion. The proximity of vertebral body's restricts shift to the right.

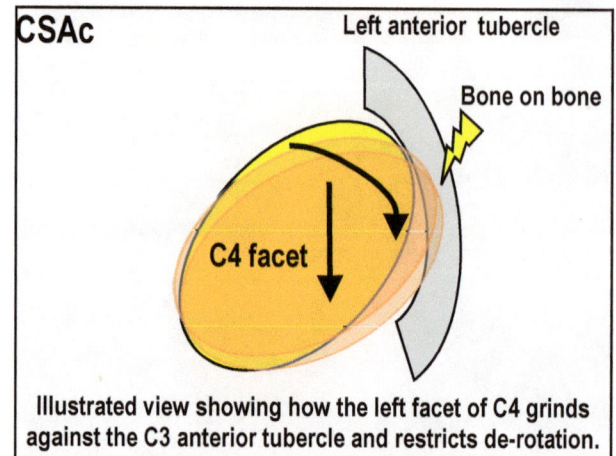

CSAc

Left anterior tubercle

Bone on bone

C4 facet

Illustrated view showing how the left facet of C4 grinds against the C3 anterior tubercle and restricts de-rotation.

140

Cervical Theory
L3-Right-Right Evolving Torsions

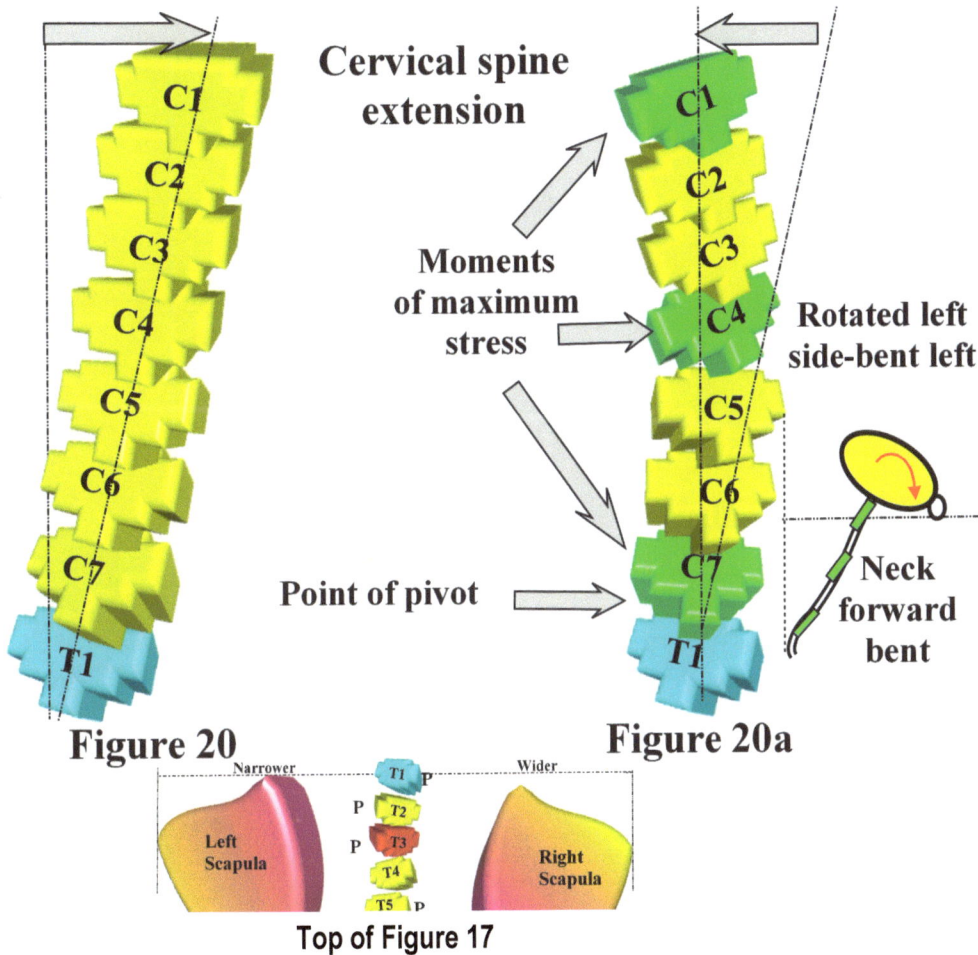

Cervical spine extension

Moments of maximum stress

Point of pivot

Rotated left side-bent left

Neck forward bent

C1 C2 C3 C4 C5 C6 C7 T1

Figure 20

Figure 20a

Narrower — Wider

Left Scapula — Right Scapula

T1 P / P T2 / P T3 / T4 / T5 P

Top of Figure 17

Figure 20 shows the vertical line that would follow on from the subluxated thoracic spine shown in **figure 17,** copied from page 131. The cervical vertebrae lean to the right and rotate right. The neck makes adjustments to counter the subluxation pattern below.

For survival, the eyes should be level and looking ahead, so with the aid of balance the skull attempts to maintain an upright position by rotating to the left.

Figure 20a shows the points of stress. Again it is a simple division of seven, with C4 in the middle taking the maximum bending and stress and the two ends, C1 and C7 taking the secondary stress.

Therefore, the Occiput-C1, C4 and C7 are forced to side-bend and rotate to the left, as shown in **figure 20a**.

Cervical
L3-Right-Right Extension Subluxation

Figure CSC shows the C1-occipital joint in the starting position shown in **figure 20** on the previous page. C1 and the occiput are separated. In this position the right eye is lower than the left and the head is turned to the right.

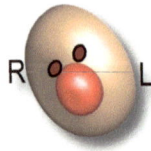

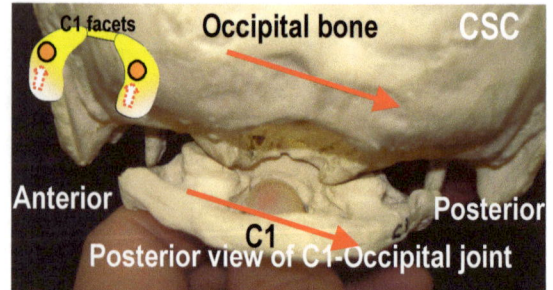

Figure CSCa shows the occipital bone rotating left as the person straightens their head and rotates left in an attempt to look forward. If the person does not straighten their head before rotating left, it is unlikely a subluxation will form. However, if the person does straighten their head first, which is the more likely occurrence, the occipital bone is forced to side-shift to the right. This derails the occipital facets from those of C1. If the person then rotates their head and forces it to the left, the joint subluxates.

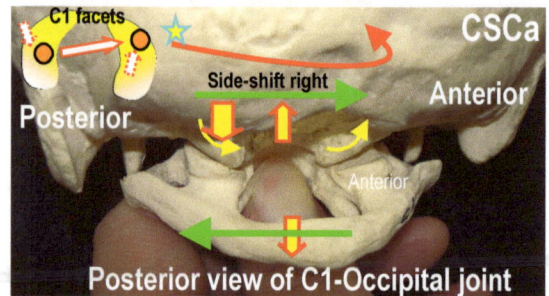

Figure CSD shows the T1-C7 joint at the starting point, as illustrated in **figure 20**. **Figure CSDa** shows what happens at the T1-C7 joint when the person straightens their head and rotates left. In straightening, C7 side-shifts to the right across the facets of T1. This approximates the left facet of C7 with the left lamina of T1. When the person then rotates their head, the posterior part of left transverse process of C7 collides with the anterior surface of the left T1 transverse process, where it lesions.

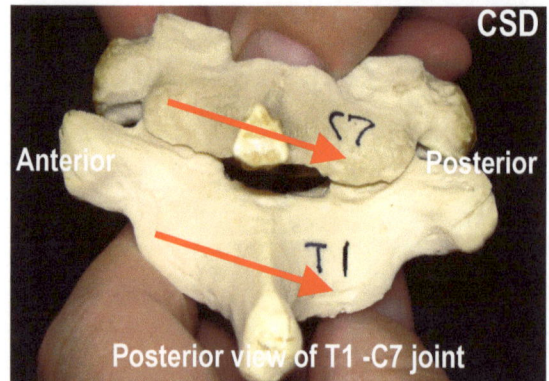

C5-C4 becomes trapped in the centre by the downward force of the rotated head.

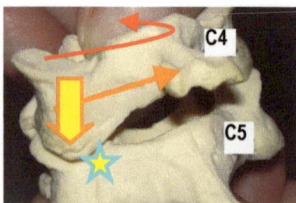

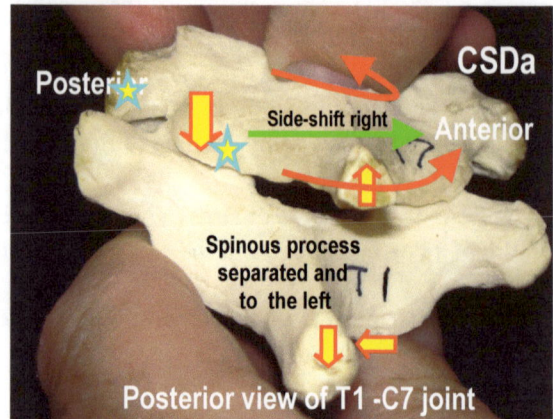

Figure CSC

- C1 facets
- Occipital bone
- CSC
- Anterior
- Posterior
- C1
- Posterior view of C1-Occipital joint

Figure CSCa

- C1 facets
- CSCa
- Side-shift right
- Posterior
- Anterior
- Anterior
- Posterior view of C1-Occipital joint

Figure CSD

- CSD
- Anterior
- C7
- Posterior
- T1
- Posterior view of T1 -C7 joint

Figure CSDa

- Posterior
- CSDa
- Side-shift right
- Anterior
- Spinous process separated and to the left
- T1
- Posterior view of T1 -C7 joint

Cervical Theory
L3-Right-Right Torsions

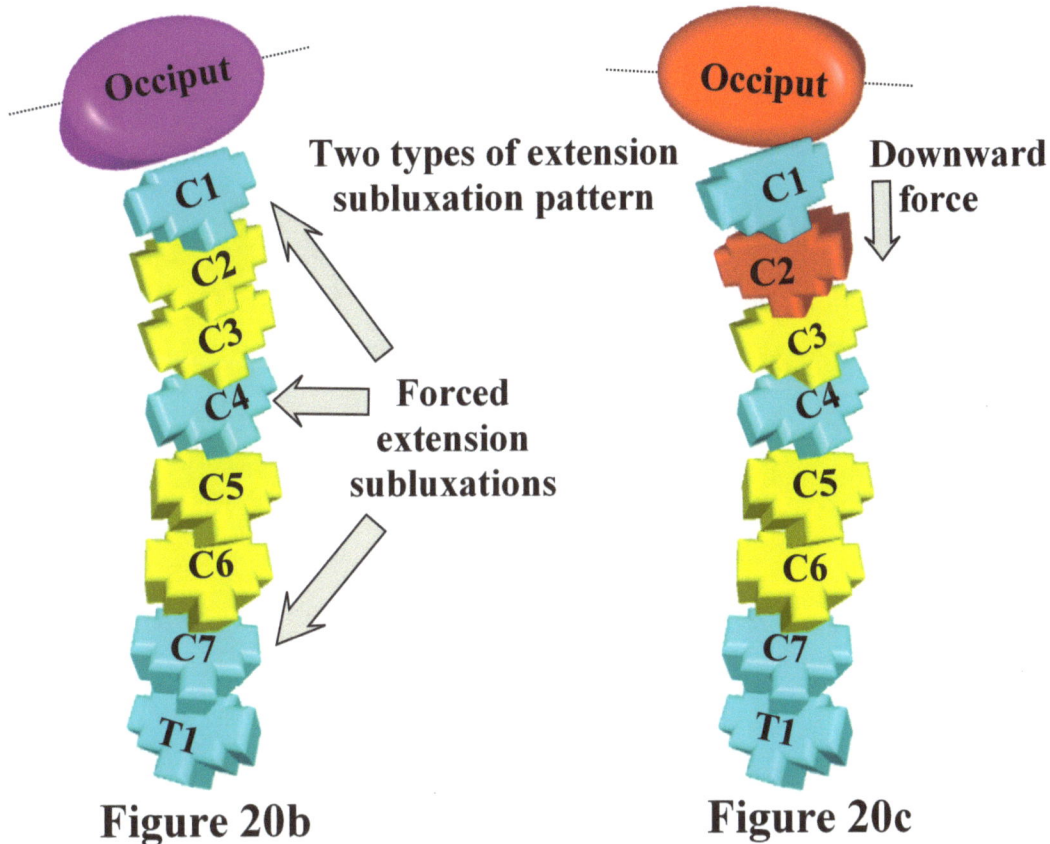

Figure 20b

Figure 20c

Figure 20b shows the extension lesions that occur at C5-4 and T1-C7 with the C1-occipital added. This causes the person to incline their head downwards and to the left as shown on the next page in **figure CSH**.

However, with these lesions locked in place, if the person attempts to rotate their head to the right, as shown in **figure CSJ** on the next page, further complications arise. Rotating to the right causes the occipital bone to tilt backwards. The C1-occipital joint, therefore finds itself in a double lock lesion.

When the occipital bone is forced to rotate right, a downward pressure is brought to bear on the right. The lesioned occipital bone and C1 have little room to manoeuvre and as a result C2 becomes compressed and in many cases lesions in flexion, as shown above in **figure 20c**.

The L3-right-right patient can present with either or both of the neck patterns shown in illustrations **figure 20b** or **20c.**

Cervical Theory
L3-Right-Right Outcome

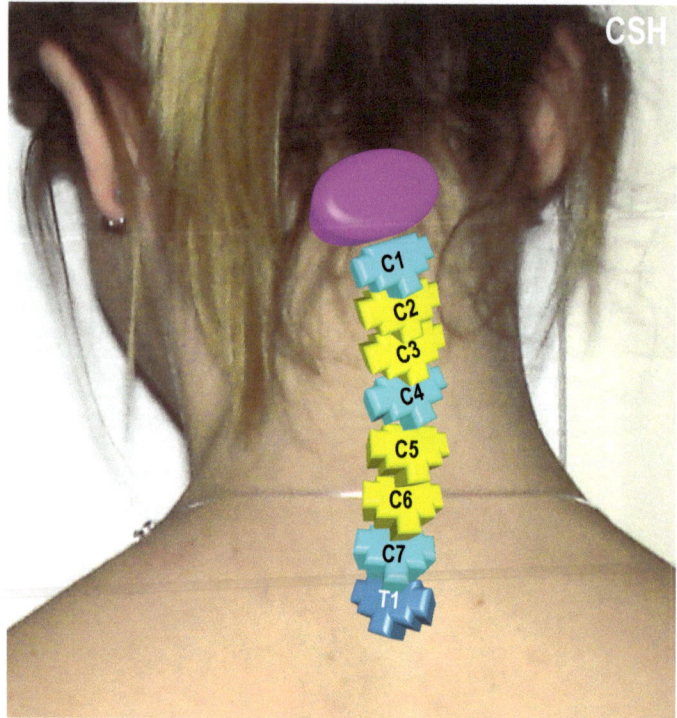

Figure CSH is a photograph of Lisa's neck with the **figure 20** illustration superimposed. Notice how the lesion pattern inclines and rotates her head to the left.

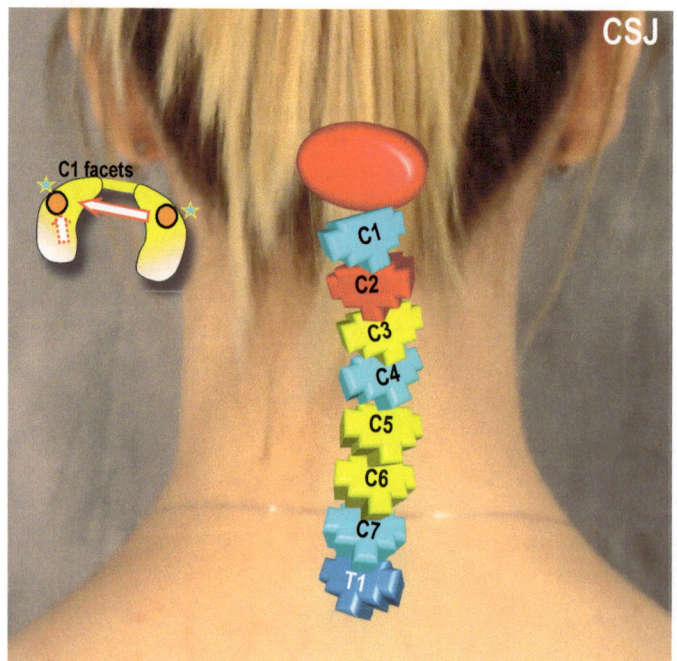

Figure CSJ shows a photograph of Lisa forcing her neck to rotate right in order to look straight ahead and level her ears.

In this photograph the lesion pattern illustrated in **figure 2** has been superimposed.

To the casual observer it could be thought that she did not have a problem with her neck alignment.

Theory
Cervical Flexion L3-Left-Right

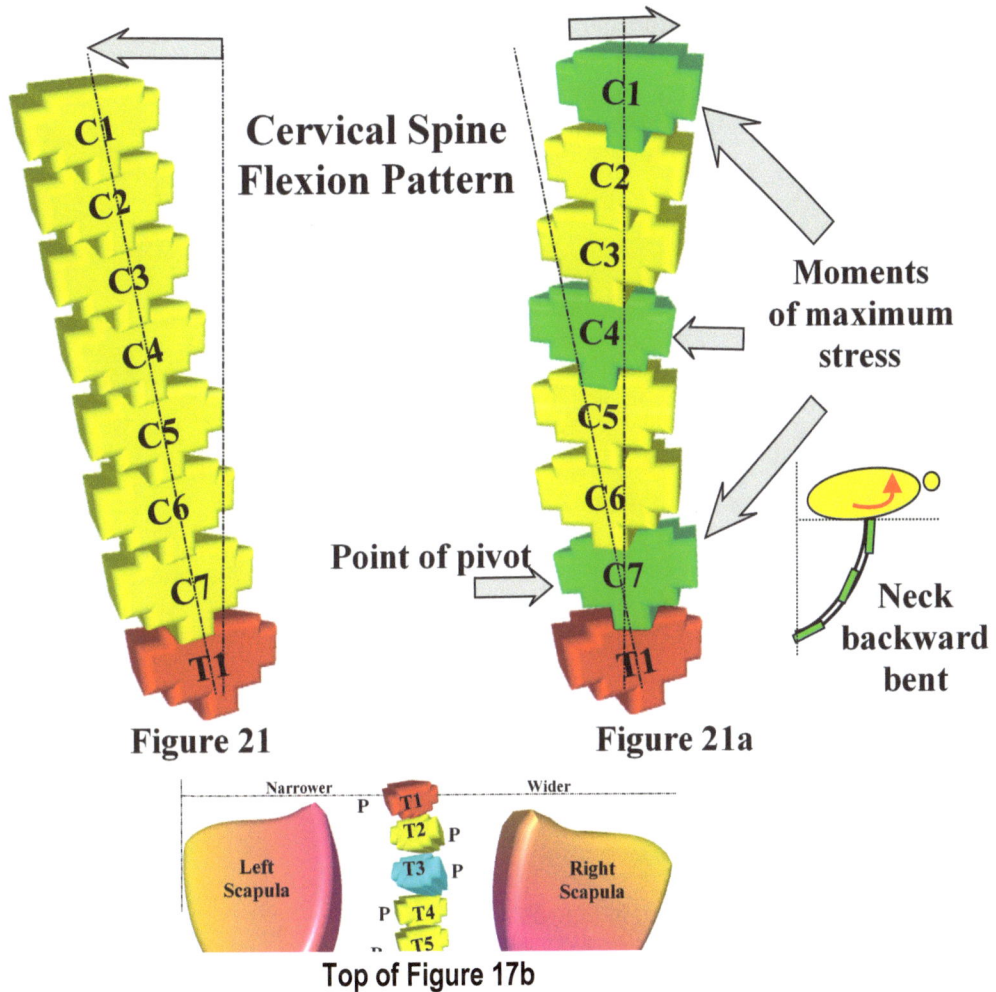

Cervical Spine Flexion Pattern

C1, C2, C3, C4, C5, C6, C7, T1

Point of pivot

Figure 21

Moments of maximum stress

Neck backward bent

Figure 21a

Narrower — Wider

Left Scapula — Right Scapula

T1, T2, T3, T4, T5

Top of Figure 17b

Figure 21 illustrates the line that would follow on from the subluxated thoracic spine shown in **figure 17b**. The cervical vertebrae lean to the left and rotate left. The neck makes adjustments to counter the lesion pattern below.

For survival, the eyes need to be level and looking ahead and so with the aid of balance, the skull attempts to maintain an upright position by rotating to the right.

Figure 21a shows the points of stress. Again it is a simple division of seven, with C4 in the middle taking the maximum bending and stress and the ends, C1 and C7 taking the secondary stress.

Therefore, the Occiput-C1, C4 and C7 are forced to side-bend and rotate to the right, as shown in **figure 21a**.

Cervical
in L3-Left-Right Flexion Subluxation

Figure CSE shows the C1-occipital joint in the starting position shown in **figure 21** on the previous page. C1 is positioned in backward bending. In this position the left eye is lower than the right and the head is rotated to the left.

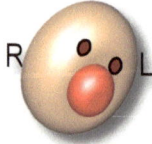

Figure CSEa shows the occipital bone rotating right as the person straightens their head and rotates right in an attempt to look forward. If the person does not straighten their head before rotating right, it is unlikely a subluxation will form. However, if the person does straighten their head initially, which is the more likely occurrence, the occipital bone is forced to side-shift to the left. This derails the occipital facets from those of C1. If the person then rotates their head and forces it to the right, the joint subluxates.

Figure CSF shows the T1-C7 joint at the starting point shown in **figure 21**. Extension with rotation in the cervical vertebrae is not possible. **Figure CSFa** shows what happens at the T1-C7 joint when the person straightens their head and rotates right, as shown in **figure 21a**. On straightening their head C7 side-shifts to the left across the facets of T1. This approximates the right facet of C7 with the right lamina of T1. When the person then rotates their head, the posterior part of the right transverse process of C7 collides with the anterior surface of the right T1 transverse process, where it lesions. **C5-C4** becomes trapped in the centre by the downward force of the rotated head.

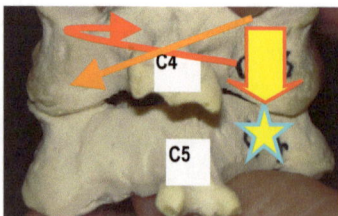

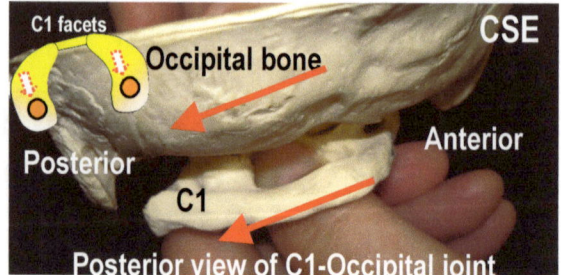

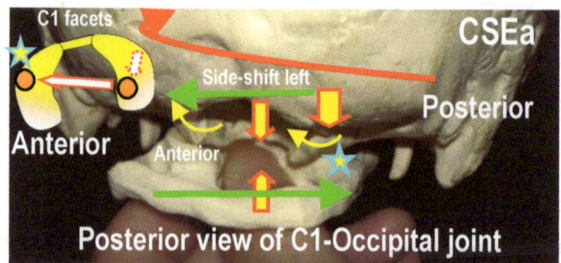

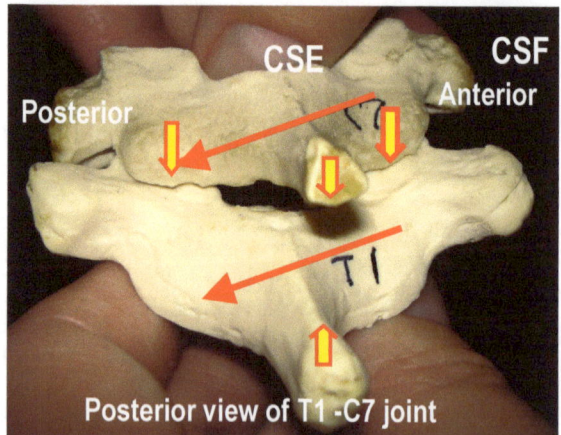

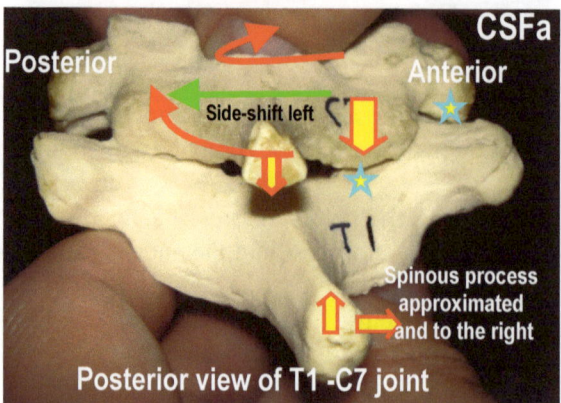

Posterior view of C1-Occipital joint

Posterior view of C1-Occipital joint

Posterior view of T1 -C7 joint

Posterior view of T1 -C7 joint

Theory
L3-Left-Right Evolving Torsions

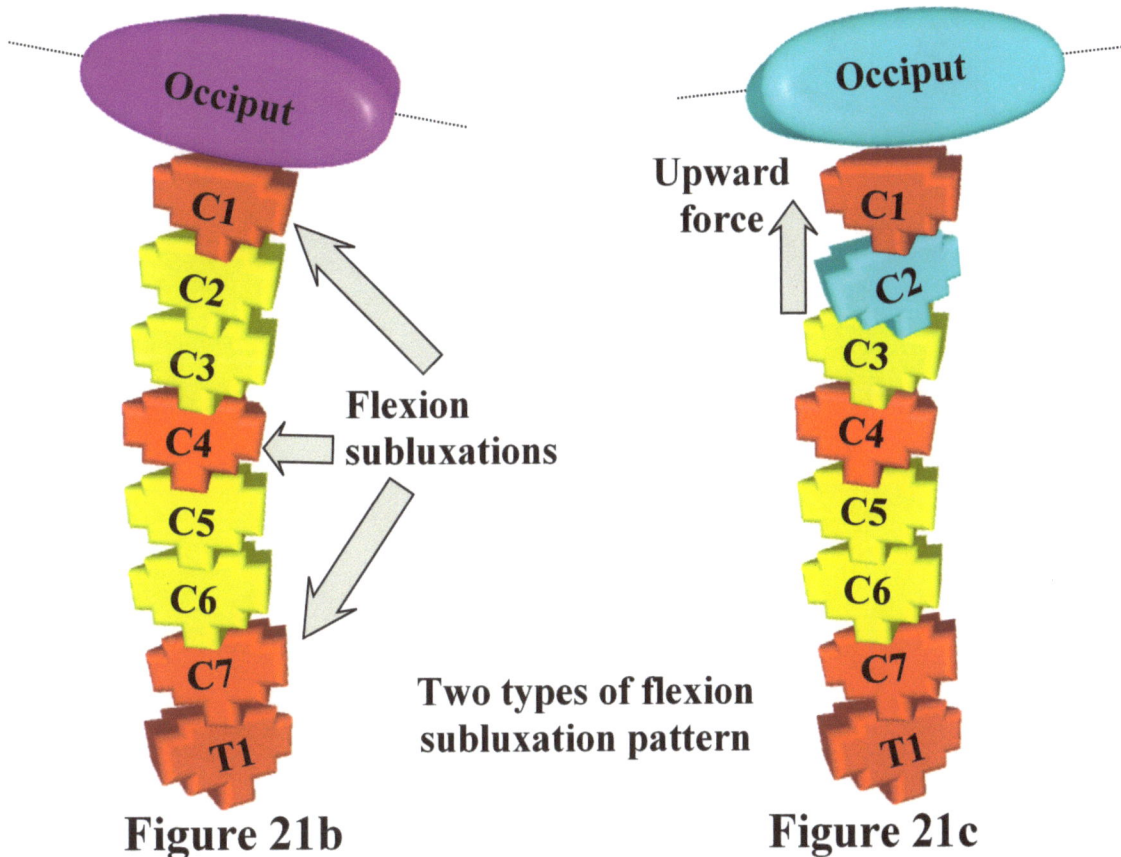

Figure 21b

Figure 21c

Figure 21b shows the flexion lesions that occur at C5-4 and T1-C7 with the C1-occipital added. This causes the person to incline their head upwards and to the right.

However, with these lesions in place, if the person attempts to rotate their head to the left as shown in **figure 12c**, further complications arise. Rotating to the left causes the occipital bone to tilt downwards. The C1-occipital joint therefore finds itself in a double-lock and becomes a lesion.

If the occipital bone is forced to rotate left, an upward pressure is exerted on the left. The lesioned occipital and C1 joints pull the left side of the next vulnerable vertebra below C1 superiorly. As a result C2 is forced to lesion in extension, as shown above in **figure 21c**.

The L3 left-right patient can present with either or both of the neck patterns shown in illustrations **figure 21b** or **21c**.

Cervical Theory
L3-Left-Right Outcome

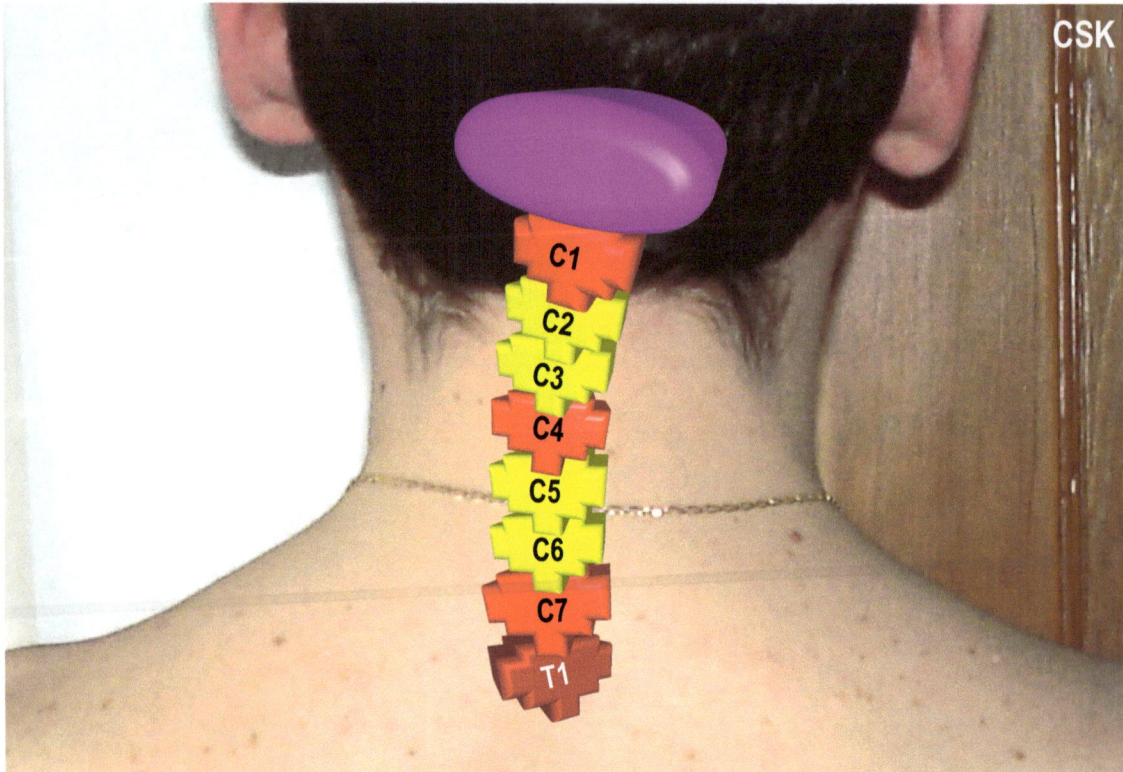

Figure SCK above is a picture of Matthew's neck with **figure 21b**, superimposed. Notice how his head rises and rotates to the right.

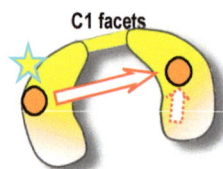

Figure CSEb

If Matthew were to turn his head left from the above position, the placement of the occipital facets acting on C1 would look like **figure CSEb**. Because the right occipital facet is not at the extremity of the C1 facet, the joint does not readily subluxate.

Therefore, it is more usual for the person with the L3-left-right lesion pattern to present as in **figure SCK**.

Chapter Eleven

Diagnosing the Two Models

Correct diagnosis is essential before treatment begins. If you get this wrong, because PPT's are so powerful, you could make your patients pain and posture worse, rather than correcting. The previous chapters detailed the mechanics behind the two lesion patterns. This chapter looks at how these patterns physically present in practice.

There are four possible lesions patterns based on how L3 becomes lesioned. The two rarest are the L3-right-left and the L3-left-left patterns. By far the most common pattern is the forward leaning L3-right-right shown in **figure IDM1**, followed by the backward leaning L3-left-right shown in **figure IDM2**.   For expediency these will be referred to as: **RR** and **LR**

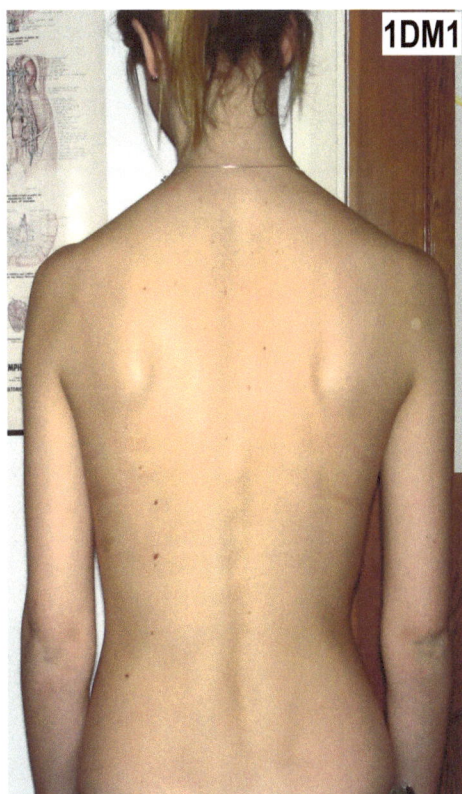

(L3)-**Right-Right** (RR)

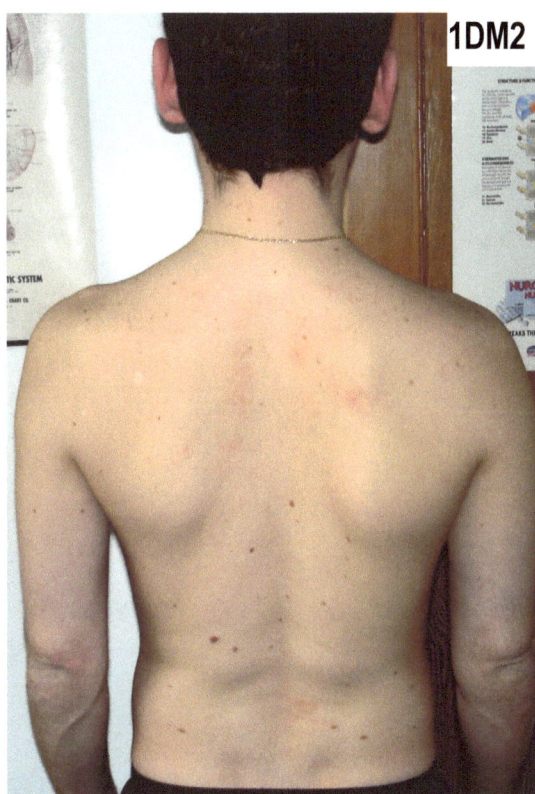

(L3)-**Left-Right** (LR)

Right-Right General Posture

Right-right posterior view.

General observation

Figure 1DM3 shows a photograph of Lisa. Her back closely approximates the R-R forward bending lesion pattern and is generally rotated to the right.

The major differential markers to look for are, as follows:

Pelvis: Her pelvis sways upwards and to the right. This causes a more shapely and medial curve at the waist line on the right in comparison to the left.

Her pelvis and torso are generally rotated to the right.

Head: Her head is side-bent left and rotated left. This is more clearly seen in **figure 1DM1** on the previous page. Her right ear is superior.

Shoulders: Her left shoulder area is generally wider with a lesser angle than her right.

Her right gleno-humeral joint is higher than on her left.

Arms: Her right arm hangs in a flexed position.

Pelvis: Her left buttock is posterior in relation to her right and the fold of the left buttock is inferior. Her pelvis is side-bent left and rotated right and side-shifted right.

Knees: Her left knee is flexed and rotates inwards as if she were taking a step forward on that leg. The right knee is angled medially.

Legs: Her left foot is turn outwards and her right inwards, see page 153. Her left leg is physiologically

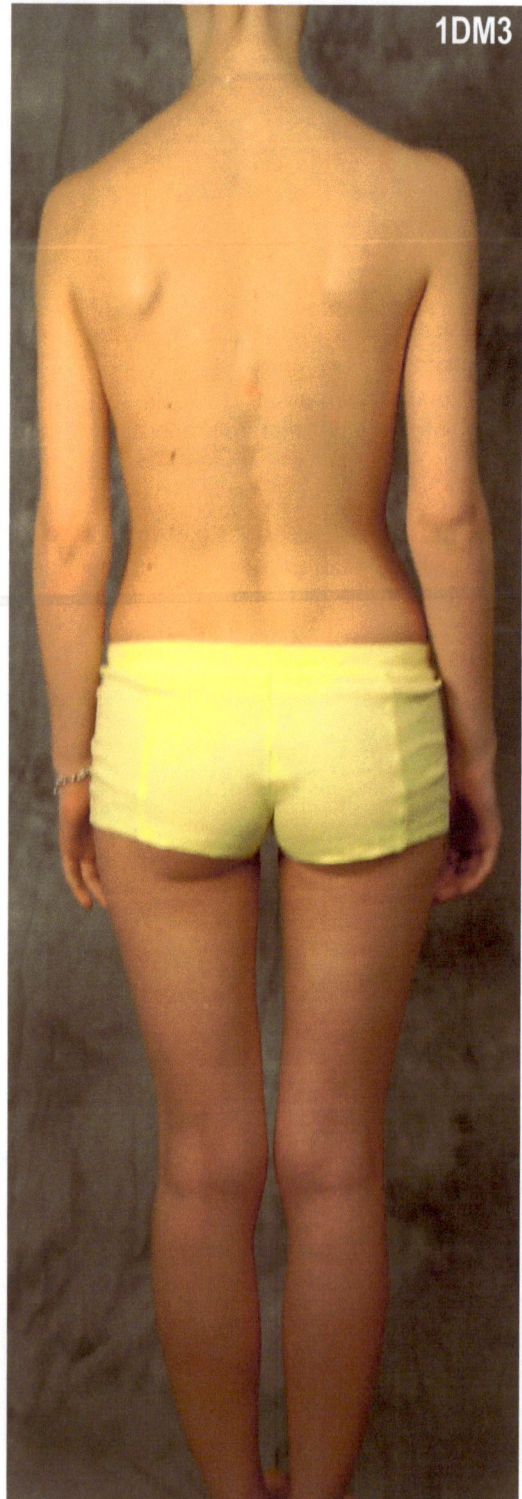

150

Left-Right General Posture

Left-right posterior view

General observation

Figure IDM4 shows a photograph of Matthew. His back closely approximates the **L-R** backward bending lesion pattern and is generally rotated to the left.

The major differential markers to look for are as follows:

Generally the L-R back looks more symmetrical then the R-R and has the appearance of standing upright.

Pelvis: His pelvis is side-bent right, side-shifted to the left and rotated to the left. This causes a more shapely and medial curve at the waist line on the left in comparison to the right. This can be seen more obviously in **figure 1DM2** at the beginning of this chapter.

Head: His head is side-bent right and rotated right. Again this is more clearly shown in **figure 1DM2**. His left ear is superior.

Shoulders: His right shoulder area is generally wider with a lesser angle than his left.

Arms: His left arm hangs straighter and more anterior than his right. His left gleno-humeral joint is higher than on his right.

Legs: His right knee is slightly flexed. The left leg will be anterior when standing and right leg physiologically shorter than the right left.

Feet: Both his right and left feet are turned outwards, see page 153.

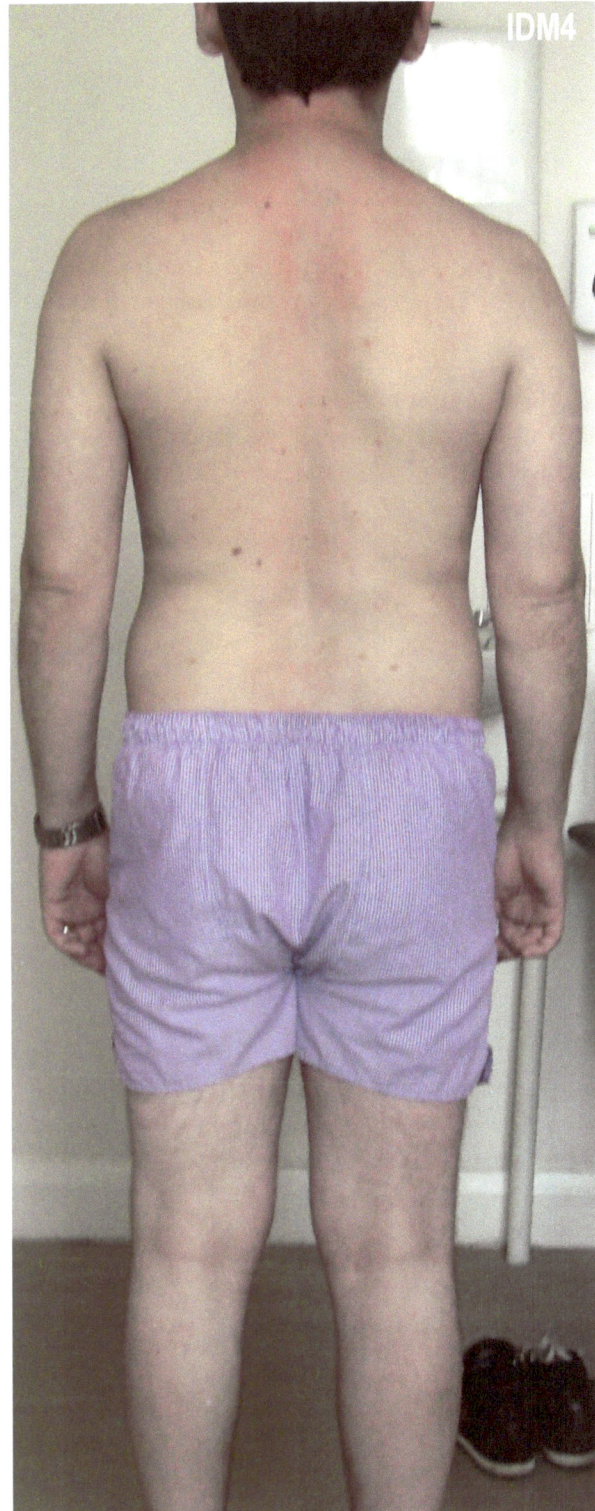

151

Right-Right and Left-Right Side-Views

Differential diagnosis

Right-Right (Expanded)

Figures IB is a side-view of Lisa's typical **R-R** torso.

Whilst she has exaggerated her posture for clarity, it can be seen that her whole posture is one of forward leaning.

Head: The chin of a **R-R,** due to the forward leaning angle of their neck, is aimed at the floor, therefore to look ahead as Lisa is doing, she has to lift her chin..

Shoulders: Both her shoulders are anterior with a convexity between.

Torso: Her upper torso is rounded and her shoulders rounded.

Left -Right (Compacted)

Figures IC is a side-view of Matthews typical **L-R** torso.

It can be seen that his whole posture is one of back-ward leaning.

Head: The chin of a **L-R**, due to the backward leaning angle of their neck, is aimed upwards, therefore to look ahead, as Matthew is doing, he has to lower his chin.

Shoulders: Both his shoulders are posterior with a concavity between.

Torso: His upper torso is flat and his shoulders square.

Forward bent posture

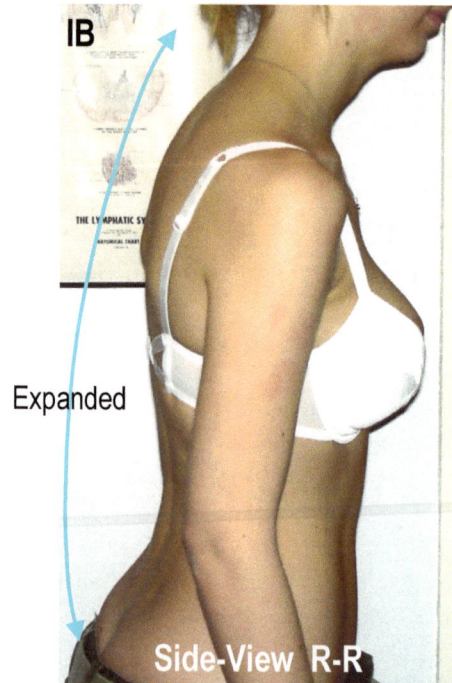

IB
Expanded
Side-View R-R

Backward bent posture

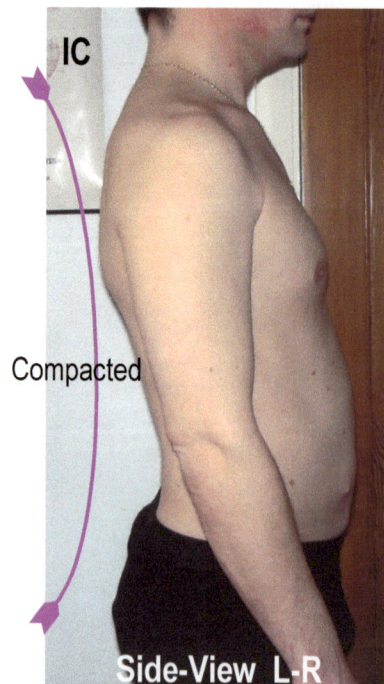

IC
Compacted
Side-View L-R

Leg Position of Right-Right and left-Right

Right-Right feet

When the person is stationary and asked to face forward, there legs and feet will position themselves as follows:

In the **R-R** lesion pattern, on standing, the right leg will be forward in relation to the left and turned inwards.

The left foot will be turned outwards and posterior in relation to the right.

Due to the outward angle, the left foot will have a flattened arch, whereas the right leg inward foot will have a raised arch. See **Figure 1F.**

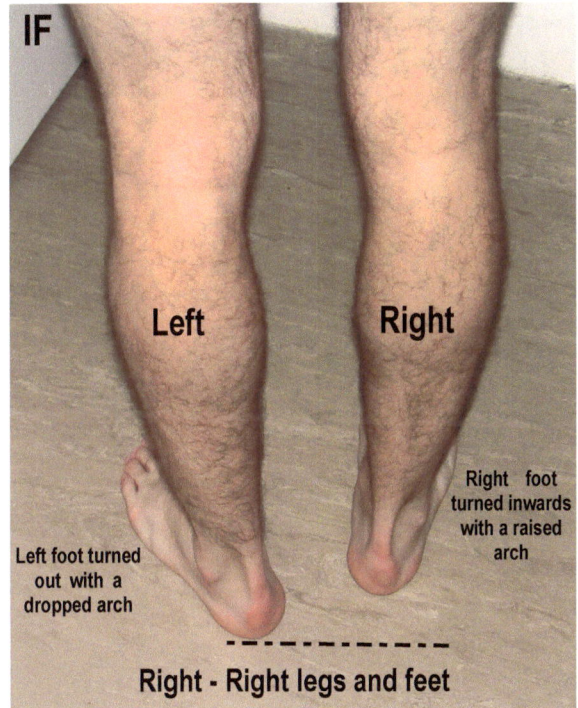

IF

Left   Right

Right foot turned inwards with a raised arch

Left foot turned out with a dropped arch

Right - Right legs and feet

Left-Right feet

The position of the feet in the L-R are far less pronounced than in the R-R. The example is exaggerated.

In the **L-R** lesion pattern the left foot will be forward in relation to the right and turned inwards with a slightly flattened arch. The right leg and foot will be turned outwards with a raised arch . See **Figure 1X.**

In some cases the right foot can become very rotated outwards.

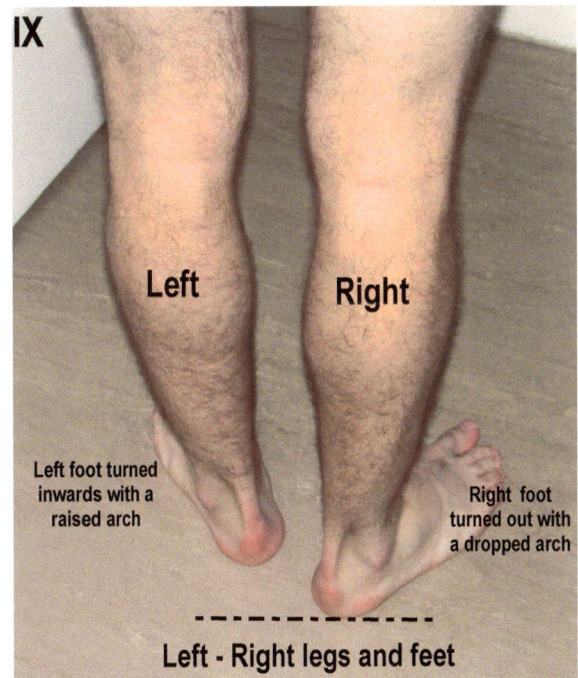

IX

Left   Right

Left foot turned inwards with a raised arch

Right foot turned out with a dropped arch

Left - Right legs and feet

Right-Right
Knees, Neck and Head

Right-right knees

Observe the tracking of Lisa's knees, shown in **figure IG**. Her left patella is twisted medially and inferiorly.

The distal end of her right thigh is angled medially and causes a medial shearing force to her right knee joint.

When weight bearing the opposing and twisting forces exerted through her legs places torsion and strain on both her hip joints and ankles.

Her left knee is anterior in comparison to her right due to mild knee flexion.

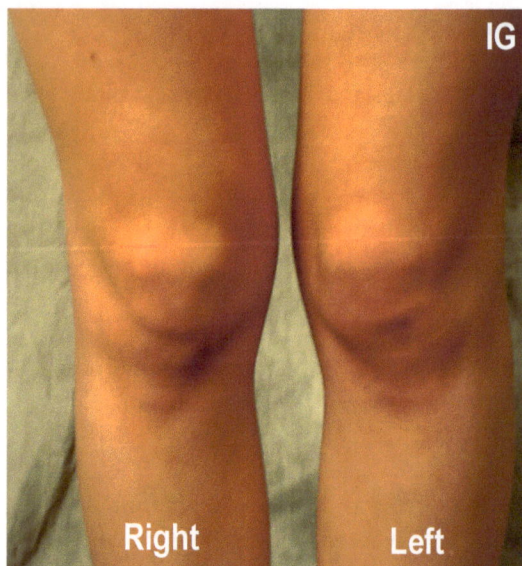

IG

Right   Left

Right-right neck and head

Figure IH is another photograph of Lisa's back. Look at the effect the angles of her shoulders and scapula have on her neck.

Notice how her left neck muscles are pulling, and that her head is rotated and side-bent to the left. This can be more easily appreciated by comparing the level and depth of her ears.

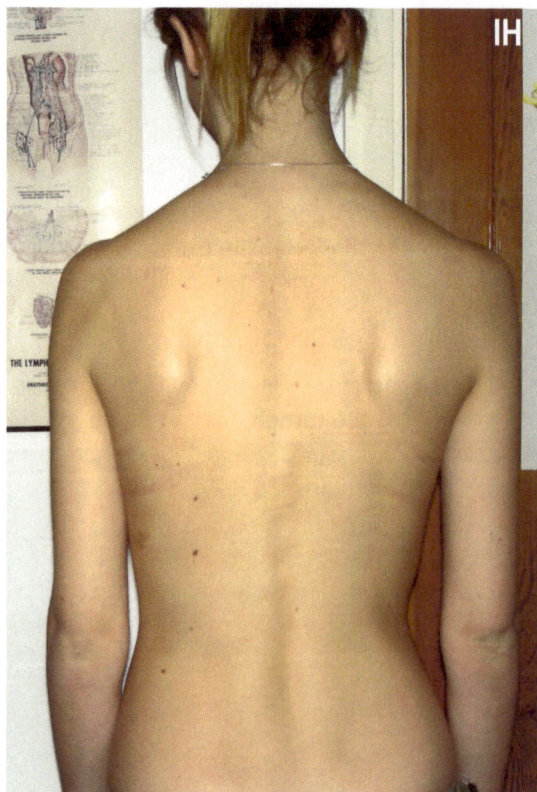

IH

Right-Right Assessment Clinical Assessment

Right-right plumb line from below

The purpose of a plumb line is to show the line of gravity. In a perfect spine the line of gravity would be down the centre of the body. When a plumb line is placed against Lisa's back as in **figure IJ**, the extent to which her upper torso leans to the left is highlighted. Observe her neck and see that the line of gravity passes to the right.

L3-right-right plumb line from above

If the plumb line is moved to the left to reflect the line of gravity that passes through the middle of her neck, it can be seen from **figure IK** that it passes through her left sacroiliac joint, her medial left knee, calf and Achilles tendon. It is these areas that take the full forces of gravity.

Right-right clinical mobility neck

Figure IL and **IM** shows Lisa turning her head as far as she can to the left and then right, without rotating her torso. (Look at her pony-tail). Refer to page 164.

The limit to which she can rotate her neck is restricted. The maximum neck rotation for a young adult thought to be approximately 60-70 degrees in both directions.

Right-right in forward bending

Figure IN shows Lisa bending forward. In this forward bending test, observe the misalignment of her thoracic rib cage. Starting from L1, note how her spine veers to the right and rotates to the left.

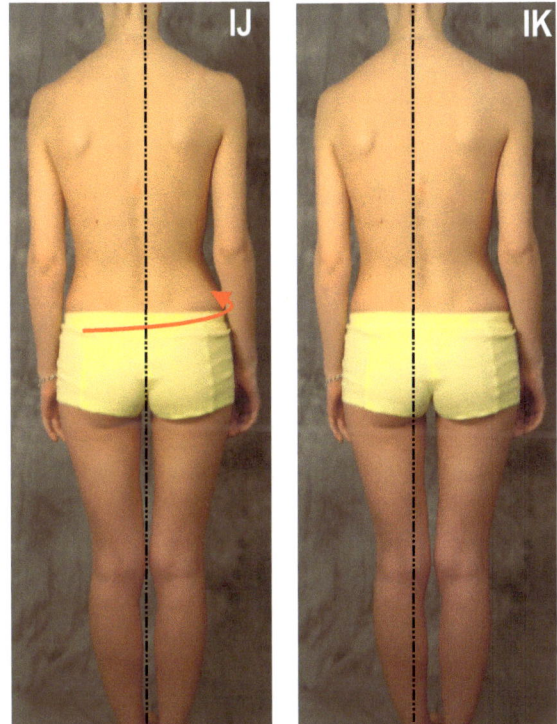

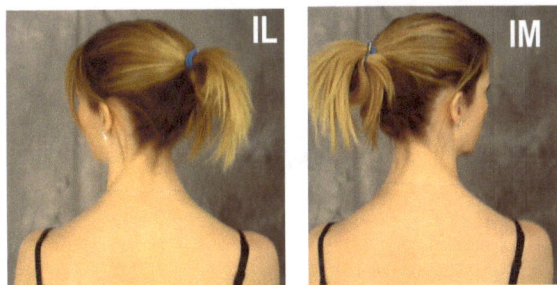

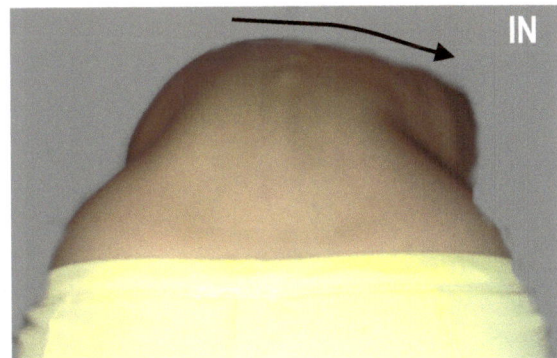

Right-Right and L3-Left-Right Photograph Comparisons

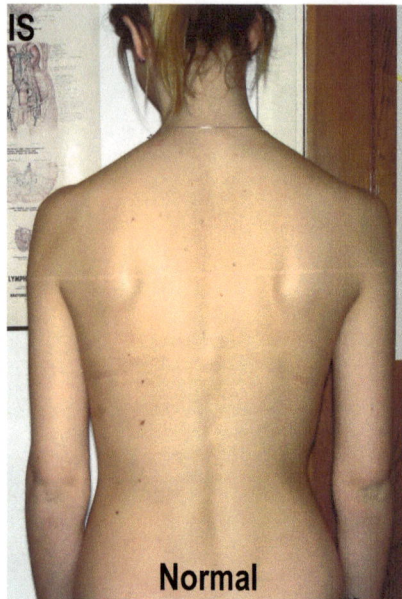

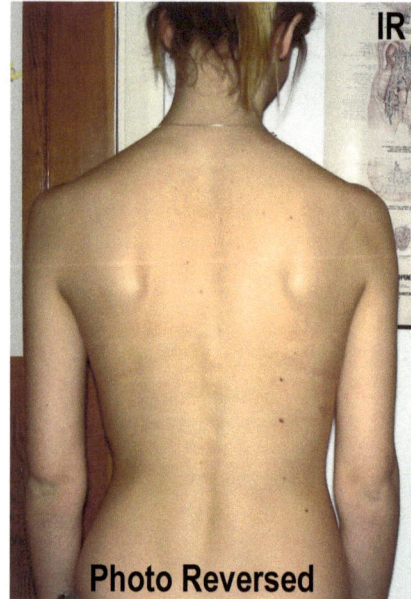

Normal

Photo Reversed

R-R normal and reversed photograph

We are so conditioned to seeing the normal **R-R** posture that our eyes see it as normal. **Figures IS** and **IR** show a photograph of Lisa's back, taken normally and then in reverse. This highlights the distorted posture and negative forces at work.

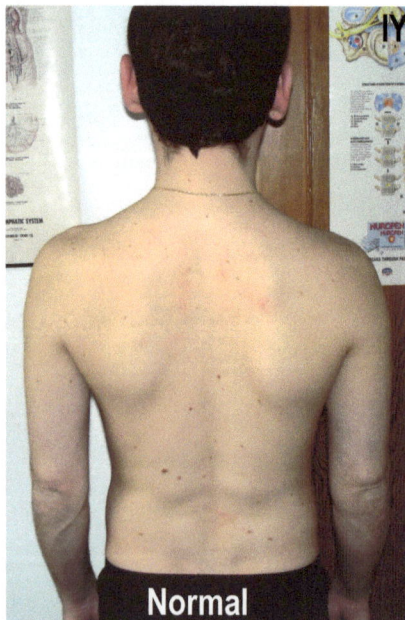

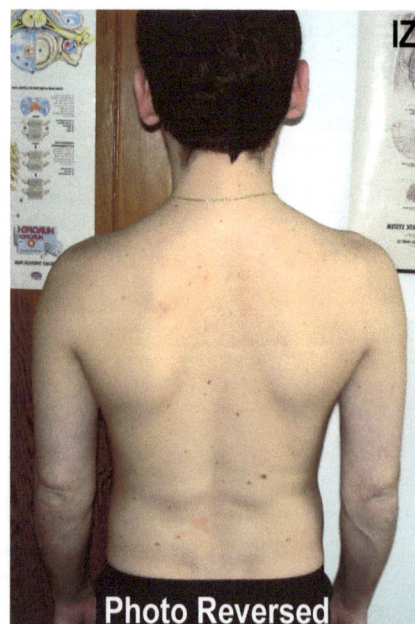

Normal

Photo Reversed

L-R normal and reversed photograph

Figures IY and **IZ** show a photograph of Mathew's back, normally and then in reverse to highlight the opposing distorted posture and negative forces at work.

Left-Right
Plumb Line

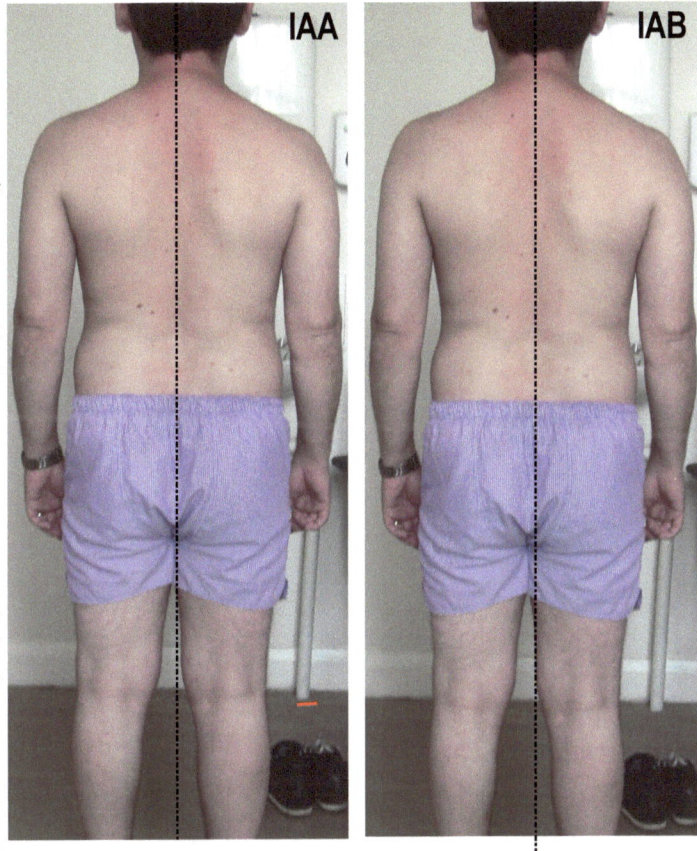

Gravity line from below

In **figure IAA** the line of gravity referenced from the midline below has been drawn in against Matthew's back. It can be seen that the line of gravity passes up the left side of his neck.

This lateral line of gravity is less than that seen in the **R-R** pattern. For this reason his shoulders are squarer.

Gravity line from above

Observe the plumb line when it is positioned to pass through the mid-line of his neck, as shown in **figure IAB**. The line of gravity passes down his body and is slightly to the right of his sacrum.

Because the line of gravity does not pass directly through the left ankle joint there is less torsion on the foot than seen in the **R-R** subluxation pattern. Unlike people with the **R-R** subluxation pattern, people with the **L-R** subluxation pattern are less likely to present with a fallen instep in their left foot.

Left-right in forward bending

Figure RD shows Matthew bending forward. In this forward bending test, we are looking at the misalignment of his thoracic rib cage. Starting from L1, note that his spine rotates to the right.

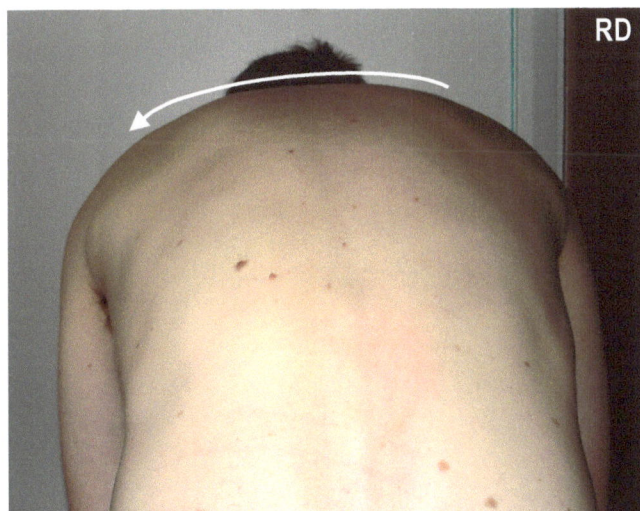

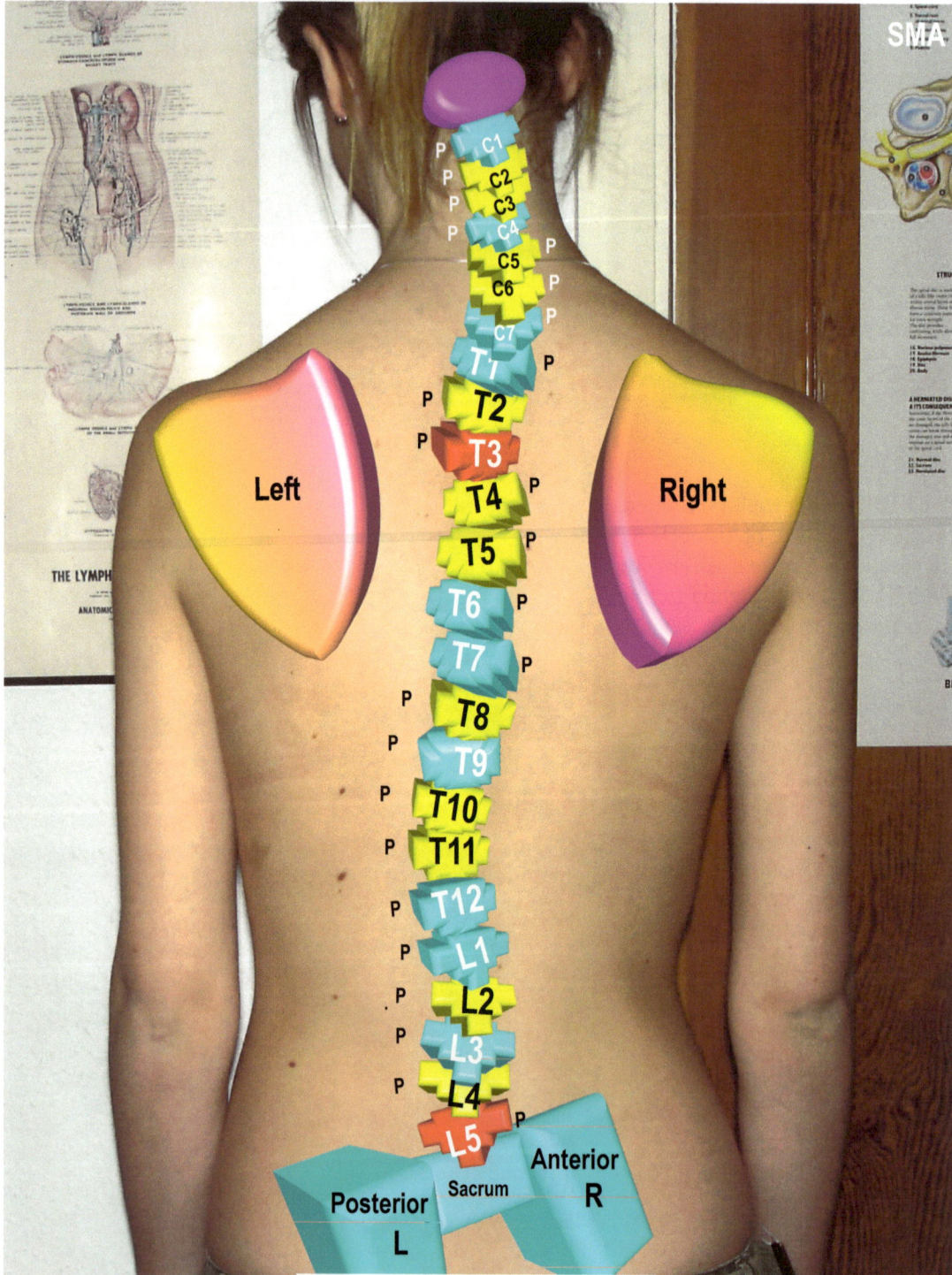

Right-Right
Lesion Pattern

SMA

C1
C2
C3
C4
C5
C6
C7
T1
T2
T3
T4
T5
T6
T7
T8
T9
T10
T11
T12
L1
L2
L3
L4
L5

Left

Right

THE LYMPH

ANATOMIC

Anterior
R
Posterior
L
Sacrum

| Flexion Lesion | Normal | Extension Lesion |

Left-Right
Lesion Pattern

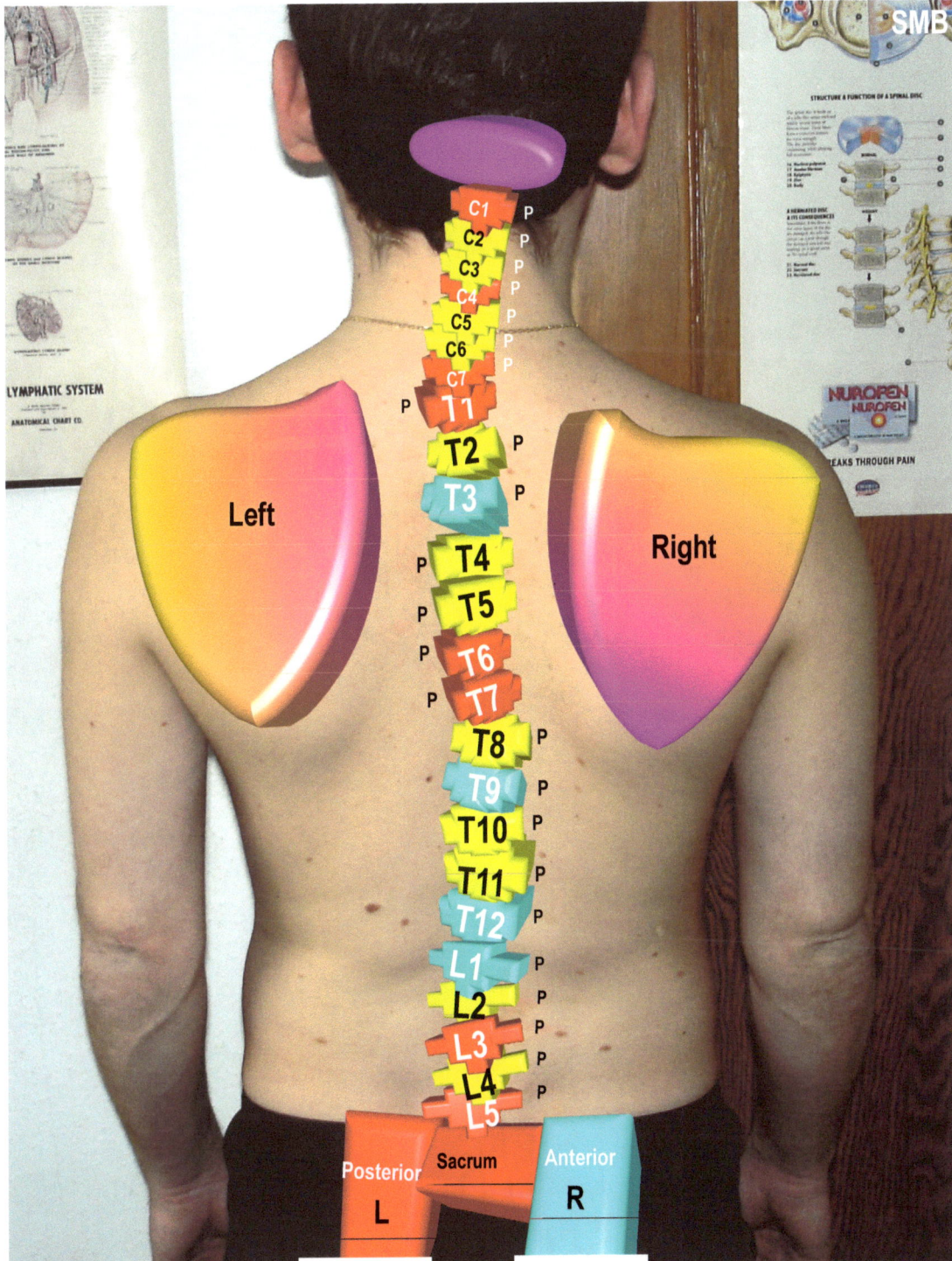

SMB

C1	P
C2	P
C3	P
C4	P
C5	P
C6	P
C7	P

P T1

Left

Right

T2 P

T3 P

P T4

P T5

P T6

P T7

T8 P

T9 P

T10 P

T11 P

T12 P

L1 P

L2 P

L3 P

L4 P

L5 P

Posterior | Sacrum | Anterior
L | | R

 Flexion Lesion   **Normal**   **Extension Lesion**

159

Palpation For Differentiation Forces and Landmarks of a Lesioned R-R pelvis

Below are the typical forces and landmarks that can be palpated in the **R-R** pelvic joints. When you are palpating use very gentle force. If you are in doubt ask your patient what they feel.

Make sure you start by levelling the ASIS's. This will be explained in this chapter. You must have a constant before you start your palpations, otherwise your findings cannot be replicated.

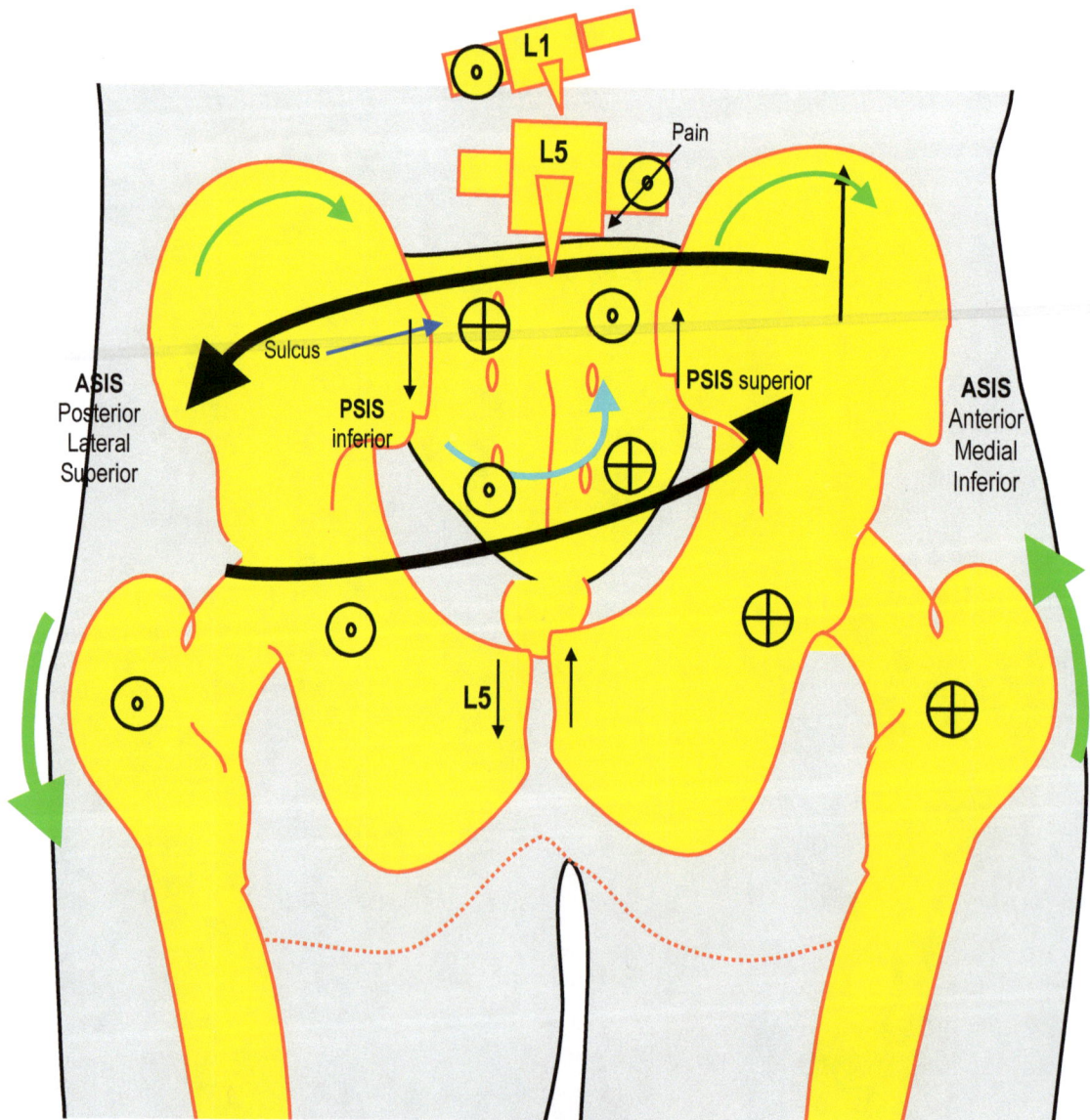

Figure IDN
Directions R-R pelvic lesioned joints
(o) Moving towards (posterior) you —— Moving away (Anterior) from you ⊕

160

Palpation For Differentiation Forces and Landmarks of a Lesioned L-R pelvis

The most obvious difference between the **R-R** and the **L-R** is the pelvic side-shift. However, you must never forget that **R-L** and **L-L** pelvis's do exist in a small number of your patients. Sods law states that they will walk into your practice.

The **R-L** pelvis can easily be mistaken for the **R-R** pelvis and **L-L** pelvis for the **L-R** pelvis, so make sure you observe your patient from the sides during your initial observation. Because PPT's are so powerful, if you make a wrong diagnosis, you can cause your patient a lot of pain. Be cautious.

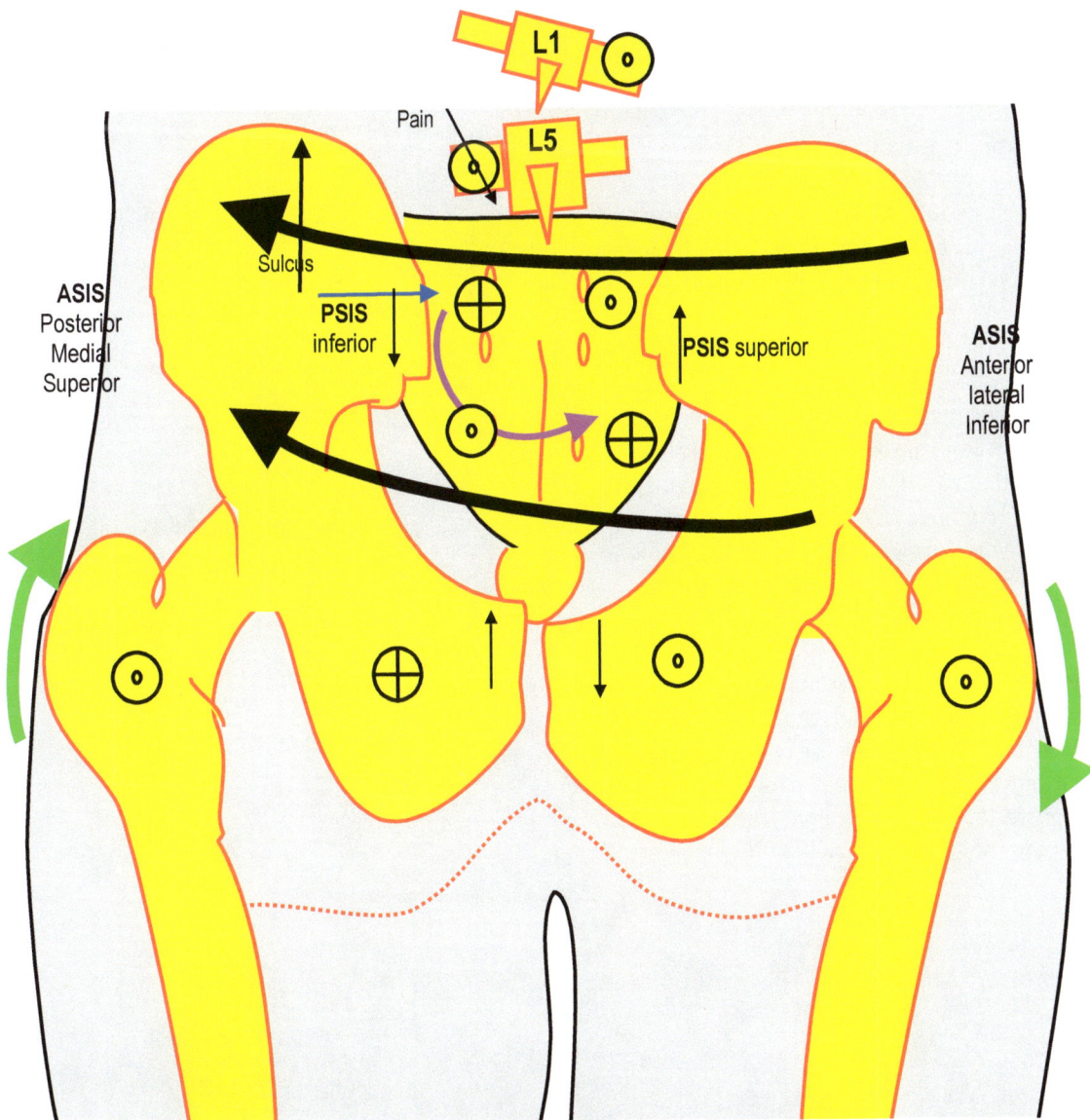

Figure IDP
Directions L-R pelvic lesioned joints
Moving towards (posterior) you —— Moving away (Anterior) from you

Preparing for Palpation
the need for a Constant

Patients have a habit of getting on your couch at an angle similar to that seen in **figure IDM 6** which is hopeless for serious palpation analysis, so watch out for this.

Figure IDM 7 shows the correct starting position.

In **figure IDM8** it can be seen that a cushion has been placed under Paul's shins. There are three reasons for this:

• To help the patient avoid foot cramps

• Most western people sit much of the time and this translates into tight hamstrings and stretched quadriceps. This compensates for this anomaly.

• It feels more comfy.

You must have a constant to base your palpation
You must have a constant before you palpate otherwise your palpation results will be meaningless. Place your index and ring fingers of both hands as shown in **figure IDM 9.** If you close your eyes you will be able to align your fingers when you bring them together.

This provides a good method of measurement. Place your fingers under each ASIS and rotate the pelvis until they are the same distance from the couch. See **figures IDM 10, 11** and **12**. This makes all irregularities show up on the posterior side of the body, where you can see and palpate them. See **figure IDM 13**.

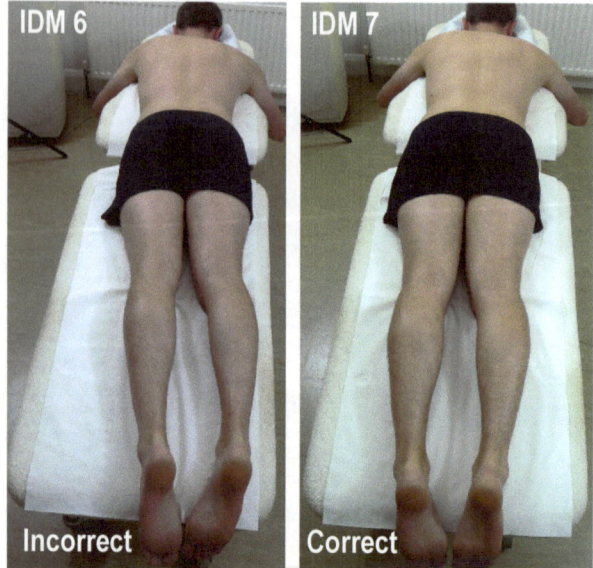

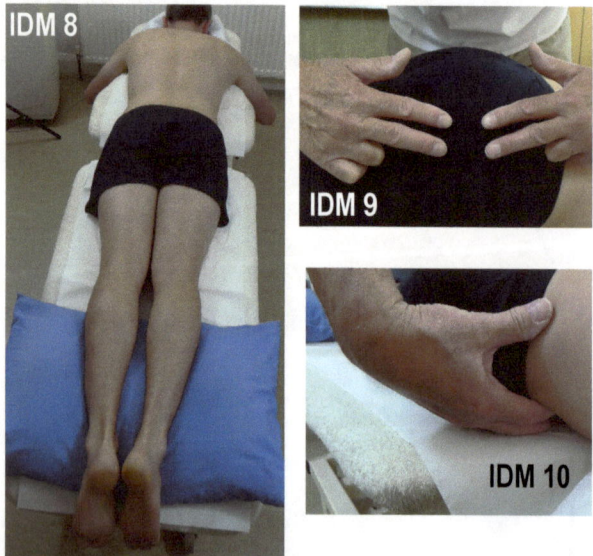

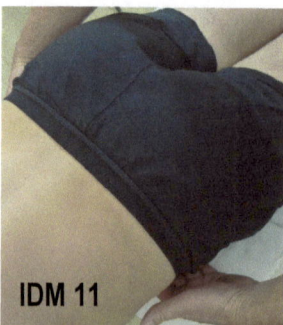

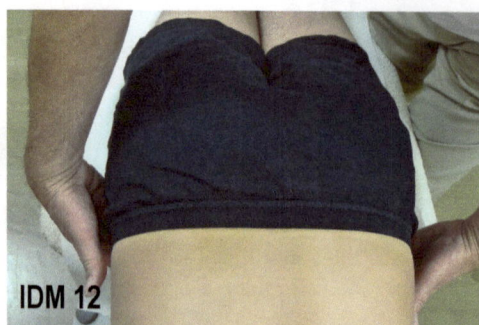

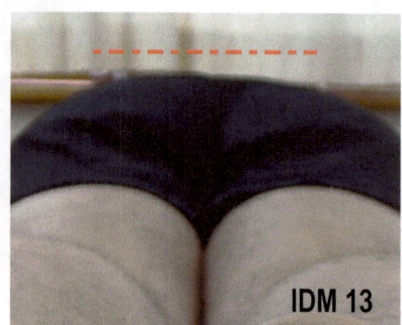

IDM 6   IDM 7

Incorrect   Correct

IDM 8   IDM 9   IDM 10

IDM 11   IDM 12   IDM 13

Palpation of hips to Assess Pelvic Lesion

Hip assessment.
The alignment of the hips will help you assess the pelvic lesion present.

Right-Right
A right-right lesioned pelvis is generally rotated to the left. See illustration **figure IDM 5a**.

The left trochanter will be posterior and medial.
The right trochanter will be anterior and lateral.

See **figure IDM5**. Stand to the side of your patient and place the pads of your thumbs on the posterior surface of the greatest trochanter's.

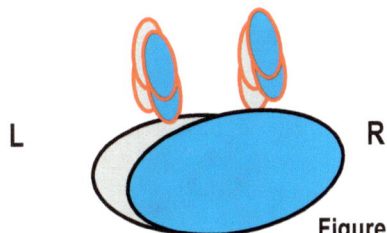

Figure IDM5a
R-R pelvis rotated right

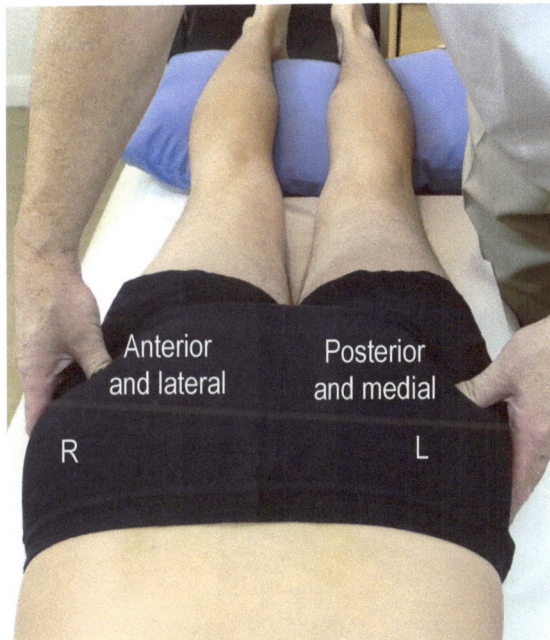

Figure IDM 5
In Right-Right left trochanter is posterior and medial.

Left-Right
A left-right lesioned pelvis is generally rotated to the right. See illustration **figure IDM 5c**.

The left trochanter will be posterior and lateral.
The right trochanter will be anterior and medial.

See **figure IDM5b**. Stand to the side of your patient and place the pads of your thumbs on the posterior surface of the greatest trochanter's.

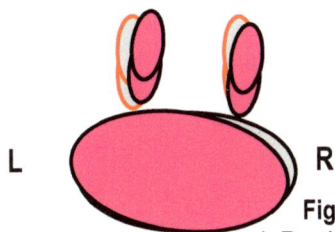

Figure IDM5c
L-R pelvis rotated right

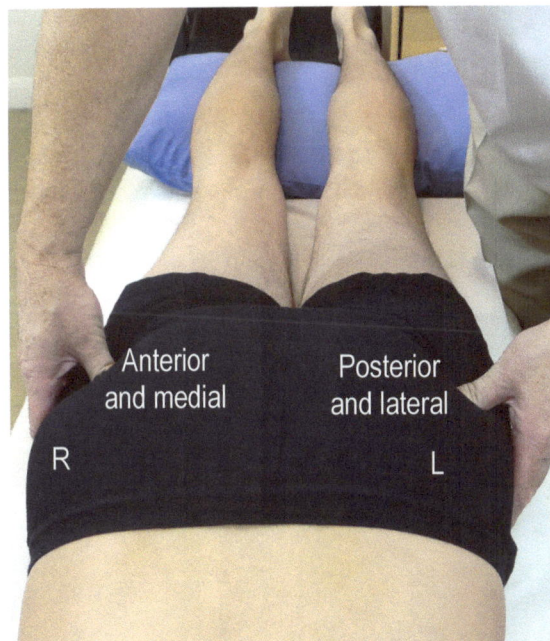

Figure IDM 5b
In Left-Right left trochanter is posterior and lateral.

Neck rotation is influenced by Pelvic Side-Shift

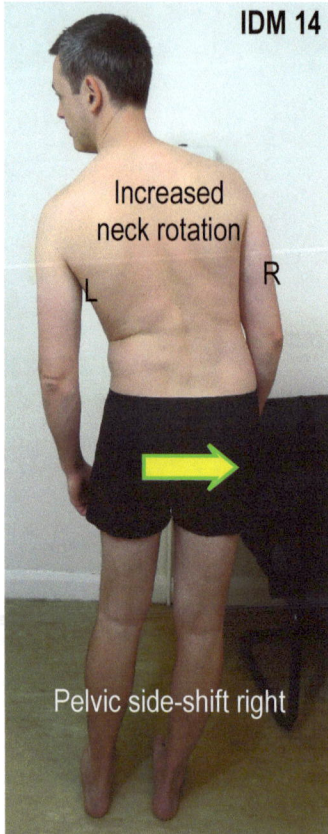

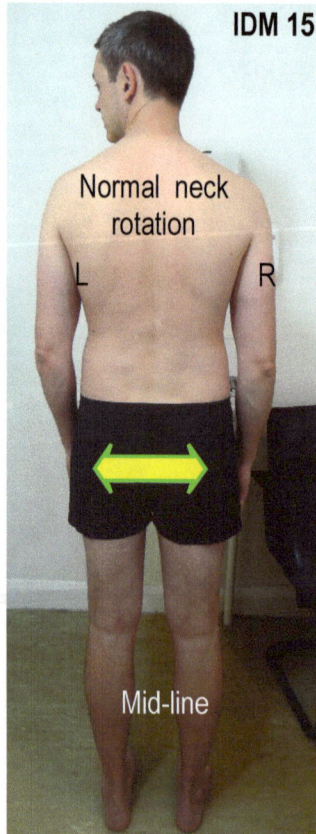

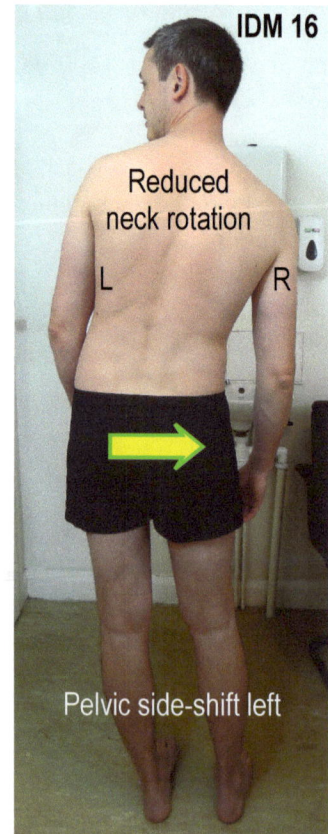

IDM 14 — Increased neck rotation — L R — Pelvic side-shift right

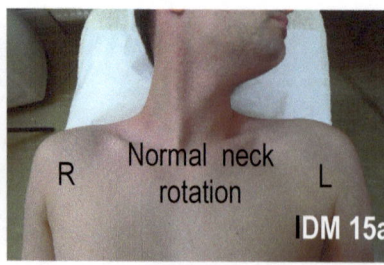

IDM 15 — Normal neck rotation — L R — Mid-line

IDM 16 — Reduced neck rotation — L R — Pelvic side-shift left

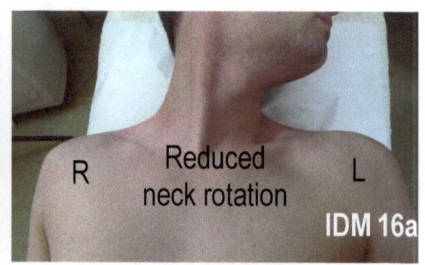

Pelvic side shift has considerable influence on neck rotation

Figures 1DM14 and **14a** show an increased neck rotation to the left when pelvic side-shift is to the right. This is seen the RR lesion pattern. Notice the neck turns inferiorly.

Figures 1DM15 and **15a** show normal neck rotation to the left when pelvic side-shift is in the mid-line.

Figures 1DM16 and **16a** show an decreased neck rotation to the left when pelvic side-shift is to the left. This is seen the LR lesion pattern. Notice the neck turns superiorly.

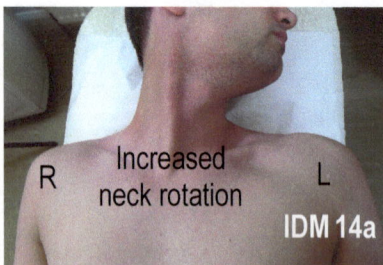

R — Increased neck rotation — L — IDM 14a — Pelvic side-shift right

R — Normal neck rotation — L — IDM 15a — Mid-line

R — Reduced neck rotation — L — IDM 16a — Pelvic side-shift left

Pelvic Palpation Indicators
Level of Hips and Rotation of L5

Palpation of hips

Figure IDM17 shows a method of determining which leg is physiologically shorter.

Do this test after you have the ASIS's constant.

A physiological short leg can be pushed in a superior direction whereas the long leg will feel comparatively fixed and stable.

In a pelvis that is **RR** lesioned it will be possible to move the left hip and surrounding tissue superiorly, as shown in **figure IDM18**.

In the **LR** lesioned pelvis the hip and surrounding tissue will move superiorly on the right but much less than would be felt in the **RR** pelvis. The **LR** pelvis is shown in **figure IDM1**.

Palpation of L5 transverse process's

In the right-right lesion pattern the right TP of L5 can be palpated and found tender and posterior, as shown in **figure IDM 20**.

In the **LR** lesion pattern the TP of L5 is found tender and posterior on the left, as shown in **figure IDM 21.**

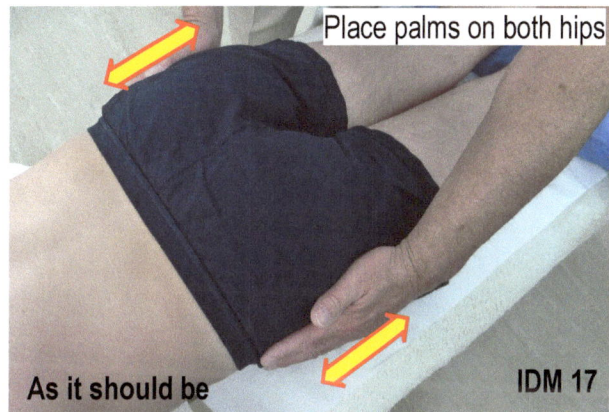

Place palms on both hips

As it should be   IDM 17

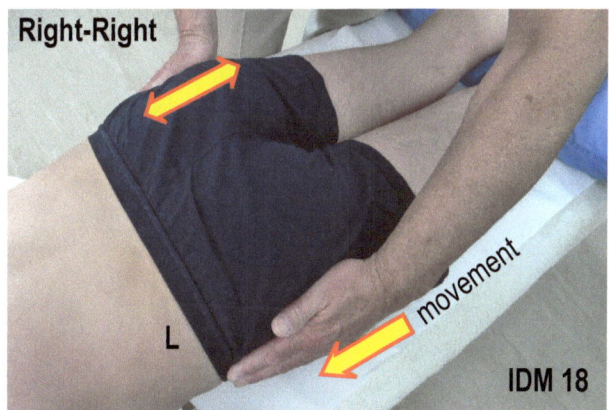

Right-Right

L

movement

IDM 18

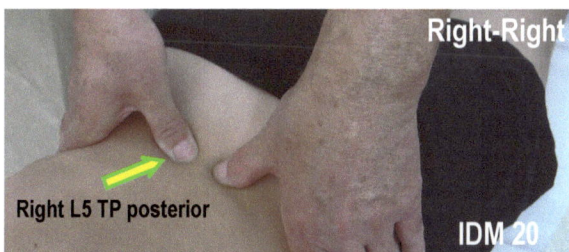

Right-Right

Right L5 TP posterior

IDM 20

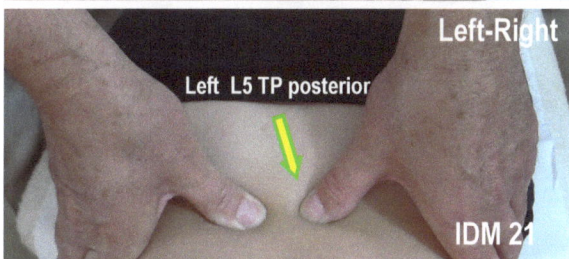

Left-Right

Left L5 TP posterior

IDM 21

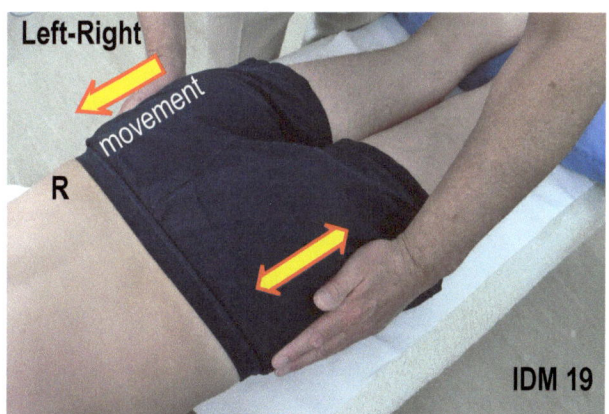

Left-Right

movement

R

IDM 19

Pelvic Palpation Indicators
Leg Length and Sacral Base Side-Shift

Assessment of the iliac crests

You must have the ASIS constant before you start. You will need to check the levels at the mid-point of the iliac crests to assess the leg length difference. Let the legs angle as the patient positions them naturally.

IDM 22

Place the palms of both hands over the iliac crests on either side, as shown in **figure IDM 22**. Make sure you stand with your head directly above the crests to get an accurate picture of the level difference.

If the left iliac crest is superior it indicates a **RR** pelvic lesion, see **figure IDM23A**.

If the right iliac crest is superior it indicates a **LR** pelvic lesion, see **figure IDM23B**.

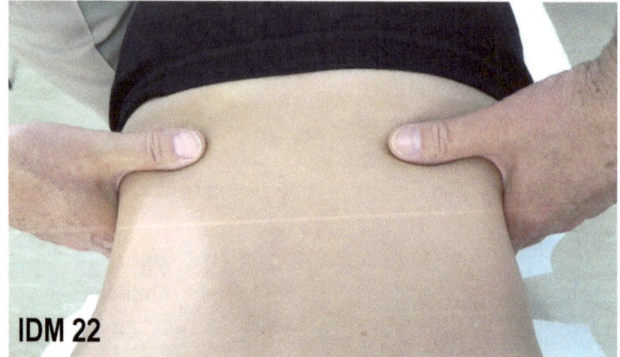

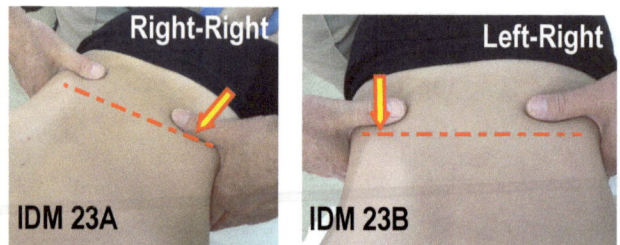

Right-Right

IDM 23A

Left-Right

IDM 23B

Assess the side-shift at the the level of apex of the sacrum

Place your palm lightly over both the apex of the sacrum and PIIS's of the Ilia, as per **figure IDM 24**.

In the **RR** pelvic lesion, your hand will follow a side-shift pattern to the left. See **figure IDM 25**

In the **LR** pelvic lesion your hand will follow a side-shift pattern to the right. See figure **IDM 26**

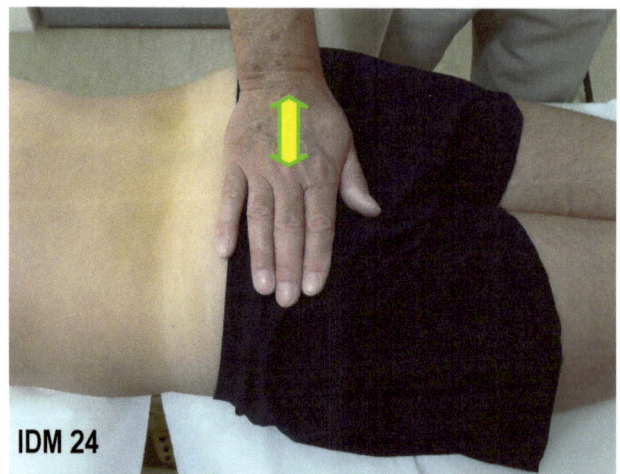

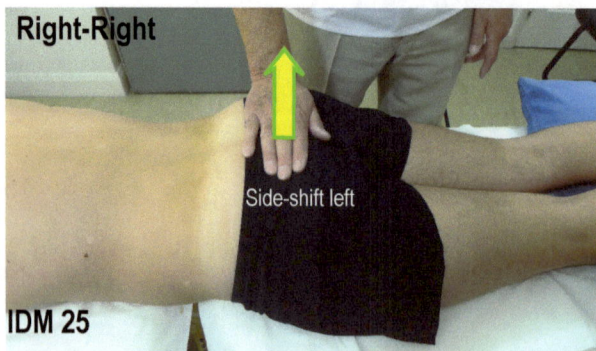

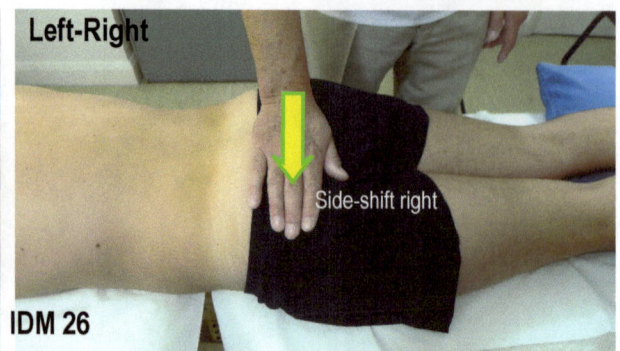

IDM 24

Right-Right

Side-shift left

IDM 25

Left-Right

Side-shift right

IDM 26

Pelvic Palpation Indicators
Pelvic Side-Shift and Side-bending

Assessment of lesioned pelvic side-shift and side-bending

Figure IDM27 shows the hand positions for testing the pelvic side-bending and side-shift in the **RR** and **LR** pelvic lesion patterns. What you are going to palpate for is the general rotation and side-shift of the pelvis as a whole and not the individual bones or joints.

The heel of your right hand is placed over the PSIS and iliac crest and your left hand hyperthenar eminence over the left PIIS.

Testing for Right-Right

With both hands placed as above, rotate and side-shift your hands to the left in an inferior direction shown by the blue arrow in figure **IDN28**. In the **RR** pelvic lesion the pelvis will rotate freely in this direction. Pelvic side-shift will be in the same direction.

Testing for Left-Right

With both hands placed as above, rotate and side-shift your hands to the left in a mildly superior direction, shown by the magenta arrow in figure **IDN29**. In the **LR** pelvic lesion the pelvis will rotate freely in this direction.

Now test the pelvis as above in the opposite direction, as shown in **figure IDM 30**. You should find the pelvis is hard to move in these directions and often very painful for the patient. If you cannot decided, ask the patient. They will tell you.

If the pelvis moves freely in this direction suspect a **LL** pelvis or **RL** pelvis.

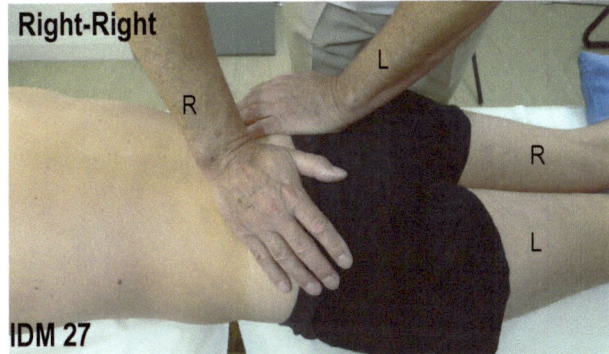
Right-Right — IDM 27

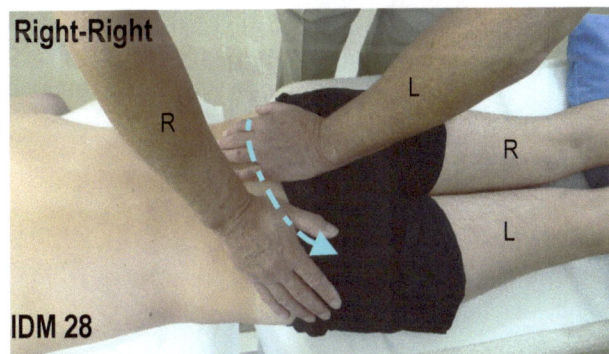
Right-Right — IDM 28

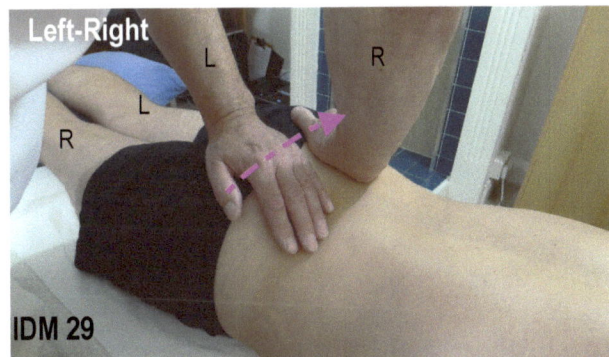
Left-Right — IDM 29

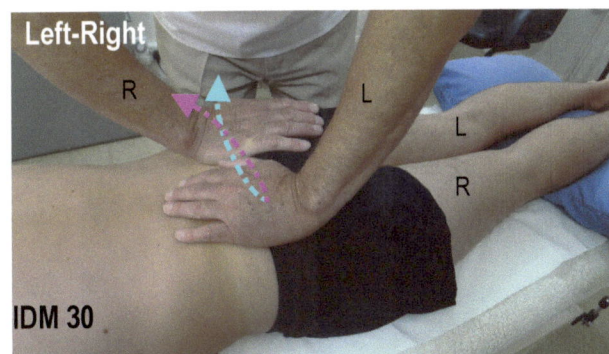
Left-Right — IDM 30

Spinal Palpation Indicators
Side-Bending at L1- Rotation of Thoracic

Assessment of lesioned L1

Starting position
Place you hand lightly but firmly over L1 as shown in **figure IDM31**

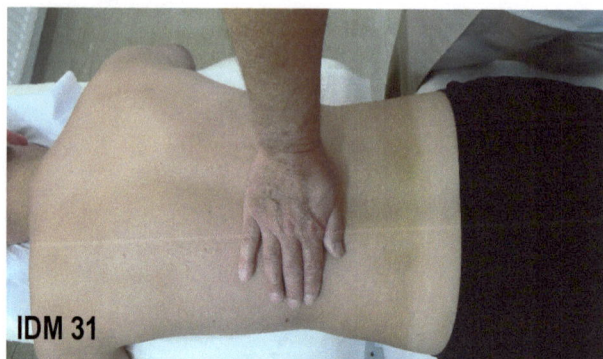

Testing for Right-Right
Side-bend your hand to the left. If L1 is lesioned in the **RR** lesioning pattern it will rotate freely in this direction as shown in **figure IDM32**

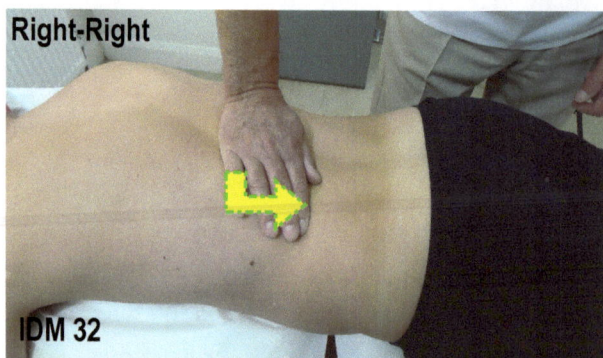

Testing for Left-Right
Side-bend your hand to the right. If L1 is lesioned in the **LR** lesioning pattern it will rotate freely in this direction, as shown in **figure IDM33**

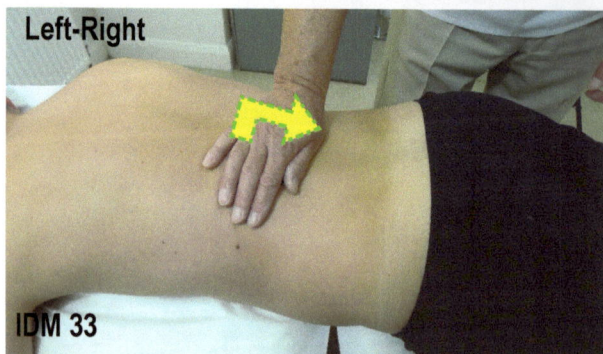

Testing rotation of thoracic vertebrae
Place your hand lightly but firmly over the spinous processes of the upper thoracic vertebrae, as shown in **figure IDM34.**

Testing for Right-Right
Rotate the spinous process of the vertebrae to the left. In the **RR** lesioning pattern the vertebrae will be rotated to the left.

Testing for Left-Right
Rotate the spinous process of the vertebrae to the right. In the **LR** lesioning pattern the vertebrae will be rotated to the right.

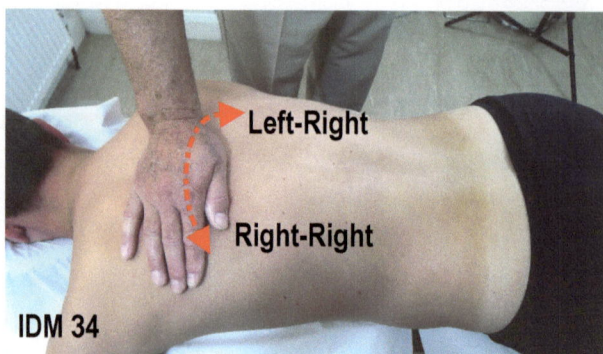

IDM 31

Right-Right

IDM 32

Left-Right

IDM 33

Left-Right

Right-Right

IDM 34

Chapter Twelve

From Spinal Mechanics to Manipulation

As we move to the next chapter on PPT manipulation, we need to ask ourselves as Osteopaths what we are trying to achieve. For me, the motivation behind all my work was to find a way to get the musculo-skeletal frame as symmetrical as humanly possible. To do this I had to put aside all the traditional spinal theories and bit-part research I had been taught and read and find out how the spine worked and locked as an integrated unit for myself. This is what the first part of this book is all about. The next part of this book is about how I applied this vital knowledge to achieve the best possible spinal symmetry, safely. I wanted to achieve this without causing the patient undue discomfort or putting them in any bizarre positions and without the crack.

A bolt and nut that are aligned are far more efficient
than a bolt with a nut that is cross -threaded

To ensure the symmetry of the skeletal system the pelvis must be level and correctly aligned. Without a symmetrical and level pelvic base, any manipulations above will be no more than a temporary fix.

Would you build a house on foundations **A** or **C** below? Because this what most human lesioned spines are balanced on.

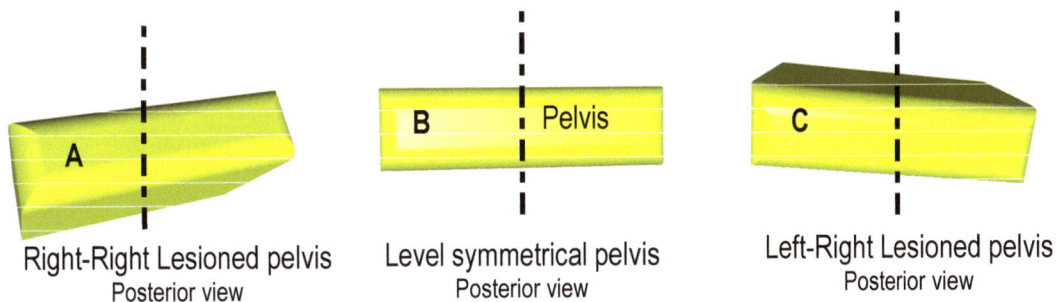

Right-Right Lesioned pelvis	Level symmetrical pelvis	Left-Right Lesioned pelvis
Posterior view	Posterior view	Posterior view

Recap on Subluxated Facets

Pelvic alignment is essential

It is essential to correct the alignment of all the pelvic joints, even when treating what might seem like an unrelated shoulder or neck problem. If you fail to do this, the corrected joints and tissue above will revert to their former state very quickly. This is basic physics.

I have collated the S/I facet subluxation illustrations from their respective chapters and placed them here on this page for easy reference.

As can be seen from the yellow stars shown on each type of subluxation, each joint is locked in several areas. The yellow stars show the areas where the facets are either locked on each other or overlapped. When manipulating, both the restricted and overlapping areas must be corrected, otherwise the joint will not articulate correctly.

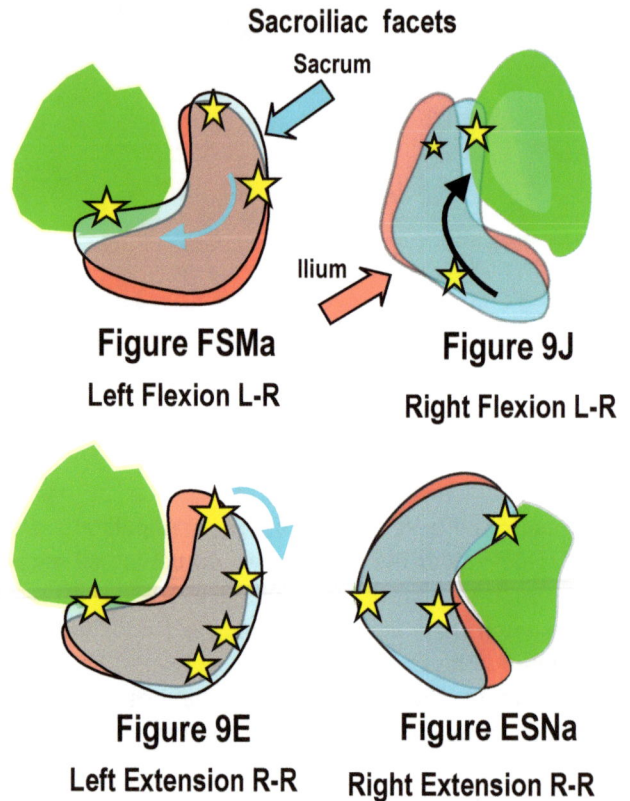

Sacroiliac facets

Figure FSMa
Left Flexion L-R

Figure 9J
Right Flexion L-R

Figure 9E
Left Extension R-R

Figure ESNa
Right Extension R-R

Facet misalignment

You would think the lesioned S/I joint would be hugely displaced by the loud clunking sound that a typical pelvic side-role manipulation elicits. But this not the case. A typical lesioned S/I joint and those above will be less than 1/20th of an inch or one millimetre out of place, often less. That is why they do not show up on X-ray,

The example illustrations above are grossly exaggerated to make their displacement easier to visualize.

The gross pelvic distortion is not caused by facet displacement alone. In fact the main cause is due to the reactive ground force that travels back up the misaligned legs. This reactive force compounds the pelvic distortion and reinforces it with every weight bearing step taken.

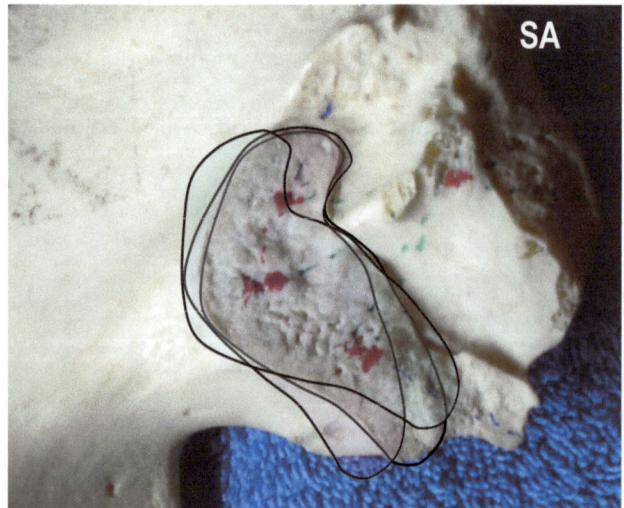

Why Manipulation?

Importance of Manipulation

Despite wishful thinking by some it is physiologically impossible to release a lesioned joint with exercise, acupuncture or medication.

Many professions claim to be able to treat back pain and each claims to have a measure of success. So what is special about manipulation as a valid treatment? **Figure SMC** is an illustration of a typical subluxated joint with an indication of the way the local ligaments and muscles would be pulled or loosened. The muscles and ligaments are stretched on the right and compressed on the left. Symmetrical muscle exercise would reinforce the lesion rather than provide release.

Figure SMD shows what happens if an attempt is made to correct the joint by selective exercise, postural alignment or muscle release. If the muscles on the right are strengthened, and therefore tightened, the joint would be forced to side-bend to the right. To the casual observer the back may give the appearance of being straighter but the joint itself will continue to be locked in lesion. Only now, it is less stable than before because of the additional side-bending.

If the left muscles are tightened, as shown in **figure SME,** the joint would side-bend to the left and compact the subluxation still further.

Figure SMF shows the same joint with the stretched muscle inflamed. If this were to be treated with Acupuncture, steroidal or non-steroidal anti-inflammatory medication the inflammation would in all likelihood reduce. But the joint would still be locked, as shown in **figure SMC.** This is because anti-inflammatory medicines cannot physically correct a lesioned joint. Lesions are physiologically reinforced by gravity every time the person stands or walks forward.

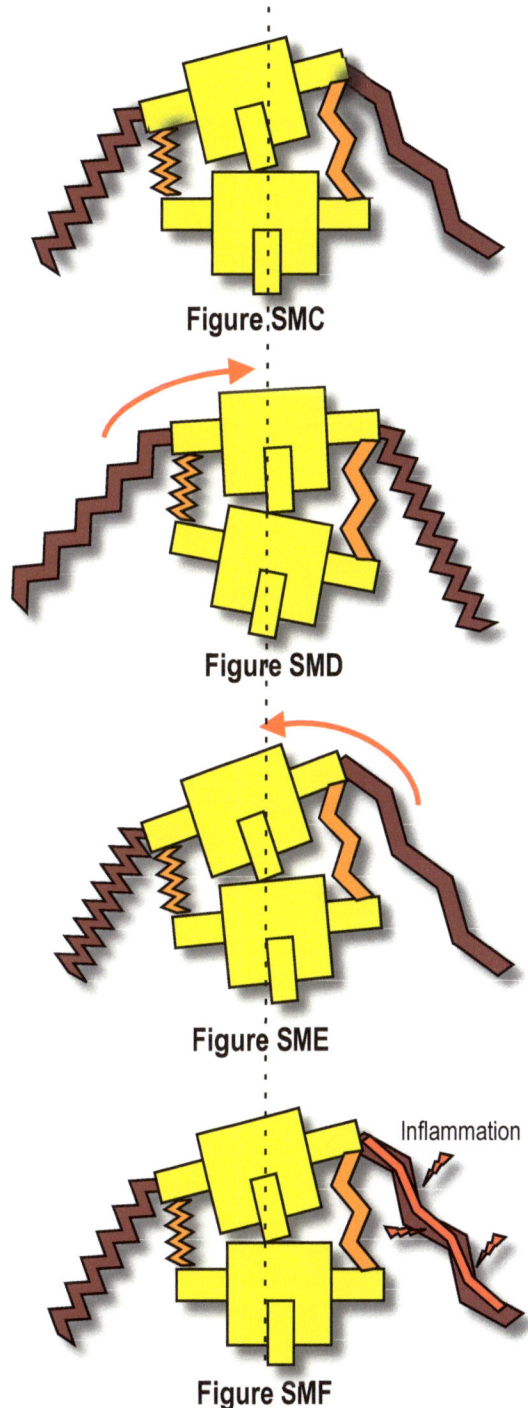

Figure SMC

Figure SMD

Figure SME

Inflammation

Figure SMF

Discussion about Manipulation

The PPT manipulator's ultimate aim with patients should be to align their musculo-skeletal frame so that their patients stand erect, symmetrical and have as much mobility as possible.

In my opinion before a manipulative procedure is performed the muscles and soft tissue should be stretched and relaxed and all the spinal joints articulated. This is done to warm up the musculo-skeletal structures for the same reasons that an athlete warms up their muscles before an activity.

On the previous page changes made by muscle-based treatments were illustrated. Muscle treatments are important but their effect is superficial compared to the changes that take place after a manipulative procedure. Joint manipulation changes the internal structure of the body and the body has to come to terms with this change. Therefore, care should be taken by the patient not to overexert themselves or exercise excessively after a manipulative procedure. It is unclear how much recovery time should be allowed but the reasons for it are understood.

Figure SMC illustrates a joint in lesion. The muscles and ligaments on the right are stretched and those on the right shortened. If this joint was to be left untreated, in time the muscles and ligaments would learn to adapt to this position.

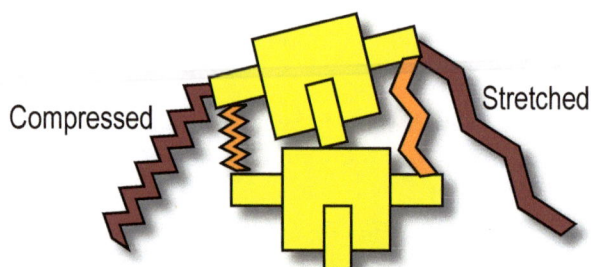

**Figure SMC
Before Manipulation**

So when the lesion is corrected, as illustrated in **figure SMG,** the muscles and ligaments on the right become slackened off and those on the left stretched. It is this stretch on the left that can leave some patients feeling sore after a treatment. Also, because the muscles and ligaments have to adjust to their corrected position, the joint is temporally weakened.

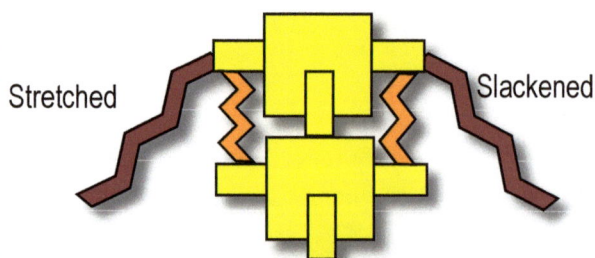

**Figure SMG
After Manipulation**

During a course of manipulative treatment, it is suggested that exercise should be light and repeated often.

From the subluxation chapters we learned that the lesioned pelvic joints lock in all the lesions above and below. Therefore, the prime objective of the professional manipulator, where the cause is not due to recent direct local trauma, is to free the sacroiliac joints before any other joints, even if the patient has presented with what appears to be a very simple and unrelated joint problem.

How the Sacroiliac Subluxation becomes Locked

Lumbar and sacrum working together

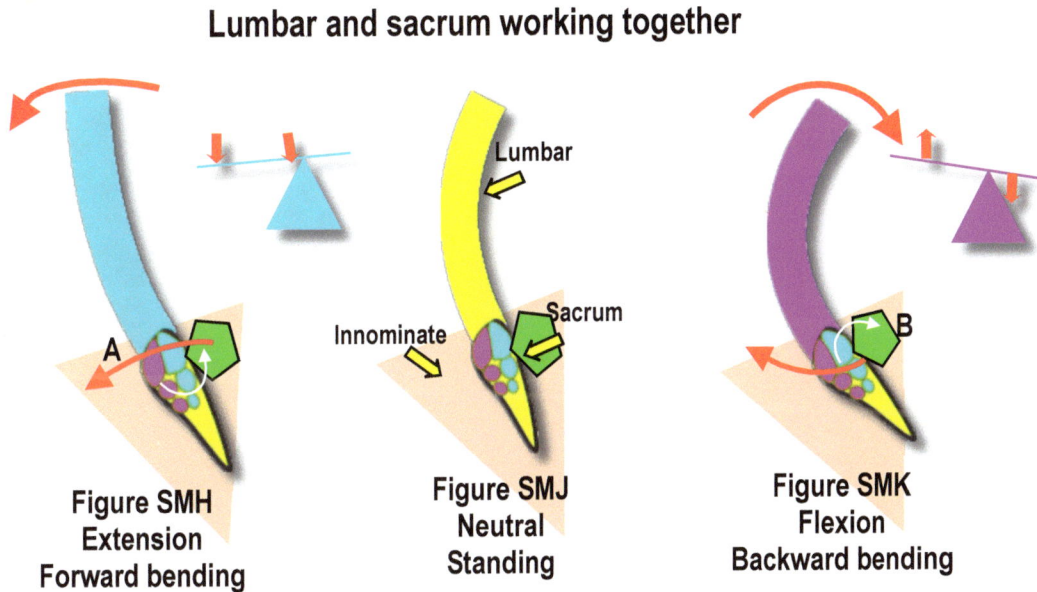

Figure SMH
Extension
Forward bending

Figure SMJ
Neutral
Standing

Figure SMK
Flexion
Backward bending

Although it is an obvious point, it needs to be reinforced that the sacrum moves as if it were an extension of the lumbar spine in the anterio-posterior plane. This is an important factor to have in mind when manipulating the sacroiliac joints effectively.

Figure SMJ illustrates the sacrum and lumbar vertebrae in neutral and is shown for reference purposes only.

Figure SMH illustrates how the base of the sacrum arcs in an anterio-inferior direction when the lumbar vertebrae are in extension.

Figure SMK illustrates how the base of the sacrum arcs in an posterio-superior direction when the lumbar vertebrae are in flexion.

The areas that take the maximum impact and lock in the flexion and extension sacroiliac subluxations are the areas between the iliac articular facets and the bony mass. There is no word for this area, so for clarity I have named it the 'Rough'.

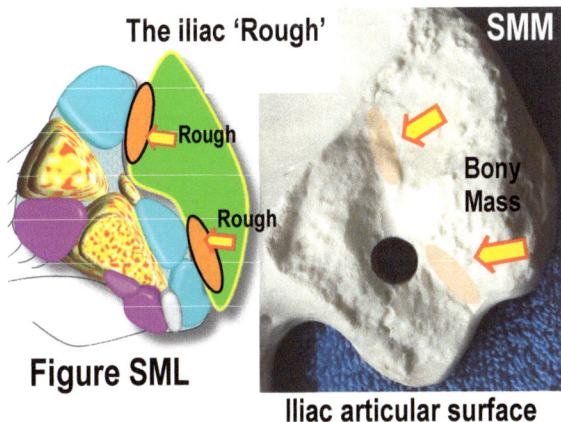

The iliac 'Rough'

Figure SML

SMM

Bony Mass

Iliac articular surface

Class 1, 2 and 3 Lesions

The articular facets of the Ilium and the sacrum are covered by synovial membranes which make the lubricated surfaces of the facets very slippery. This membrane is illustrated in **figure SMN.** With such a highly slippery surface it is unlikely that this area of the joint gets restricted in a sacroiliac lesion.

The area termed the 'rough' is the most probable site for locking to take place.

There three classes of subluxation

Class 1 Bone locked against bone

Class 2 Bone locked partially against bone

Class 3 Bone locked by surrounding forces

Figure SMO is an illustration of the upper facets of a typical thoracic vertebra. The downward force created by the inter-costal muscles forces the inferior edge of the facet of the vertebra above against the bone below and into the rough. Thoracic subluxations of this type are therefore classified as; class 1.

Figure SMP illustrates the area on the lamina of a typical thoracic vertebra where the inferior edge of the facet of the vertebra above becomes locked in a typical extension (backward bending) subluxation. Because this is not a self-tightening subluxation, it is classified as; Class 2

Figure SMQ illustrates the synovial membrane that covers the facets of a typical lumbar vertebra. As can be seen, the surface is smooth all over, therefore there is no 'rough'.

The lumbar subluxations of this type become locked in by the converging contorted forces from the sacroiliac and thoracic lesions. For this reason, lumbar vertebra lesions below L1 are classified as; class 3.

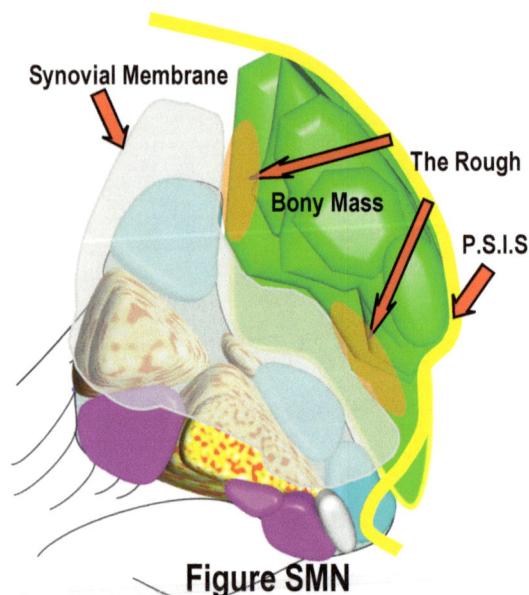

Figure SMN

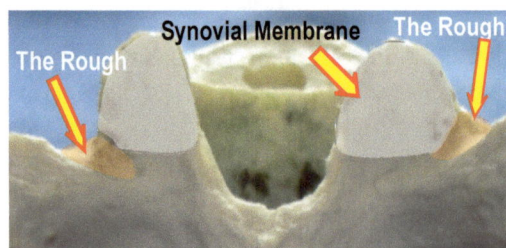

Figure SMO

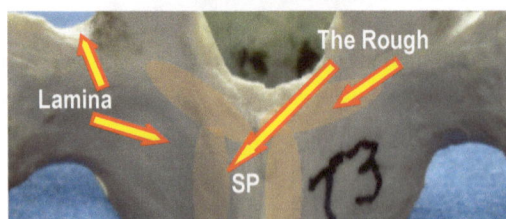

Figure SMP

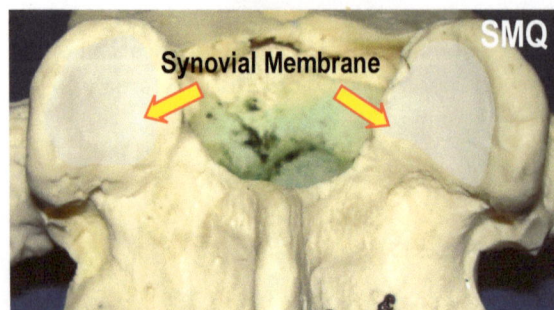

SMQ

The Mechanics of a
Thoracic Flexion Lesion

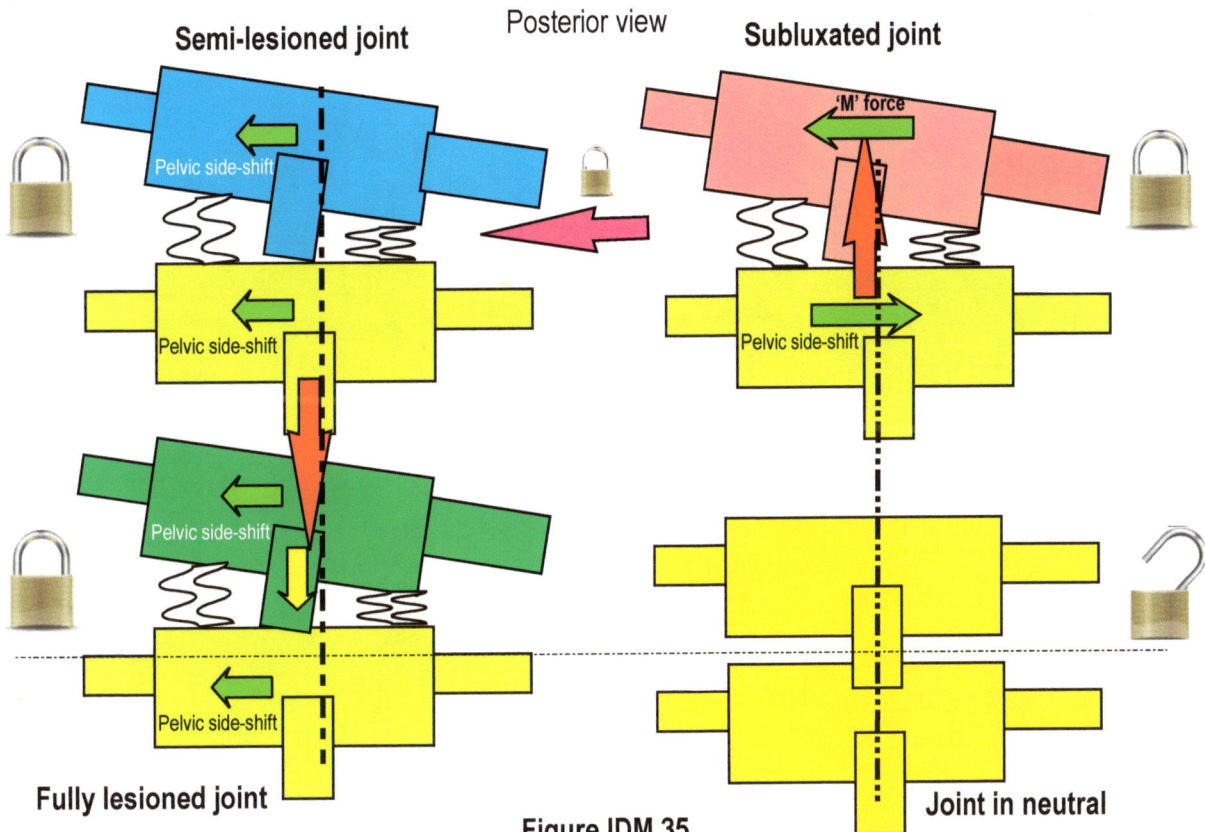

Figure IDM 35
Illustration showing the mechanics of a thoracic flexion lesion

It is important to understand when manipulating what you are correcting and so to make it easier to understand **figure IDM35** illustrates the mechanics behind a typical thoracic flexion lesion.

• The **yellow** joint is a typical thoracic in neutral.

• The **faded red** vertebra is shown in forward bending in relation to the faded yellow vertebra below. The joint is subluxated with side-bending and rotation to the right. This locks the joint.

• The **blue and faded yellow** joint is the subluxated joint, when it is forced as a whole (both vertebra locked together in subluxation) to the left by pelvic side-shift to the left, a state of semi-lesion is imposed over the subluxated joint.

• The **green and faded yellow** shows the semi-lesioned joint in its fully lesioned position when pelvic side-shift remains to the left with the joint forced inferiorly, such as when the person leans backwards.

Conventional gapping techniques aim at removing the bony subluxation whereas PPT's aim at removing the lesion. In a none-weight-bearing environment the subluxation will fall away when the lesion is corrected. That is why there is no click.

The Mechanics of a Thoracic Extension Lesion

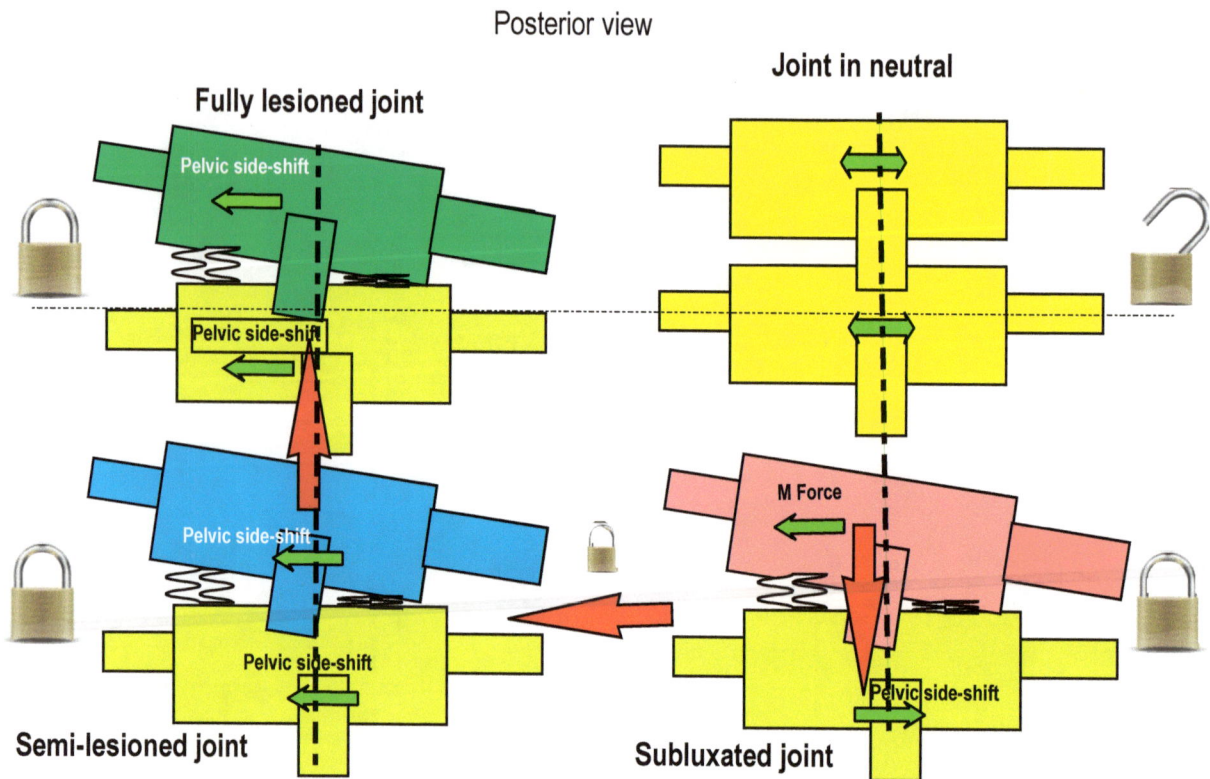

Posterior view

Fully lesioned joint

Pelvic side-shift

Pelvic side-shift

Joint in neutral

Pelvic side-shift

Pelvic side-shift

Semi-lesioned joint

M Force

Pelvic side-shift

Subluxated joint

Figure IDM 36
Illustration showing the mechanics of a thoracic Extension lesion

Figure IDM36 shows the mechanics behind a typical thoracic extension lesion.

• The **yellow** joint is a typical thoracic in neutral.

• The **faded red** vertebra is shown in backward bending in relation to the faded yellow vertebra below. The joint is subluxated with side-bending and rotation to the right. This locks the joint.

• The **blue and faded yellow** joint is the subluxated joint when it is forced as a whole (both vertebra locked together in subluxation) to the left by pelvic side-shift to the left. This imposes a state of semi-lesion over the subluxated joint.

• The **green and faded yellow** shows the semi-lesioned joint in its fully lesioned position when pelvic side-shift remains to the left with the joint forced superiorly, such as when the person stands upright or leans forward.

Chapter Thirteen

PPT
Manipulation

PPT stands for <u>P</u>assive <u>P</u>atient <u>T</u>echnique and I originated and developed PPT manipulation simply by reversing the forces that created osteopathic lesions. The word passive came from one of my patients who asked me if I would do that 'passive' technique on him again.   That was how the passive part of the name came about. The 'patient' part came from the fact that the technique is applied to patients.

PPT's are quiet manipulations. When a joint lesions, most often it does not make any sound, and therefore, the correction should make little to no sound.

Because PPT's have such a small trauma footprint on the body each joint from the iliosacral to the uppermost thoracic can be manipulated many times in one treatment session without destabilizing the back or causing undue distress to the patient.   This theoretically provides the Osteopath with the potential to get their patients backs free of pain, straighter and more mobile quicker than was ever physiologically possible before and this is born out in practice.

A professional Osteopath needs a professional couch. The couch best suited to PPT manipulation is one where the cranial and distal portions can be lowered and raised like the one shown in **figure PPT1** and **PPT1a**.

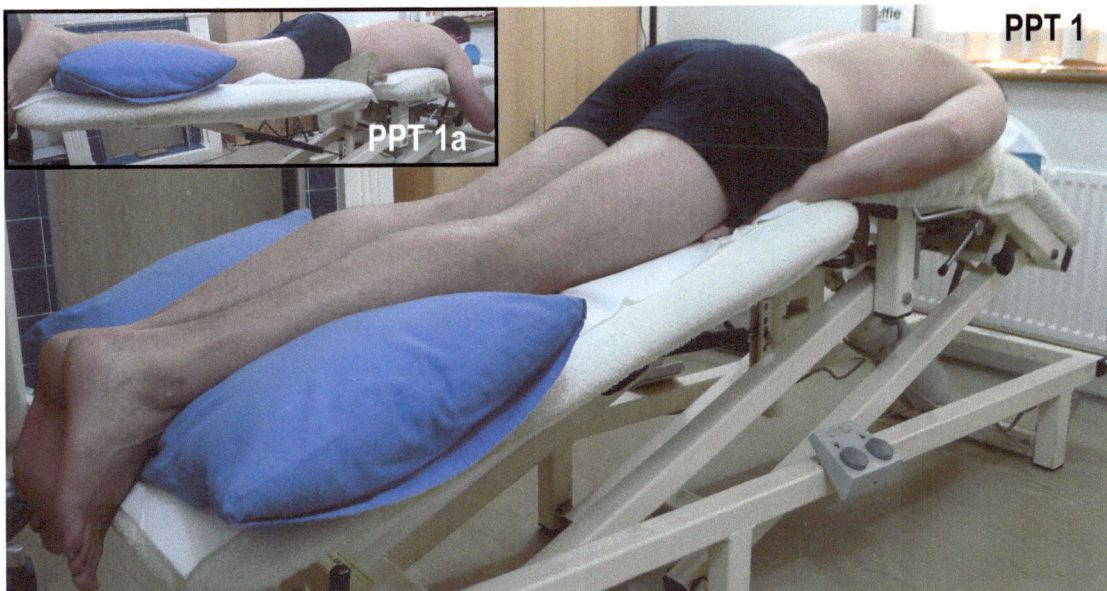

The Principle Behind PPT Manipulation

When the body is in the mid-line it is at its strongest because the latero-medial and superio-inferior forces are equal.

When the patient relaxes on the couch, because gravity is taken out of the equation the superio-inferior forces are mostly ineffectual. This means the strength of the 'M' forces (balance/muscles) is considerably reduced.

If the patient's pelvis is moved to one side of the couch as shown in **figure PPT2** the equilibrium of the latero-medial forces are dynamically changed. The pelvic side-shift is still a powerful force but it no longer has to interact with the 'M' forces so vehemently.

When the pelvis is positioned to the right as shown in **figure PPT2** the muscle and joint soft tissue on the right are stretched and tight. Conversely the joints, muscle and soft tissue on the left are relaxed and pliable.

Left side
Because the energy has already been expended to get the pelvic side-shift to the right, very little energy is needed to push the left side bones, muscles and soft tissue towards the right. Conversely resistance is felt when pushing them from right to the left.

Movements superiorly and inferiorly are made easier on the left.

Right side
The right side is the more powerful side, pushing bones, muscles and soft tissue towards the left offers a greater resistance. The upside to this is that manipulations on this side offer more power.

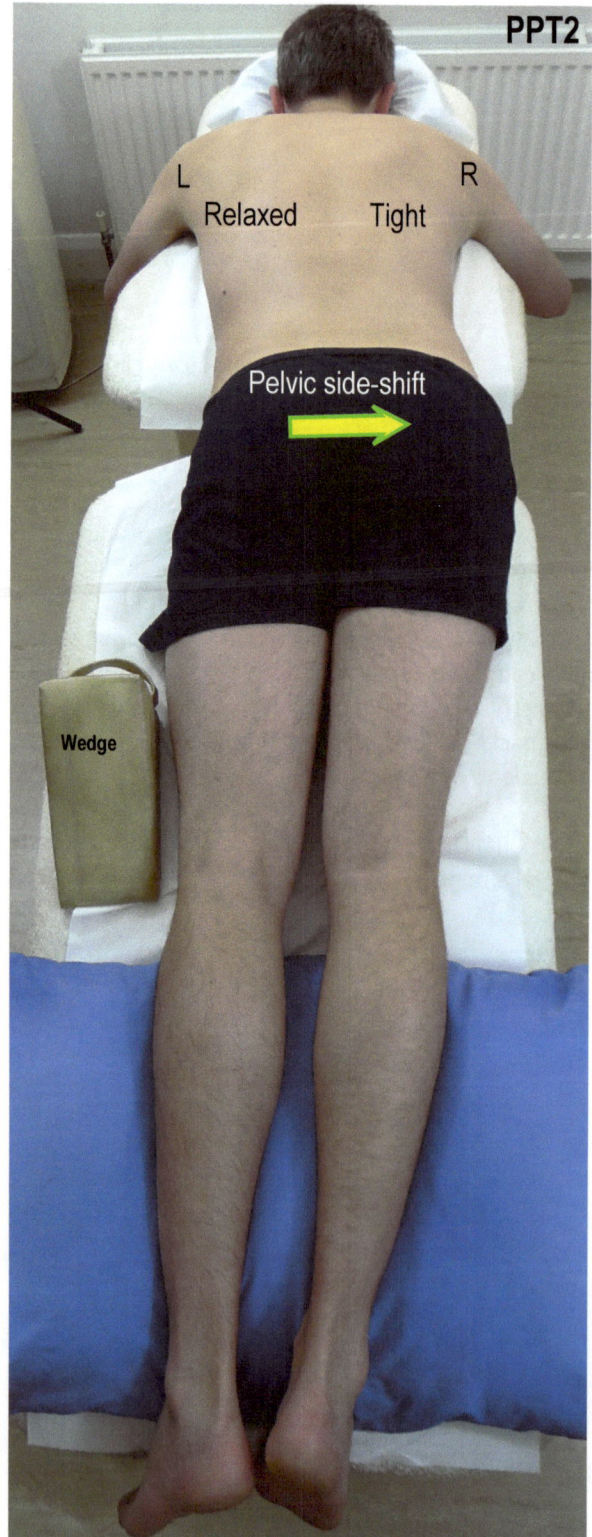

PPT2

L R
Relaxed Tight

Pelvic side-shift

Wedge

Notes on the Order of Correction and What is Meant by a Pass

When you have your diagnosis it is prudent to remove all of the lesions in the hips, knees and feet before moving on to correct the pelvis and spine. There is a set sequence for correcting the sacroiliac and iliosacral lesions and it is based on the adage. "First in, last out".

Right-Right

Start by correcting the pelvic lesions then the iliosacral on the left and then the sacroiliac lesion on the right. Be sure to remove the right L5 rotation immediately after you have corrected the right sacroiliac joint. You may need to repeat later in the session for optimum alignment.

Side-shift your patient's pelvis to the right, then work on the right side and correct the lumbar lesion from L1 down to L4. Then work your way from the upper thoracic vertebrae to correct all the lesions all the way down to the lumbar lesions . This is called a 'pass'

There could be some joints that you have difficulty correcting. Don't force anything because the joint is in all likelihood held captive by forces created by another lesion or a group of lesions elsewhere. Ignore for a moment.

Now side-shift the patients pelvis to the left and do a full 'pass' on the left side starting from the upper thoracic vertebrae downwards. The joints should be much looser now and any lesioned joints should now be easy to correct. This is the beauty of being able to manipulate every joint two to four times in a single session.

You may want to use the more powerful thoracic techniques shown on page 189 to be more thorough in removing all the thoracic lesions.

This type of treatment offers a level of alignment and mobility previously not available to Osteopaths.

When you have finished, align the ASIS's with your fingers and make sure that the transverse process's of L5 are parallel in the anterio-posterior plane.

Left-Right

The procedure for the right is similar but there are differences. Start by correcting the pelvic lesion then the sacroiliac on the right, followed by the iliosacral on the left. You may need to repeat later in the session for optimum alignment.

Be sure to remove the left L5 rotation immediately after you have corrected the left sacroiliac joint. Sometimes when you push down on the apex of the sacrum during your sacroiliac correction you inadvertently push the base on the left posteriorly. Watch out for this, it can cause your patient pain (This is something that can also occur in the right-right correction).

Now do your 'passes' starting on the left side which is the reverse on the right-right. Due to the low trauma footprint you can make as many passes up and down the spine as you like. In both the right-right and left-right patterns correct the cervical vertebrae last.

Correcting an
Iliosacral Lesion on the Left Side

This technique is best performed after your pelvic alignment correction techniques to get best results but it can be done singularly. This applies to **RR** and **LR** patterns.

• The patient should be in a prone position on the couch with their head and feet in the midline.

• The distal end of the couch can be raised or flat. Raised provides more leverage but is not essential.

• A pillow is placed under the patients shins.

• The patients pelvis should be side-shifted to the left. See **figure PPT4**

• Place a wedge under the head of the femur on the left to act as an axle. See **figures PPT3** and **PPT7**. In this position the ASIS is free to rotate anteriorly. See illustration **PPT6**.

• Make sure the patients feet are approximately aligned in a neutral position. See **figure PPT5**.

With the patients body positioned as in **figure PPT3** the left sacroiliac/iliosacral joints are made malleable and aligned in readiness to correct the iliosacral and sacroiliac lesions.

Stand to the right of your patient level with their pelvis. Firmly push (not thrust) the PSIS with the heel of your hand in a superio-latero-anterior direction. You will feel a very slight feeling of give if you have done this correctly. There is usually no click, at the worst there is a minute tick like sound.

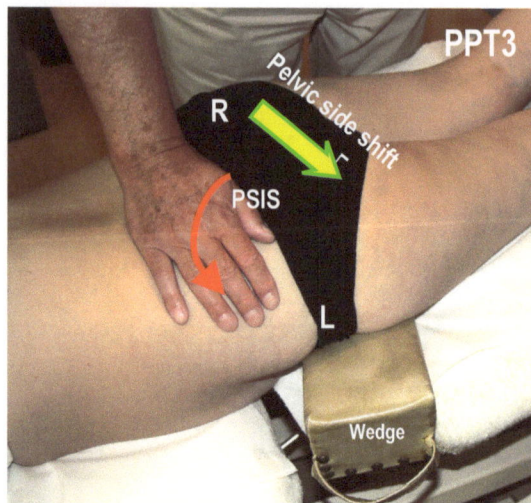

PPT3

Left Iliosacral correction on the left

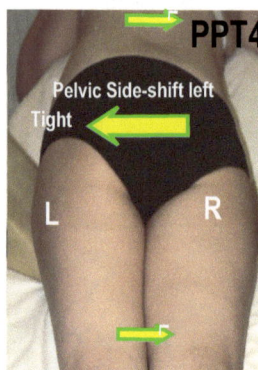

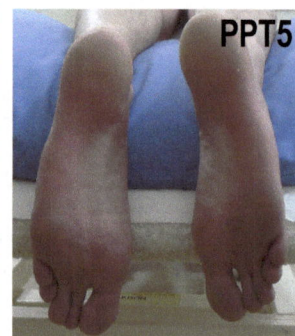

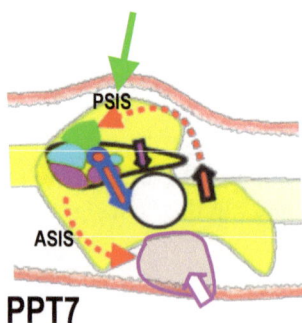

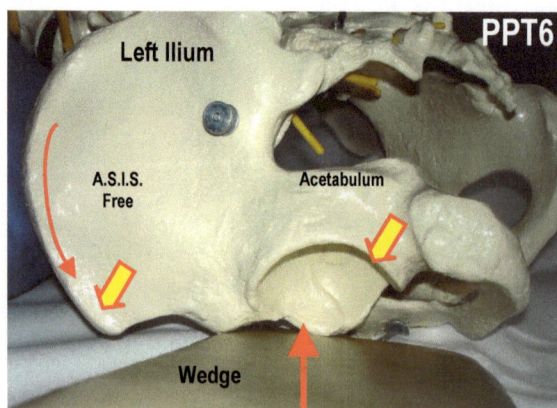

PPT4

PPT5

PPT7

PPT6

Correcting a
Sacroiliac Lesion on the Right Side

In the right sacroiliac lesion the base of the sacrum on the right is posterior in relation to the Ilium over the S/I 'F' facet. This technique applies to **RR** and **LR** patterns.

In the **LR** pattern this manipulation is corrected first followed by the left. In the **RR** the right side follows after left side Iliosacral has been manipulated.

• Your patient should still be in a prone position.

• Side-shift the patient's pelvis to the right, as shown in **figure PPT13**.

• If you have a professional couch lower the distal end for best results. If not, you can proceed with a flat couch. Place a wedge under the right ASIS, as shown in **figure SMQd.** This ensures that when pressure is applied in an anterior direction to the right side of the sacral base, the wedge under the ASIS will block the anterior movement of the ilium.

• **Figures PPT14 and PPT15** show the area to the right of the base of the sacrum over the 'F' facet where your PPT pressure will be applied.

• **Figure PPT16** shows the manipulation itself. The procedure is a follows:

Stand to the left of your patient, level with their pelvis and place the thenar eminence of your right hand on the right side of the base of the sacrum, just medial to the 'F' facets. Feel for the superior or inferior momentum of the sacrum.

Next, lean forward from the hips on the base of the sacrum. If the momentum of the sacrum was inferior make the angle of your correction anterio-superior. If it was superior, make your correction in an inferio-anterior direction.

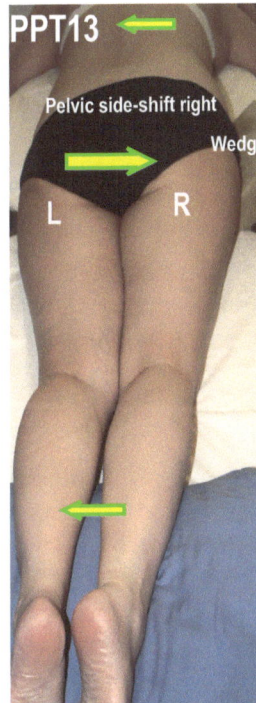

PPT13

Pelvic side-shift right

Wedge

L   R

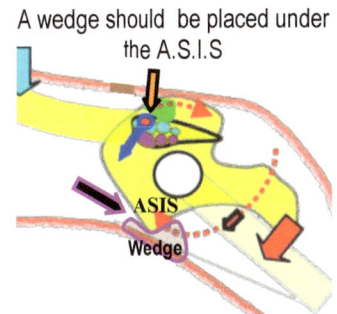

A wedge should be placed under the A.S.I.S

ASIS

Wedge

Figure SMQd

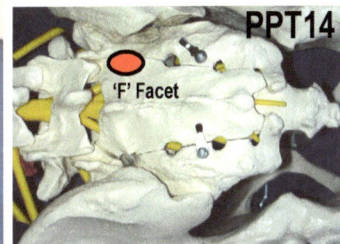

PPT14

'F' Facet

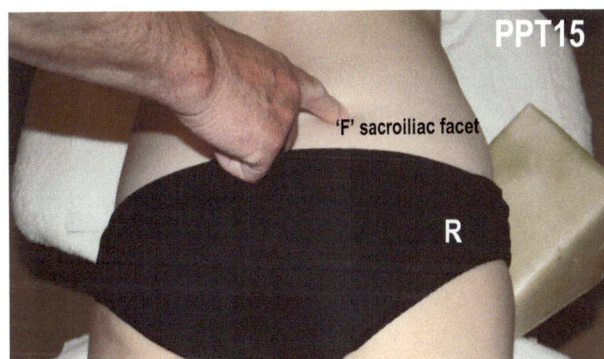

PPT15

'F' sacroiliac facet

R

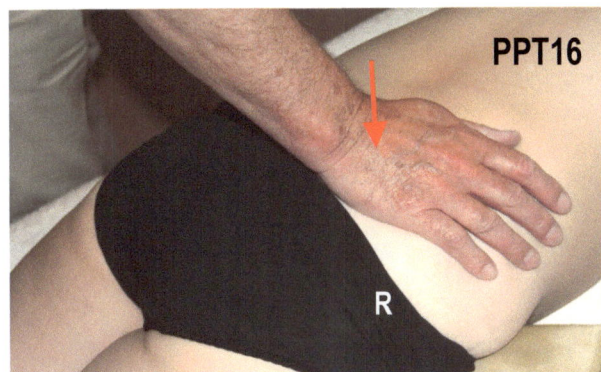

PPT16

R

Correcting Pelvic Compensation in the L3-R-R Lesion Pattern

There are three locks in a pelvic distortion syndrome

To recap, the majority of pelvic displacements start with a sacroiliac lesion on one side which creates an iliosacral lesion on the other side. The sacral and iliac lesions in every case distort the angle of the hips and legs. Therefore, when reactive forces return up the legs, with the original sacroiliac and iliosacral joints locked in their lesioned position, the upward gravitational forces distort the position of the pelvic-innominate's further. What's more, every time a leg becomes weight bearing all of the pelvic lesions are reinforced and create a buckling compensation in the pelvic joints. These are the lesions we need to release first.

Left leg adjustment RR

In the R-R Pattern the left buttock is posterior. The left leg is physiologically longer than the right with the left leg and foot turned outwards which creates hip and knee tracking problems and a flat instep. The pelvic side-shift is to the right. To remove the pelvic compensation:

The Patient is placed in a flat prone position with their pelvis side-shifted to the right. See **figure PBR1**. Stand at the foot of your couch, see **figure PBR2**, and lift the patient's left leg by the amount the left leg trails the right when standing straight, see **figure IF on page 153**. Draw the raised left leg with the foot turned out leg laterally until you feel the sweet spot of give. Pull the left leg until the buttocks are level, then lower the foot. See **figure PBR2**.

Right Leg adjustment RR

In the right-right pattern the right leg is the physiologically shorter than the left and the leg, knee and hip are turned inwards creating a raised arch.

Remain standing at the foot of the couch. Both legs should now be flat on the couch. See **figure PBR3**. Clasp your patients right ankle and move it medially until you find the sweet spot. Make sure the right foot is turned inward and that the buttocks are still level. Push the right leg superiorly a fraction. If the buttocks are not level repeat both procedures.

Left Leg Compensation RR

Place a wedge under the left hip. Stand to the right of your patient and place the heel of your hand on the PSIS and draw it in an inferior arc. This will loosen the tension within the left pelvic lesions. See **figure PBR4**.

Right Leg Compensation RR

Place a wedge under the right hip. Stand to the left of your patient and place the heel of your hand on the PSIS and ease it in a superior arc. This will loosen the the tension in the right pelvic lesions. See **figure PBR5**.

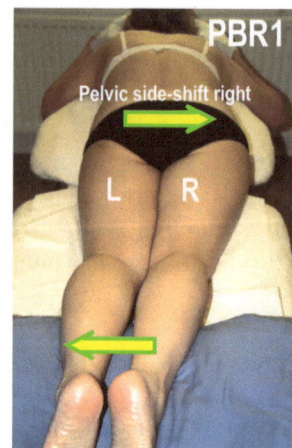

PBR1
Pelvic side-shift right
L R

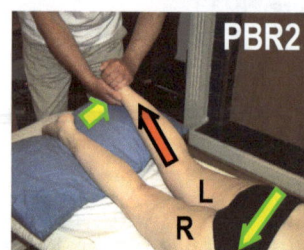

PBR2
L
R

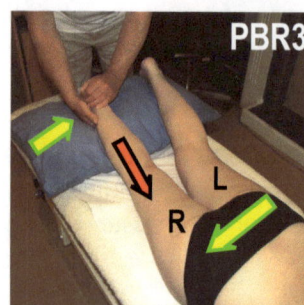

PBR3
L
R

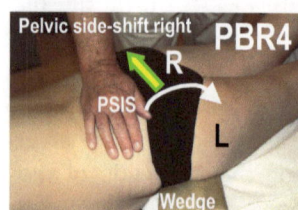

Pelvic side-shift right
PBR4
R
PSIS
L
Wedge

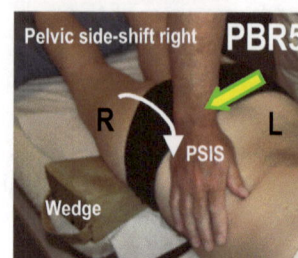

Pelvic side-shift right
PBR5
R
L
PSIS
Wedge

Correcting Pelvic Compensation in the L3-L-R Lesion Pattern

A note on compensation lesions

These compensation lesions can be seen as the complete opposite to the way the sacroiliac and iliosacral needs to be corrected to remove the lesions. However, if you fail to loosen them as a precursor to your manipulation, you will find it very hard to get the pelvis fully aligned and mobile.

Left leg adjustment L-R

In the L-R Pattern both the right and left buttocks are posterior. The right buttock being the more posterior. The legs are similar in length and the hips, knees and feet resemble normal tracking. Pelvic side-shift is to the left. This type of locking is more severe than in the R-R lesion pattern.
To remove the pelvic compensation:

The Patient is placed in a flat prone position with their pelvis side-shifted to the left. See **figure PBL1**. Stand at the foot of your couch, see **figure PBL2**, and take hold of the patient's right leg. Lift the lower leg or ankle by the height the posterior right leg is in relation to the left, as shown **page 153 figure 1X**. Then draw the right leg laterally until you feel the sweet spot of give. Then pull the right leg until you see the buttocks become level then put the leg back on the pillow. See **figure PBL2**.

Right Leg adjustment L-R

Remain standing at the foot of the couch. (Both legs should now be flat on the couch) See **figure PBL3**. Clasp your patients left ankle or lower leg and move it medially until you find the sweet spot. Push the left leg superiorly a fraction. Make sure that the buttocks are still level. If the buttocks are not level repeat both procedures.

Left Leg Compensation L-R

Place a wedge under the left hip. Stand to the right of your patient and place the heel of your hand on the PSIS and draw it in an inferio-anterior arc. Be gentle. This will loosen the tension within the left pelvic lesions. See **figure PBL4**.

Right Leg Compensation L-R

Place a wedge under the right hip. Stand to the left of your patient and place the heel of your hand on the PSIS and ease it in a superio-anterior arc. This will loosen the the tension in the right pelvic lesions. See **figure PBL5**.

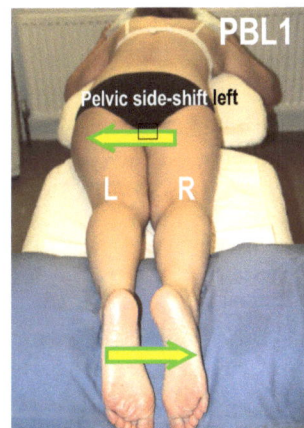

PBL1 — Pelvic side-shift left — L R

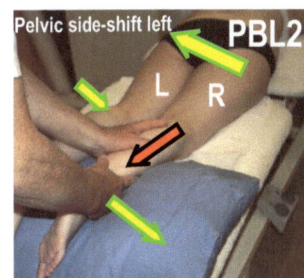

PBL2 — Pelvic side-shift left — L R

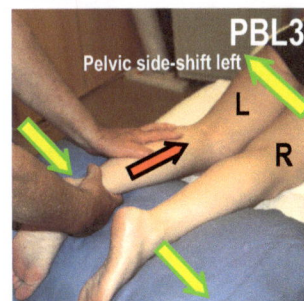

PBL3 — Pelvic side-shift left — L R

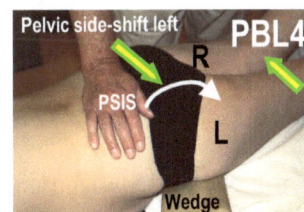

PBL4 — Pelvic side-shift left — R L — PSIS — Wedge

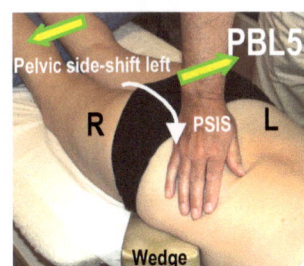

PBL5 — Pelvic side-shift left — R PSIS L — Wedge

Correcting the Pelvic Balance in the Right-Right Lesion Pattern

Correct the position of the legs and feet.

When you have finished correcting the R-R compensation lesions shown on the previous pages, your patient should be relaxing on the couch in a similar position to that shown in **figure PBB1**.

Left leg correction

Bring the left leg medially whilst gently pulling the left leg inferiorly and internally rotate the left foot to a position you judge to be neutral. See **figure PBB2**. Watch out that the buttocks remain at the same height.

Right Leg correction

After correcting the position of the left leg, bring the right leg along side the left. As you do this taking hold of the lower right leg or ankle and gently push the right leg superiorly. At the same time externally rotate the right foot so it sits in the position you judge to be neutral. See **figure PBB2**. Observe that the buttocks have remained at the same height.

Next correct the lesions

With the legs and buttocks aligned side-shift the pelvis to the left and place a wedge under the left hip and correct the left iliosacral lesion according to the procedure shown on **page 180**.

Next side-shift the pelvis to the right with the wedge under the ASIS and correct the sacroiliac lesion with the procedure shown on **page 181**.

Take the wedge away and place the patient in the mid-line. Check that the spine is not affecting alignment of the pelvis, by following the method shown on **page 162 figures DM9 and 10.** Then check that the buttocks are level.

The buttocks and all the pelvic joints should now be aligned and mobile, if not, repeat the whole process.

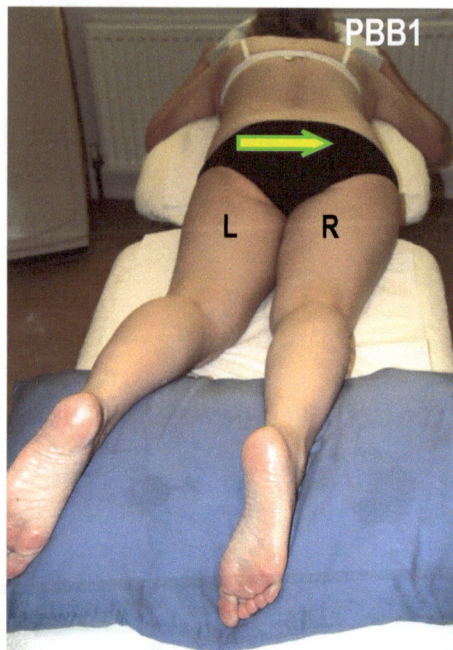

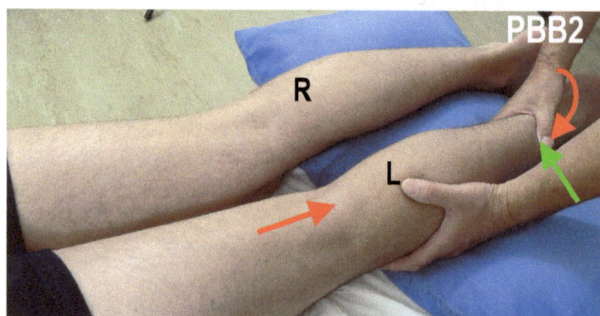

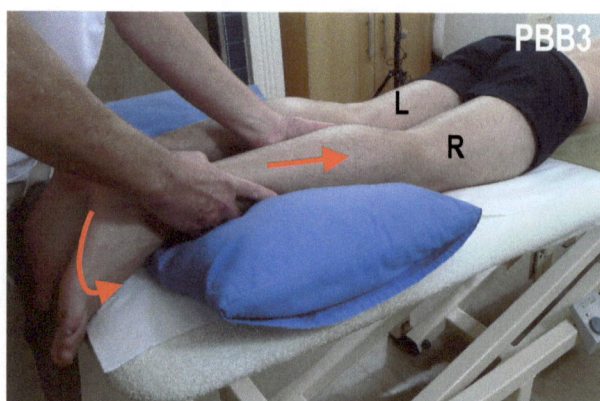

Correcting the Pelvic Balance in the Left-Right Lesion Pattern

Correct the position of the legs and feet.

When you have finished correcting the L-R compensation lesions shown on the previous pages, your patient should be relaxing on the couch in a similar position to that shown in **figure PBB4**.

Right leg correction

Take hold of the leg and gently pull the right leg inferiorly whilst externally rotating the left foot. You have to judge the correct neutral position. See **figure PBB5**. Observe the buttocks to ensure they have remained at the same height.

Left leg correction

After correcting the position of the left leg, take hold of the lower right leg or ankle gently push the right leg superiorly. At the same time internally rotate the right foot so it sits in the position you judge to be neutral. See **figure PBB6**. Again make sure the buttocks remain at the same height.

Next correct the lesions

With the legs and buttocks aligned side-shift the pelvis to the right and place a wedge under the right ASIS and correct the right sacroiliac lesion according to the procedure shown on **page 181**.

Next side-shift the pelvis to the left and correct the iliosacral lesion with the procedure shown on **page 180**.

Take the wedge away and place the patient in the mid-line. Check that the spine is not affecting alignment of the pelvis, by following the method shown on **page 162 figures DM9 and 10.** Then check that the buttocks are level.

The buttocks and all the pelvic joints should now be aligned and mobile, if not, repeat the whole process.

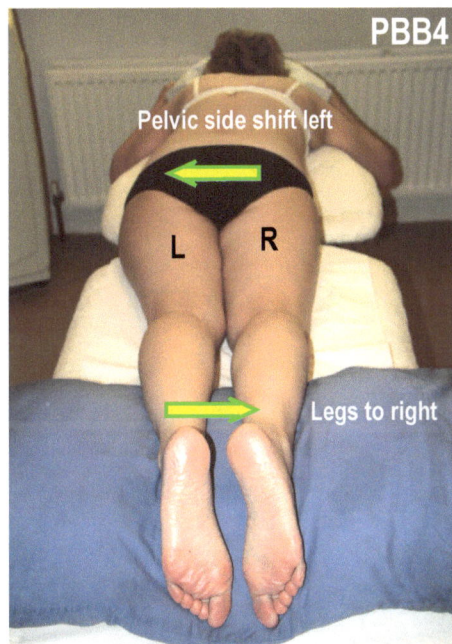

PBB4
Pelvic side shift left
L   R
Legs to right

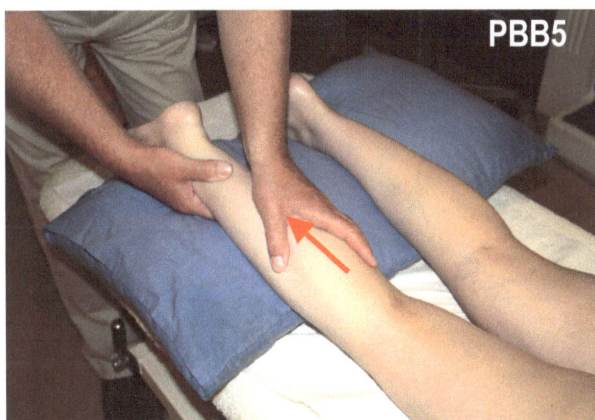

PBB5

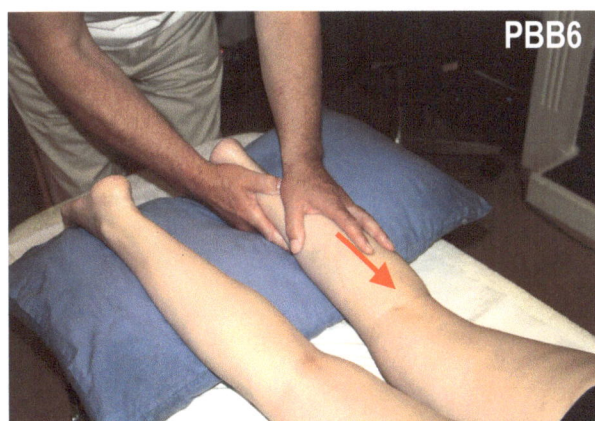

PBB6

Correcting the Pelvic Balance in a Compound Lesion Pattern

Compound lesions

Sometimes your patient will arrive at your practice with an un-recognizable and painful lesion pattern. The asymmetry will be because the pelvis has endured a set of lesions on top of one of the two main types of lesion pattern described in this book. In this case you will have to initially wing it to unlock the overlaying lesions. Here are some guidelines that might help.

Assess and treat your patient

With your patient in a prone position and in the mid-line, follow the procedure on **page 162 figures DM9 and 10** to find your pelvic constant.

Stand at the foot of the couch and assess which buttock is posterior. The posterior buttock is usually the leg you will need to pull but to double check this by following the procedure on **page 165 figure IDM 17**.

The momentum of the leg is inferior and matches with the posterior buttock this is more simple. Do not correct the foot position. Side-shift the pelvis to the opposite side of the inferior leg then pull the leg and move it laterally. Find the sweet spot and pull. Release the compensation lesion on that side by taking the innominate the way it is going. On the opposite side, the convexity, gently push the leg superiorly and move from side to side to find the sweet spot and ease superiorly. After correcting the compensation lesion on that side, side-shift the pelvis to that the opposite side and correct the iliosacral lesion. Then side-shift the pelvis to the opposite side and remove the sacroiliac lesion. Next time your patient arrives for their next treatment you should be able to identify the underlying lesion pattern.

Further complications

If the momentum of the leg is inferior but does not match to the posterior buttock, ignore the buttocks and be guided by the leg momentum.

Do not correct the direction of the feet. On the inferior leg move the leg medially and laterally with a slight pull to find the sweet spot then gently pull that leg. Carry out the same procedure on the opposite leg with a mild upward pressure. Move the leg medially and laterally to find the sweet spot and when you have found it gently push superiorly. Next, release the compensation lesions by placing your hand on the innominate to feel which direction of the inclination. If it moves superiorly easier than inferiorly, ease it superiorly etc. Next, side shift the pelvis to the side that had the inferior leg and place a wedge under that hip and ease the PSIS superiorly. Change the pelvic side-shift to the opposite side and place wedge under the ASIS and ease the base of the sacrum anteriorly.

It is not recommended that you work on the underlying lesion pattern on the initial session. Let gravity do its work, so ask your patient to have their follow up treatment within two to three days.

Momentum: The flow of energy
Sweat spot: An area where there is the maximum flexibility.

Correcting a Lumbar Rotation Lesion

L5 lesion in right-right lesion pattern

L5 is rotated to the right in the right-right lesion pattern. The right TP of L5 will be posterior on the right and the SP inferior. When a right-right patient presents they will usually exhibit pain over the right TP of L5. The knee drop mobility test produces pain and restriction over the right side of L5 when the left knee is flexed. See **figure PPT 24**. The right lumbar muscles will be tight and stretched and the right L5 TP and surrounding area tender.

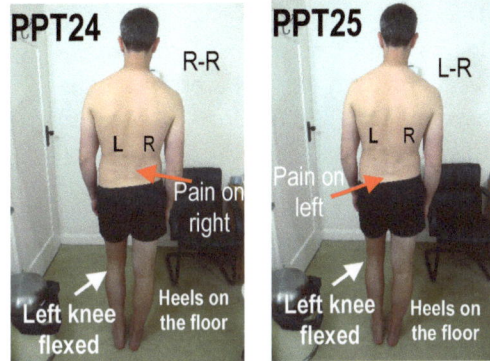

PPT24 R-R
L R
Pain on right
Left knee flexed
Heels on the floor

PPT25 L-R
L R
Pain on left
Left knee flexed
Heels on the floor

L5 should be corrected directly after the right side of the sacroiliac has been corrected. The distal end of the couch should remain in the lowered position with the wedge under the right ASIS, and the pelvis side-shifted to the left, as per **figure PPT26**.

Place the thenar eminence of your right hand over the right TP of L5 as per **figure PPT26** and then gently lean from your pelvis on the TP in an anterio-lateral arc whilst drawing the L5 SP towards you. As this is a tender area, make your adjustment quick. You will feel the L5 vertebra de-rotate under you hand.

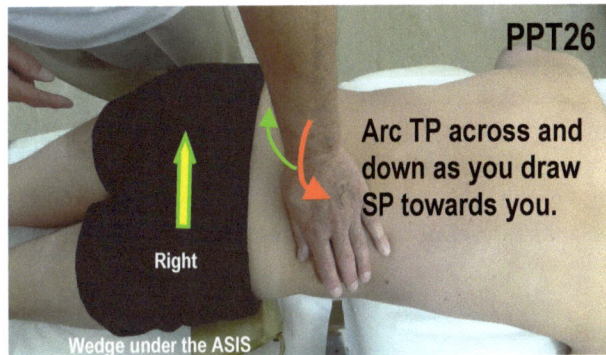

PPT26
Arc TP across and down as you draw SP towards you.
Right
Wedge under the ASIS

L5 lesion left-right lesion pattern

L5 and L3 will be rotated left, therefore the left TP's will be posterior. Their SP's will be inferior. In the left-right pattern the patient presents with pain and muscle tightness over the left TP of L5. The right knee drop test elicits pain over the left TP of L5. See **figure PPT25**.

This lesion should be corrected directly after the left iliosacral/sacroiliac joints have been corrected. The position of the couch and pelvic side-shift should remain the same except that the wedge needs to be placed under the left ASIS.

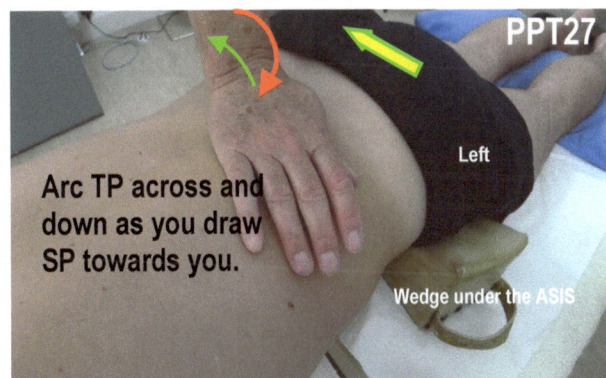

PPT27
Arc TP across and down as you draw SP towards you.
Left
Wedge under the ASIS

Place the thenar eminence of your right over the left TP of L5 as per **figure PPT27**, then gently lean from the pelvis over the TP and arc it in an anterio-lateral direction whilst pulling the SP of L5 towards you. You will feel the L5 vertebra de-rotate under you hand. Do the same for L3.

All lumbar rotation lesions can be manipulated like this. You can also use the same technique as used for removing thoracic rotation lesions. However, the above are more convenient in the lumbar area.

Correcting a Lumbar Side-Bending Lesion

Lumbar extension lesion

We are going to use L3 as an example. In the extension lesion pattern the 'M' force is side-bending. Therefore, this is the force we need to remove. This method can also be used for all lumbar lesions including L1.

The distal end of the couch is dropped as per **figure PPT28**, this will stretch the lumbar lesions and make them easier to manipulate. If you do not have a professional couch you can do this on a flat surface.

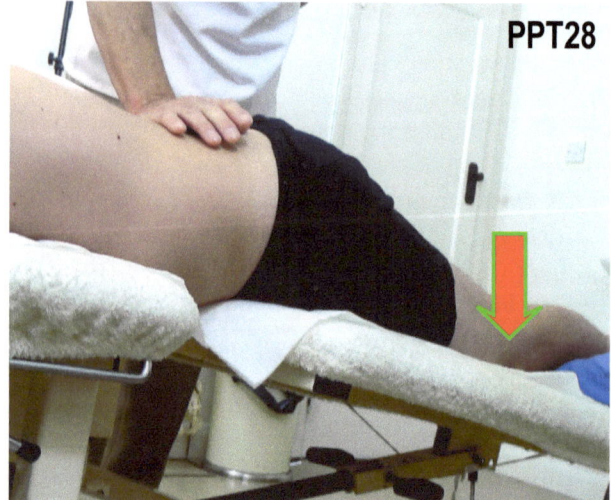

Figure PPT29 is a photograph of a typical L3/4 R-R extension lesion. On palpation the side of the SP can be felt protruding on the left. It can be moved slightly in a superior direction but feels restricted when inferior movement is attempted.

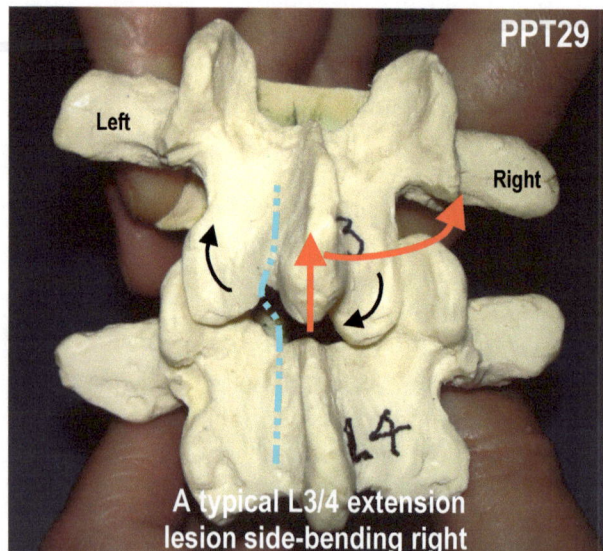

PPT28

L3 side-bending correction

Place the thenar eminence of your right hand against the right SP of L3 as per **figure PPT30** and then gently lean from your pelvis and move the SP in a superior direction then both side-shift and arc L3 to the right as per **figure PPT29**. As always, make your adjustment quick. You will feel the L3 vertebra de-side-bend and free under you hand.

Your thrust should be vertical followed by the angle of the articulation which is an arc.

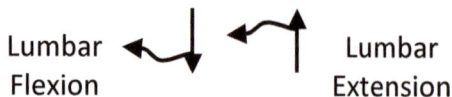

Lumbar Flexion   Lumbar Extension

Notes

You will need to use more pressure to correct lumbar lesions than thoracic lesions. Never force!

The arc follows the arc of the pelvic side-shift which has a pendulum action action at this level.

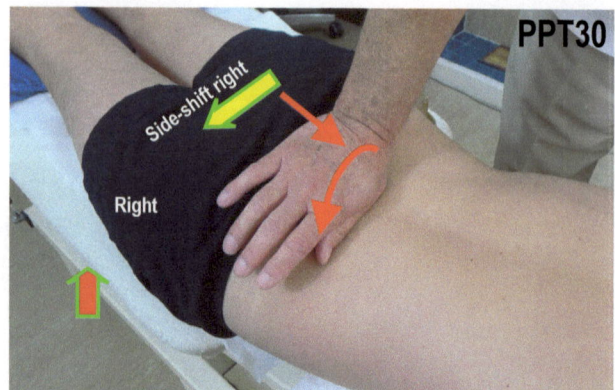

PPT29

Left

Right

A typical L3/4 extension lesion side-bending right

PPT30

Side-shift right

Right

Correcting a Side-Bending Lesion in Thoracic Flexion

Lesion: Side-bent right in thoracic flexion

The couch and arms should be in the position shown in **figure PPT 1** at the start of this Chapter. The patient places their hands under their thighs and the proximal and distal ends of the couch are lowered to stretch the back.

Figure PPT31 illustrates a typical mid-thoracic flexion (forward bending) lesion with the 'M' force side-bent right. The left side of the T6   SP is left and superior.

Figure PPT32 illustrates how to palpate for a thoracic lesion. Place the medial side of your right thumb against the left side of the SP and feel for the protruding bulge. Then keeping your thumb in the same position test it for superior and inferior movement. In the flexion lesion the SP can be moved in a superior direction and is resistant in an inferior direction.

Figure PPT33 illustrates the PPT correction. The correction shown here is for a T8 flexion lesion with rotation and side-bending to the right.

Stand to the left of the patient, level with T8 and place the thenar   eminence of your right hand firmly on the protruding side of the spinous process.

Gently push the spinous process superiorly and then medially to the right (no arc). Do this in one fluid movement.

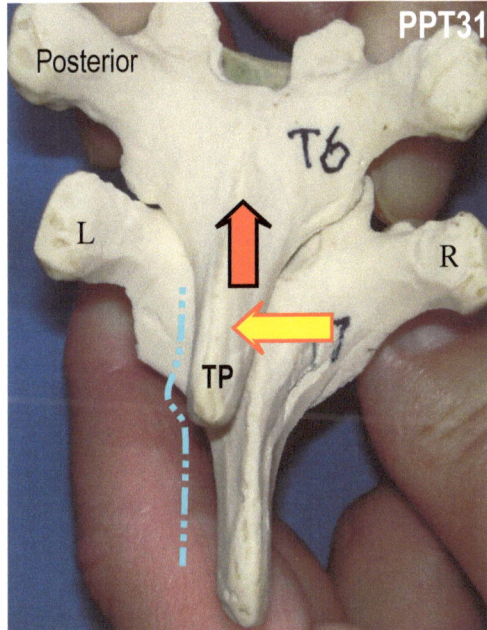
PPT31

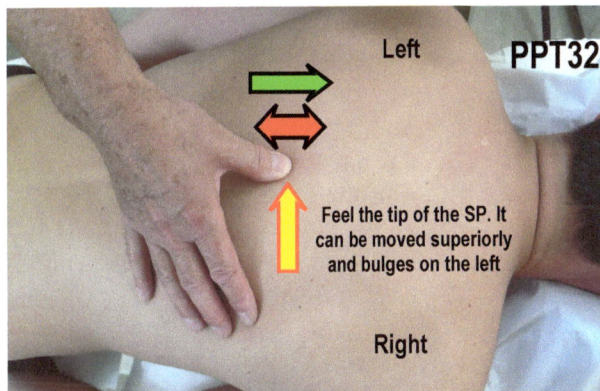
PPT32
Feel the tip of the SP. It can be moved superiorly and bulges on the left

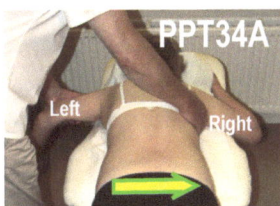
PPT34A

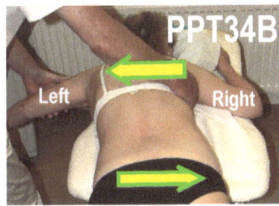
PPT34B

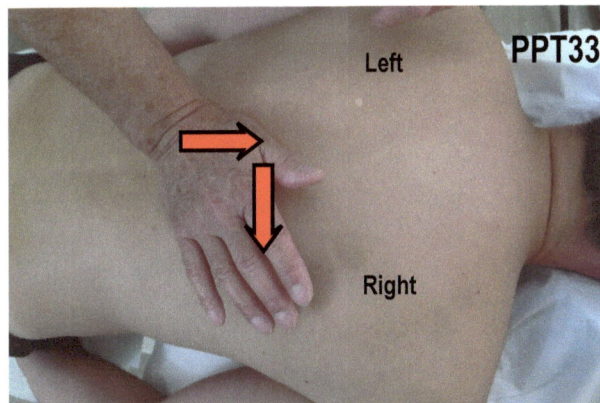
PPT33

The pelvis should be side-shifted to the right as shown in **figures PPT34 A and B** and above and the torso should be side-bent to the left as per **figure PPT34B**.

Correcting a Side-Bending Lesion in Thoracic Extension

Lesion: Side-bent right in thoracic extension

The couch and arms should be in the position shown in **figure PPT 1** at the start of this Chapter. The patient places their hands under their thighs. Technically this is a 'complicated lesion'.

Figure PPT35 illustrates a typical upper mid-thoracic extension (backward bending) lesion. The spinous process of T3 is inferior and to the left.

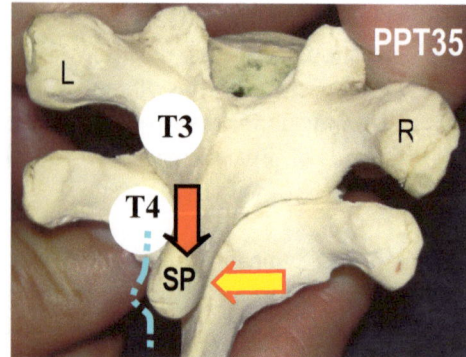

Figure PPT36 illustrates how to palpate for a thoracic extension lesion. Place the medial side of your right thumb against the left side of the SP and feel for the protruding tip. It is usually felt as a small bulge. Then keeping your thumb in the same position test superior and inferior movement. In the extension lesion the spinous process will move in an inferior direction and resist in a superior direction.

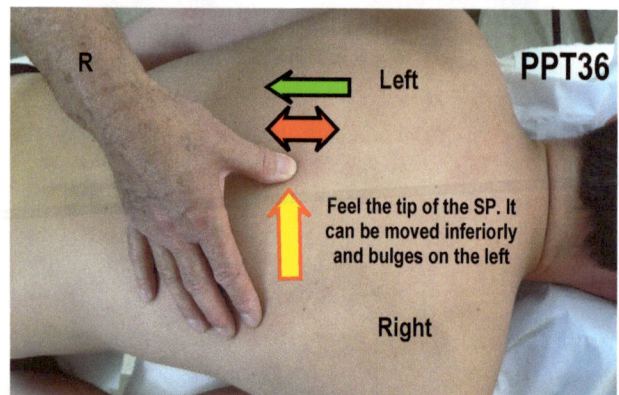

Feel the tip of the SP. It can be moved inferiorly and bulges on the left

Figure PPT37 illustrates the PPT correction. The correction shown is at T8 and is for an extension lesion with side-bending to the right. The pelvis and torso should be side-shifted to the right, as shown in **figure PPT34B**. Stand to the left of your patient, level with T8 and place the thenar eminence of your right hand firmly on the protruding side of the spinous process. Then gently push the spinous process inferiorly and then medially to the right in one fluid movement (no arc). Let your energy come from your pelvis.

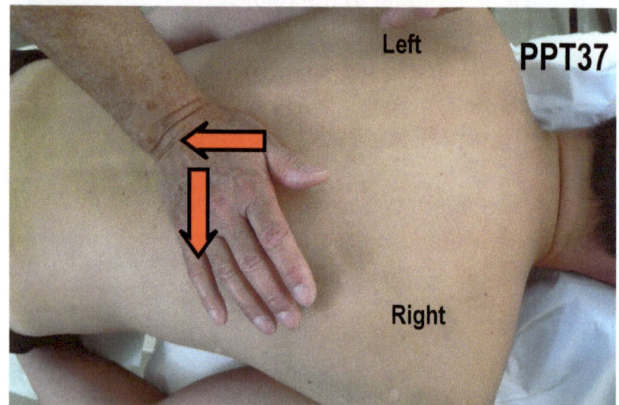

Sometimes extension lesions can be difficult to correct in the upper thoracic area. A good method of making the joint more malleable before your adjustment is to exaggerate the lesion first, as shown at T3 in **figure PPT38**. Place the thenar eminence of your right against the right side of the SP and the hyperthenar eminence of the left hand to its left and ease the lesioned vertebra to the left and inferiorly. Do not press anteriorly.

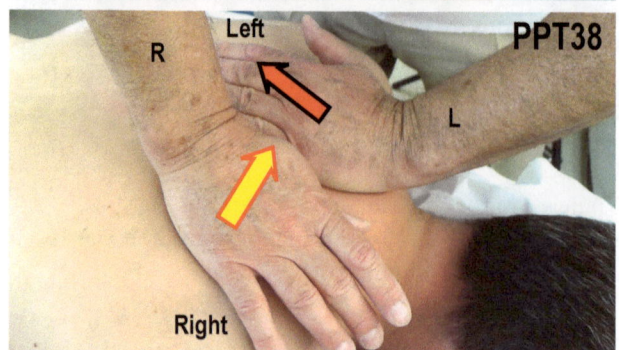

Correcting a Rotation Lesion in Thoracic Extension and Flexion

Lesion rotation right in thoracic extension

The couch and arms should be in the position shown in **figure PPT 1** at the start of this Chapter. The patient places their hands under their thighs.

Figure PPT38a illustrates how to palpate for a thoracic rotation lesion. Place the medial side of your right thumb against the left side of the SP and feel for the protruding tip. It is usually felt as a small bulge. Then keeping your thumb in the same position test for superior and inferior movement. Next check the AP levels of the TP.

In the extension rotation lesion the spinous process will move in an inferior direction and resist in a superior direction and the left TP will be posterior.

Figure PPT38b illustrates the PPT correction. The correction shown is at T6 and is for an extension lesion with side-bending and rotation to the right. The left TP will be posterior. The pelvis and torso should be side-shifted to the right, as shown in **figure PPT34b**.

See **figure PPT 38c**. Stand to the left of your patient, level with T6 and place the hyper-thenar eminence of your left hand firmly against the left side of the protruding SP and posterior TP. Gently push the SP inferiorly and to the right. At the same time lean on the left TP and carefully push it anteriorly. These movements should all be carried out in one fluid movement

In the flexion correction the spinous process is eased superiorly before the de-rotation. That is the only difference.

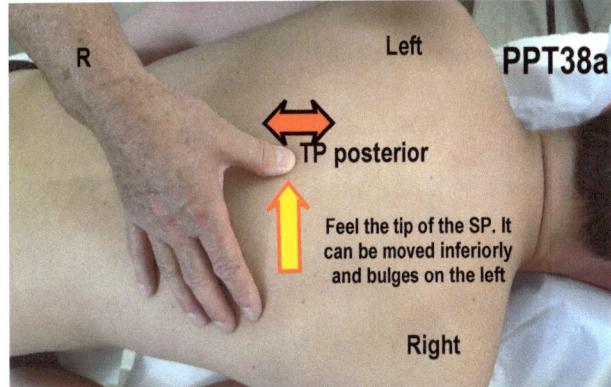

R   Left   **PPT38a**

TP posterior

Feel the tip of the SP. It can be moved inferiorly and bulges on the left

Right

Test for side-bending of the spinous process and the anterior-posterior position of the transverse process

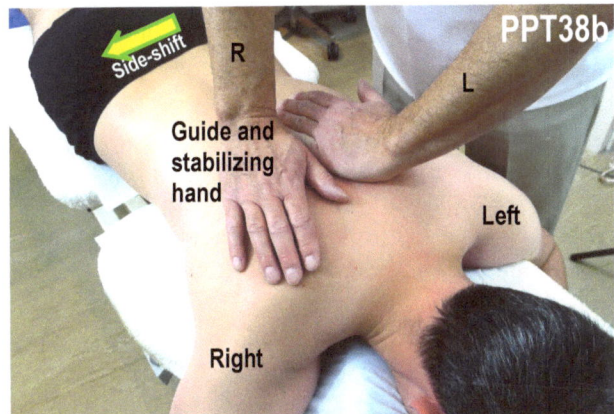

Side-shift   R   L   **PPT38b**

Guide and stabilizing hand

Left

Right

Position your hands side-by side with the pelvis side-shifted to the right to make the left side malleable

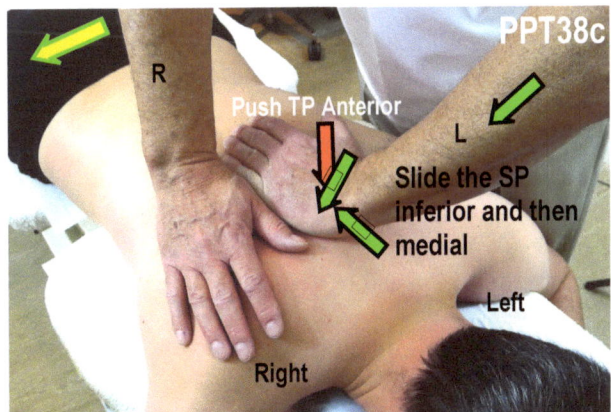

R   **PPT38c**

Push TP Anterior   L

Slide the SP inferior and then medial

Left

Right

191

Correcting a Cervical Lesion
Safety First

Safety before manipulation

It has been reported that there is a theoretical one and a half million to one risk that you could kill or cause a stroke when you manipulate a neck. So it is essential you take as much precaution as you can to avoid endangering your patient. I have spoken to many an Osteopath about this and there does not seem to be any standard test, so I will explain the way I do it.

When taking your case history look for inflammatory conditions that effect the neck such as those from the Rheumatoid family, or stenosis or a history of heart attacks or strokes etc. This list goes on and most Osteopathic courses cover this subject in some detail. Safety is an Osteopathic priority.

I have only ever come across one case where I refused to treat the neck. The patient had thought she was having strokes and went to our local AE and then her GP who both told her that it was in her mind and she was perfectly OK. I did the following compression test and she could not hold her arms straight and felt odd. I stopped treatment immediately and referred her straight back to AE with a note explaining to them that she had failed the compression test.

With your patient in the mid-line ask them to raise their arms in the air, as per **figure PPT39**. Then ask them to close their eyes to cut out their visual reference. Stand behind your patient's head and place your hands on either side of their head and gently compress their neck. Ask the patient how they feel. If they are OK keep the compression on their neck and rotate their head in both directions. Observe whether their hands waver. When they open their eyes ask them if the world is still. If they feel strange or moved their arms, do not proceed. See **figure PPT40**.

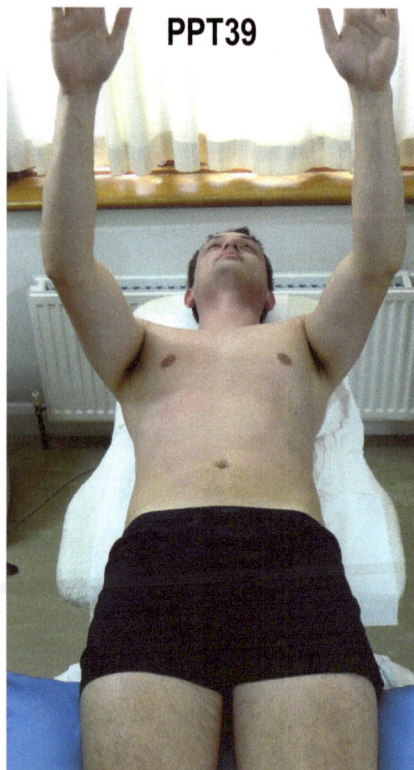
PPT39

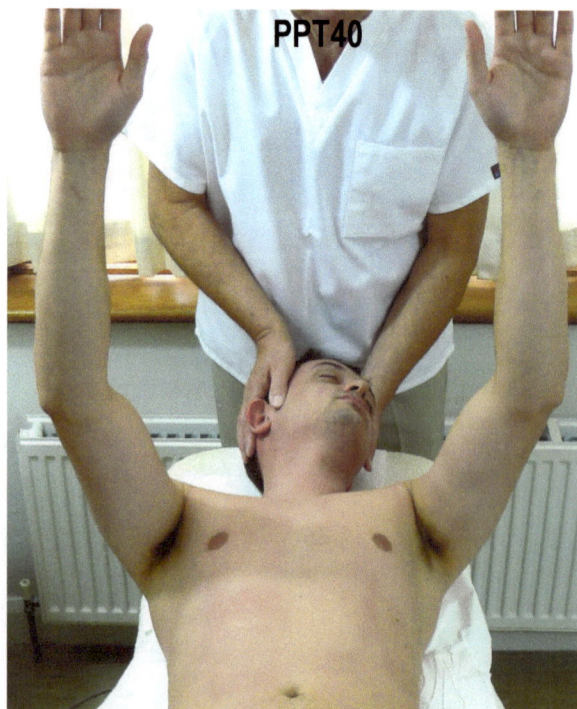
PPT40

Correcting a Cervical Lesion using the PPT Method

C3 Rotated and side-bent to the right

On palpation there will be a facet bulge to the right at C3. Side-bending to the right will be free and blocked to the left here. See **figure PPT45**.

Your patient should be supine with their pelvis side-shifted to the right, as per **figure PPT40**, their knees supported by a pillow. This will make the left side of their neck malleable. Do not place a cushion under their head as this will tighten the cervical joints and hinder your manipulation.

Stand behind your patient's head and extend your index finger, as per **figure PPT41**. Place the middle crease of the index finger of your right hand under the spinous process of C3 with the distal pad against the side of the C3 facet bulge. See **figures PPT42** and **PPT42a**.

Check whether the SP moves superiorly or inferiorly. See figure **PPT43** and **PPT 43a**. Take the vertebra the way it wants to go and gently raise your index finger in an anterior direction to introduce cervical flexion (backward bending). This will unhook the joints fixation. Now draw the pad of your finger to the right as per **figure PPT44**. There is a very slight feeling of give and that is it, the joint will release with no trauma or clunk. It really is as simple as that.

In very tight lesions around C6-7 it can help if you lift the head slightly and stretch the neck as you make your manipulation. Stretching the neck slightly in neutral can also aid the release of a tight C1-Oc.

This technique works efficiently 80% of the time.

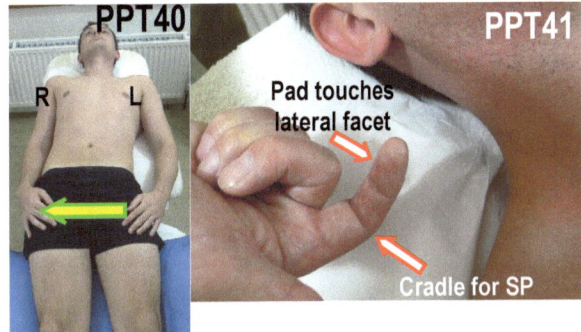

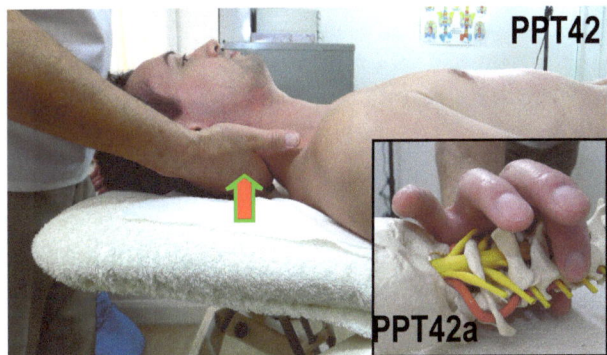

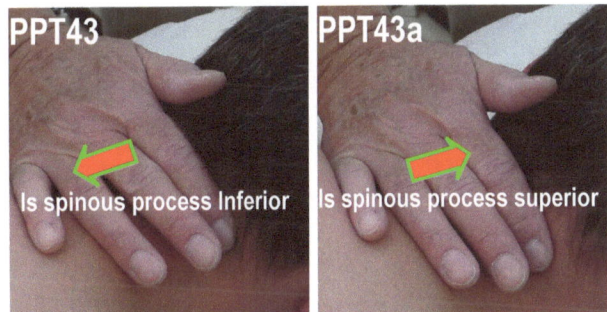

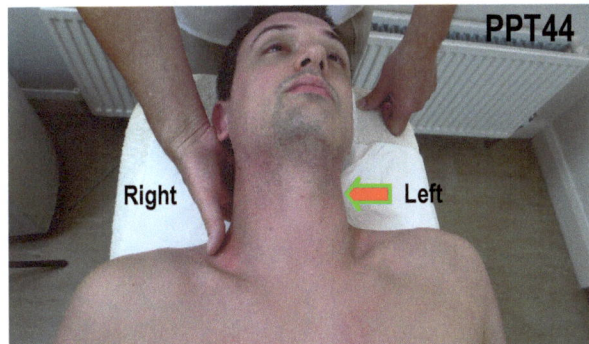

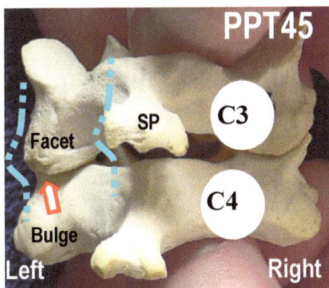

PPT40

R   L

PPT41

Pad touches lateral facet

Cradle for SP

PPT42

PPT42a

PPT43

Is spinous process Inferior

PPT43a

Is spinous process superior

PPT45

SP

Facet

C3

C4

Bulge

Left   Right

PPT44

Right   Left

Correcting a Classical Cervical Lesion Applying the PPT Principle

I do not recommend this technique as it is crude.
If you can, always use the neck technique on the previous page. The technique is safer and works more efficiently and your patients will like you a lot more.

C3 Rotated and side-bent to the right
This technique is basically a safety modification and improvement on the 'classical' and 'classical advanced' neck techniques. It is shown here for completeness only.

By side-shifting the pelvis to the left, rotation of the neck to the right is greatly reduced. This asset is used to cut out excessive rotation during classical neck manipulations and makes them safer. See page 164 for more explanation.

Palpation
On palpation there will be a slight facet bulge at C3 on the left.

When testing rotation and side-bending, the neck will be free to rotate and side-bend to the right and blocked to the left at C3. See **figure PPT45a**.

Technique
Your patient should be supine with their pelvis side-shifted to the left. Their knees should be flexed with the aid of a pillow under them. This position will tighten the left side of the patients neck and relax the right.

Stand behind your patients head and place the lateral border of your left index finger against the left facet bulge of C3. Use your finger as a fulcrum and side-bend the patients neck left at C3 until it tightens to its limit. See **figure PPT45b**.

With your finger still on the facet bulge of C3 use it as a fulcrum to rotate the patients head to the right. This is a high velocity thrust technique and causes a loud clunk as it gaps the joint. See **figure PPT45c**.

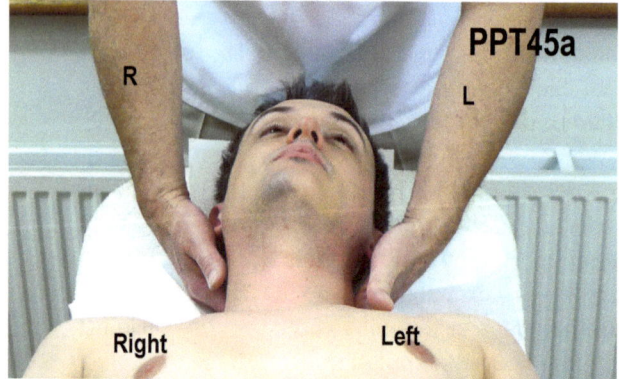

PPT45a

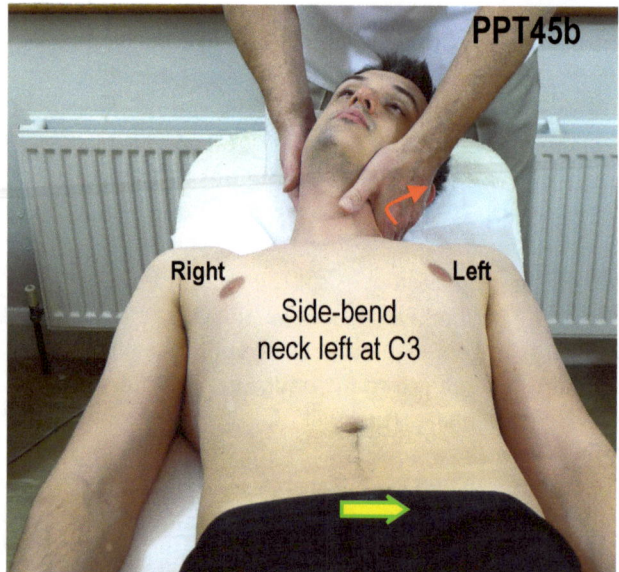

PPT45b

Side-bend neck left at C3

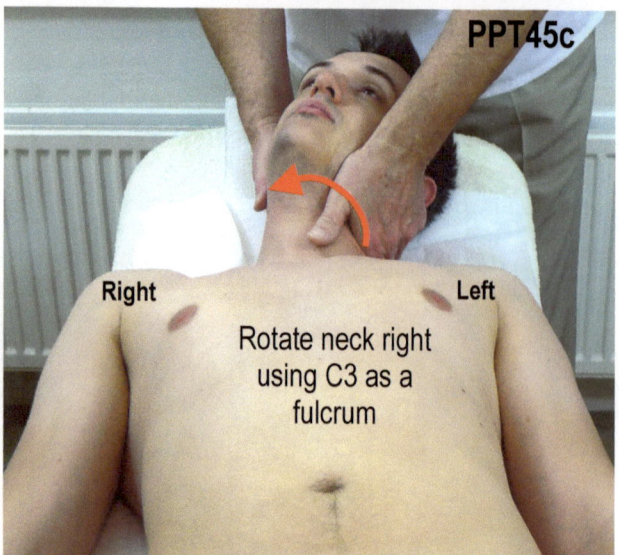

PPT45c

Rotate neck right using C3 as a fulcrum

Working with Pelvic Side-Shift

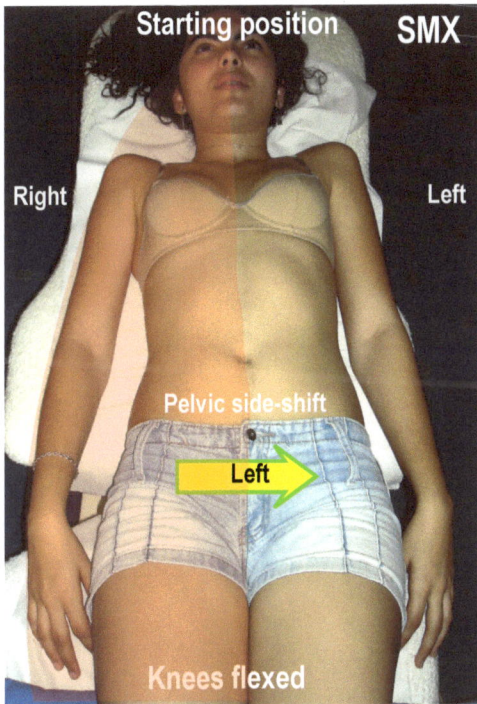

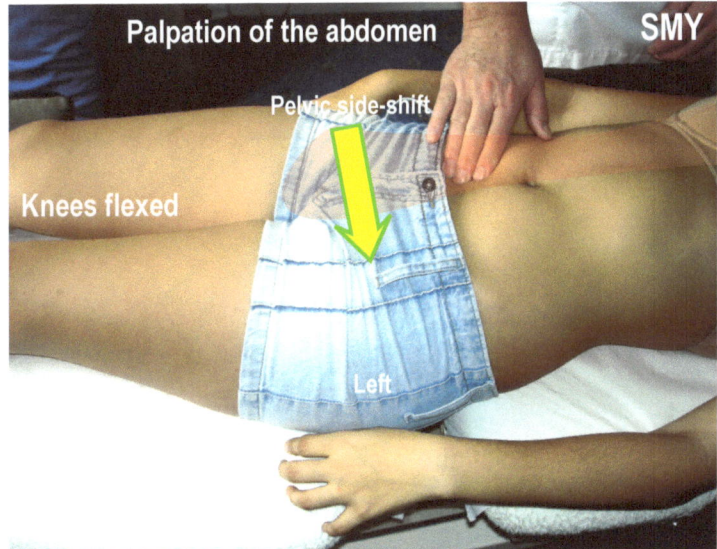

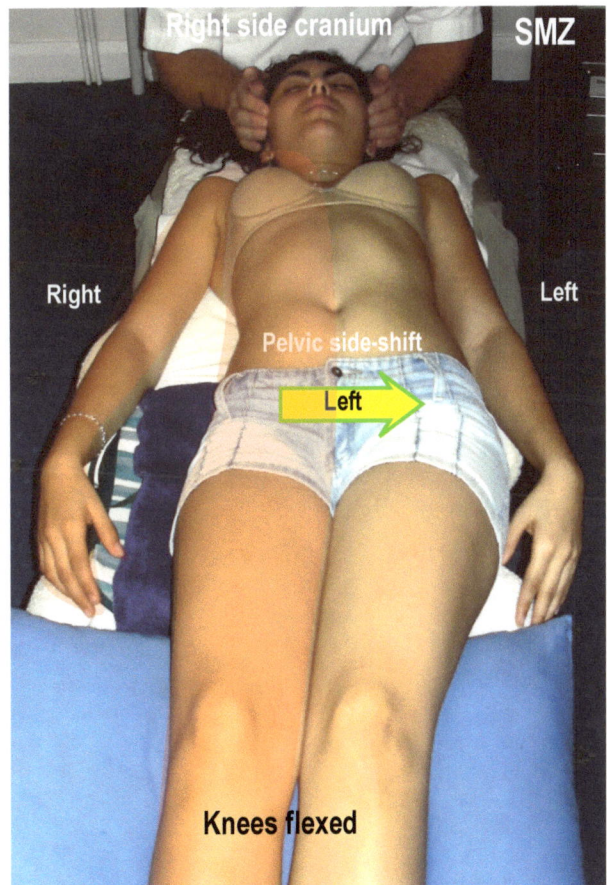

Starting position SMX

Right   Left

Pelvic side-shift

Left

Knees flexed

Palpation of the abdomen SMY

Pelvic side-shift

Knees flexed

Left

Right side cranium SMZ

Right   Left

Pelvic side-shift

Left

Knees flexed

Position: When treating or palpating the anterior right side of the body, as shown in **figure SMX**, it makes a significant difference if the pelvis is side-shifted to the left. This is because the side-shift relaxes the soft tissue on the right.

Medical Palpation: When performing medical abdominal examinations on the right as shown in **figure SMY**, visceral definition is more clearly defined if the patient flexes their knees with pelvic side-shifted to the left.

Cranial Osteopathy: Cranial bones on the right are made more malleable when the knees are flexed with pelvic side-shifted to the left, as shown in **figure SMZ**.

Side-shift should not be taken to the limit.

195

Miscellaneous Supine Techniques

Below are photographs of examples of the many assessment, articulation and manipulative procedures that can be made easier and more efficient using pelvic side shift.

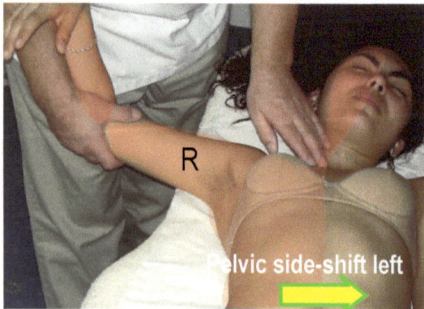

Clavicle articulation

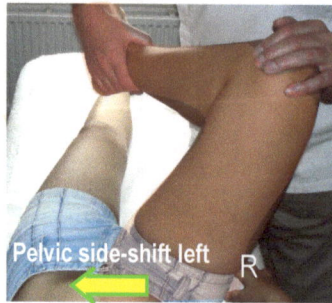

Hip articulation

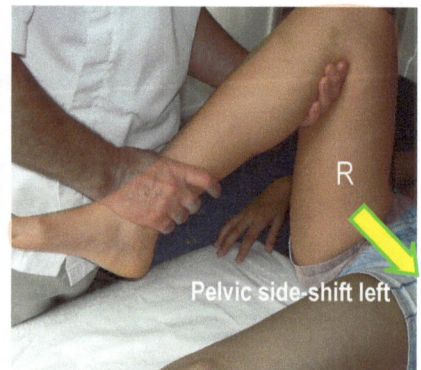

Knee assessment

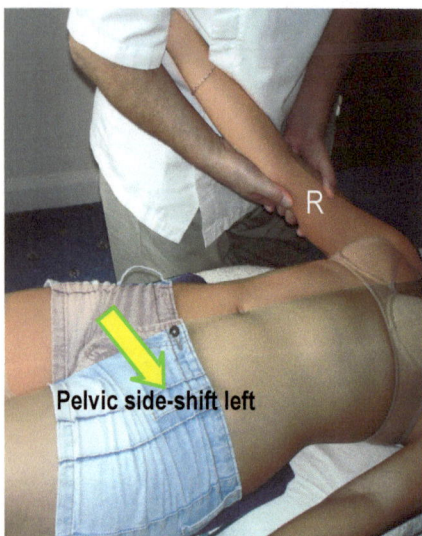

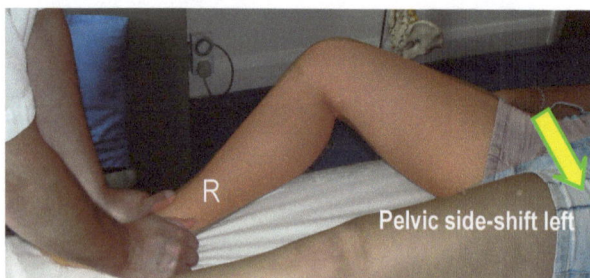

Elbow manipulation

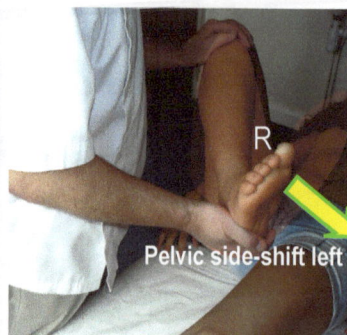

Hip assessment

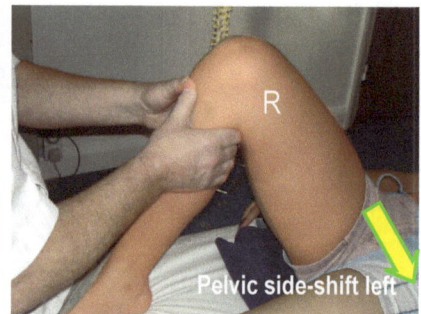

Knee assessment

Ankle manipulation

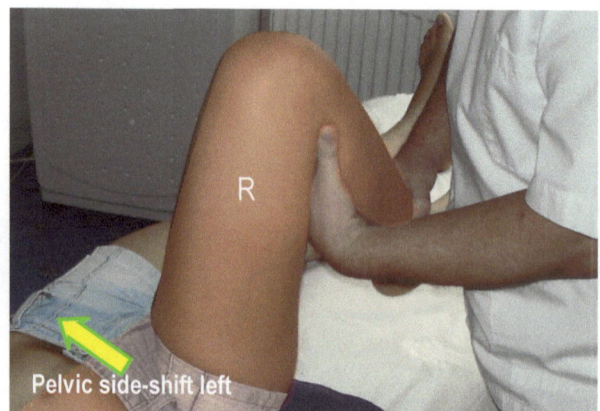

Knee manipulation

Manipulation Strategy

The benefits of PPT manipulation

In classical gapping type manipulation when faced with the thoracic curves illustrated in **figure PPT46** the manipulator will choose to correct either points **A, C** and **E** or points **B** and **D** in their efforts to iron out the curves.

The problem with that approach is that points **B** and **D** are locked in by points **A, C** and **E**. Whilst conversely points **A**, **C** and **E** are locked in by points **B** and **D**.

Points **B** and **D** will be easy to manipulate and give the quickest pain relief but points **A, C** and **E** will be much more difficult to manipulate.

If you do not release points **A, C** and **E** by the time your patient walks out of your door, points **B** and **D** will be in lesion again.

PPT approach

With PPT's, because there is very little trauma when the joints are manipulated, you are free to manipulate the same joint or set of joints several times.

To stop the joint lesions tightening on each other, start by straightening the joints at the mid-point between the lesions and work your way outwards and towards the lesions as per **figure PPT47**. This way, by the time you have got to the deeper lesions they will be in less conflict with each other and be easier to correct. Do not force.

Make a couple of passes on both sides of the spine and the lesions will fall away with little effort and stay in place.

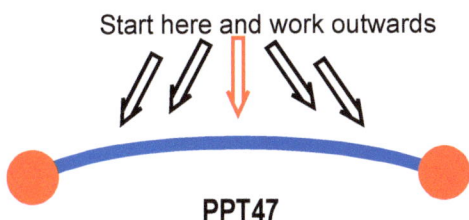

Start here and work outwards

PPT47

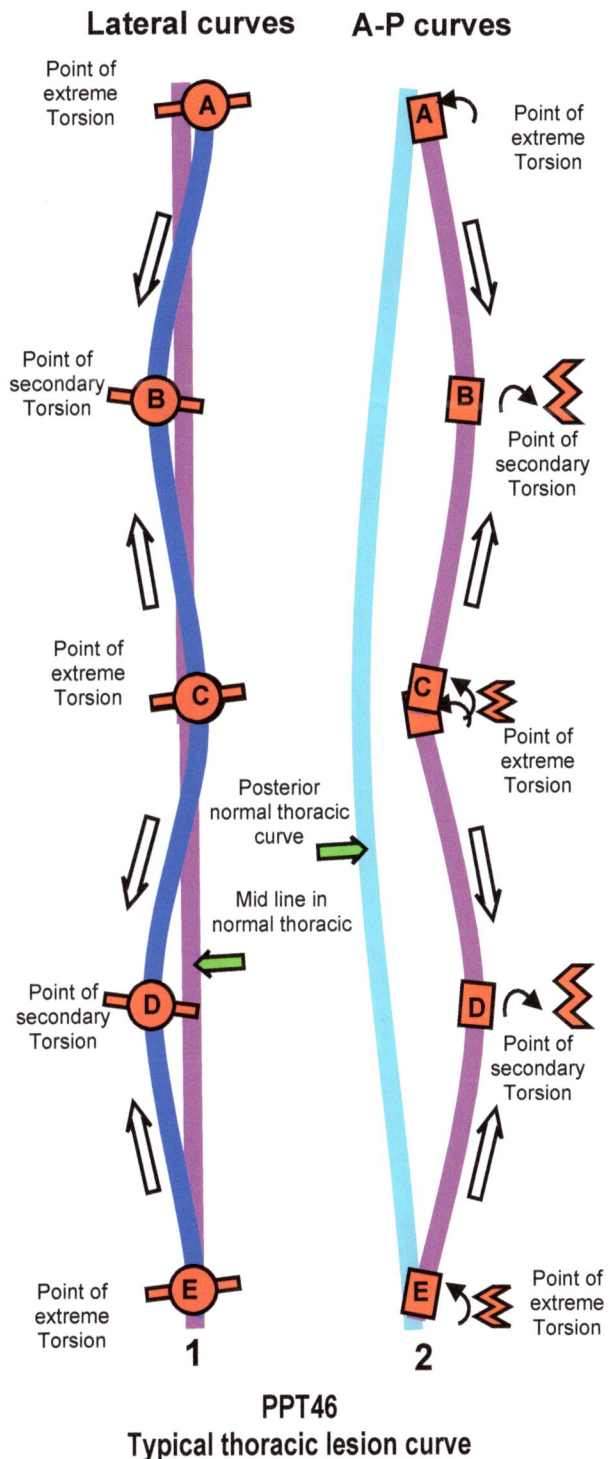

Lateral curves

Point of extreme Torsion — A

Point of secondary Torsion — B

Point of extreme Torsion — C

Posterior normal thoracic curve

Mid line in normal thoracic

Point of secondary Torsion — D

Point of extreme Torsion — E

1

A-P curves

A — Point of extreme Torsion

B — Point of secondary Torsion

C — Point of extreme Torsion

D — Point of secondary Torsion

E — Point of extreme Torsion

2

PPT46
Typical thoracic lesion curve

197

Knee Differentiation and Correction

Knee - spine differentiation

When a patient presents with a knee problem you need to be able to differentiate whether the cause is due to a knee problem or the spine.

A simple way to do this is to put your patient in a supine mid-line position as per **figure PPT 48** and rotate the knee. Test for restriction. If there is a restriction ease the knee medially and/or laterally, as shown in figure **PPT49** and then repeat the test. If the leg rotates freely in one of these positions the problem is coming from a rotated pelvis or spine.

If the source is not the spine, the problem could be due to an anterior fibular head, or an Ankle lesion.

PPT48

PPT49

PPT50

Head of fibula

Correcting an anterior fibula head

See **figure PPT50**. The fibula head is located inferior and lateral to the knee.

To correct a left knee anterior fibula head, ask your patient to side-shift their pelvis to the right. This makes the left knee malleable.

Place the thenar eminence of your right hand over the anterior border of the fibular head and apply a slight anterior pressure. Now move the knee towards the patients chest, as per **figure PPT52.** The closer you get to the chest the more malleable the knee becomes. You will feel the fibula head ease back into place with no further pressure applied to the fibula head.

Ask the patient to align their pelvis back in the mid-line and retest the knee rotation in the mid line. You should find it now rotates normally. If not check the ankle joints.

There is no thrust or click in this fibula technique. Most patient's are unaware that their fibula lesion has been corrected.

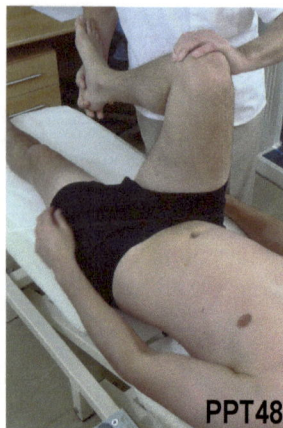

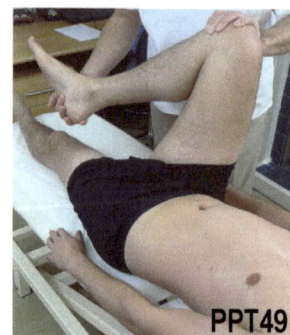

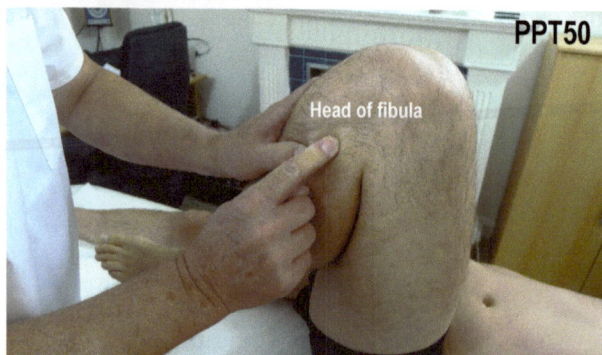

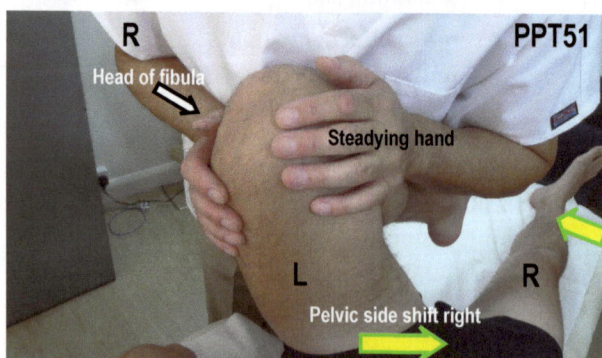

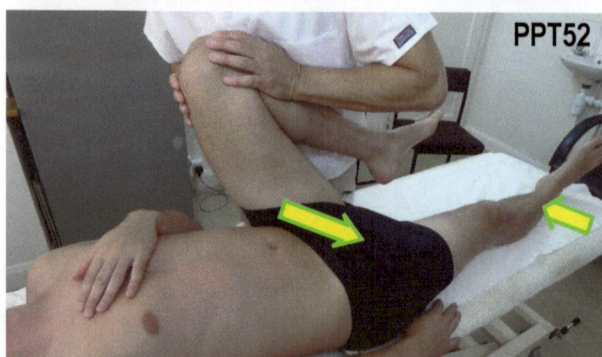

R   PPT51

Head of fibula

Steadying hand

L   R

Pelvic side shift right

PPT52

Chapter Fourteen

Physiology of the Rib Cage

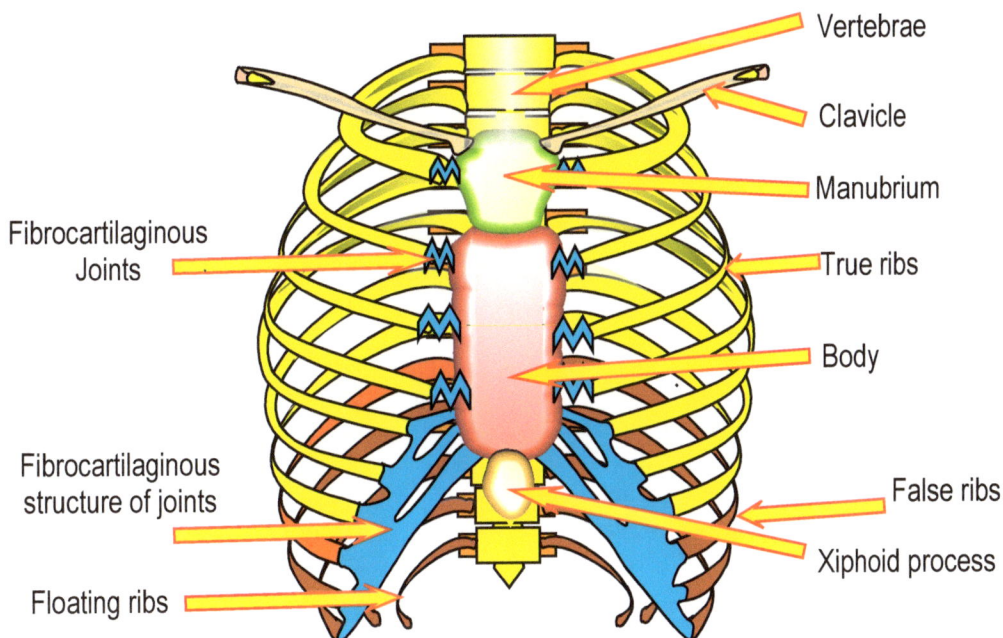

Figure 2A
The Rib Cage

Labels: Vertebrae, Clavicle, Manubrium, True ribs, Body, False ribs, Xiphoid process, Fibrocartilaginous Joints, Fibrocartilaginous structure of joints, Floating ribs

There are twenty four ribs; twelve on each side of the spine. Of these twelve, seven are called 'true' ribs and five 'false'. At their anterior the seven 'true' ribs, shown in **figure 2A** coloured yellow attach via cartilage to the Manubrium and Body and provide an element of stability to the upper vertebrae. Of the 'false' ribs, coloured red, three attach to the lowest part of the anterior rib cage via the hanging cartilage. The last two ribs (11/12) have no anterior attachment and because of this they are named, 'floating ribs'.

Names have been added to the illustration of the ribs cage in **figure 2A** for reference. In most anatomy books the height of the Manubrium is shown level with the third vertebra however, it has been lowered slightly in my illustrations to show a little more of T3.

The Xiphoid process, the Body and the Manubrium are known collectively as the Sternum.

The Rib Cage
Breathing

Breathing is a vital function of the body and the rib cage in conjunction with the diaphragm plays an important part in this function. Below is a brief recap on the action taken by the rib cage.

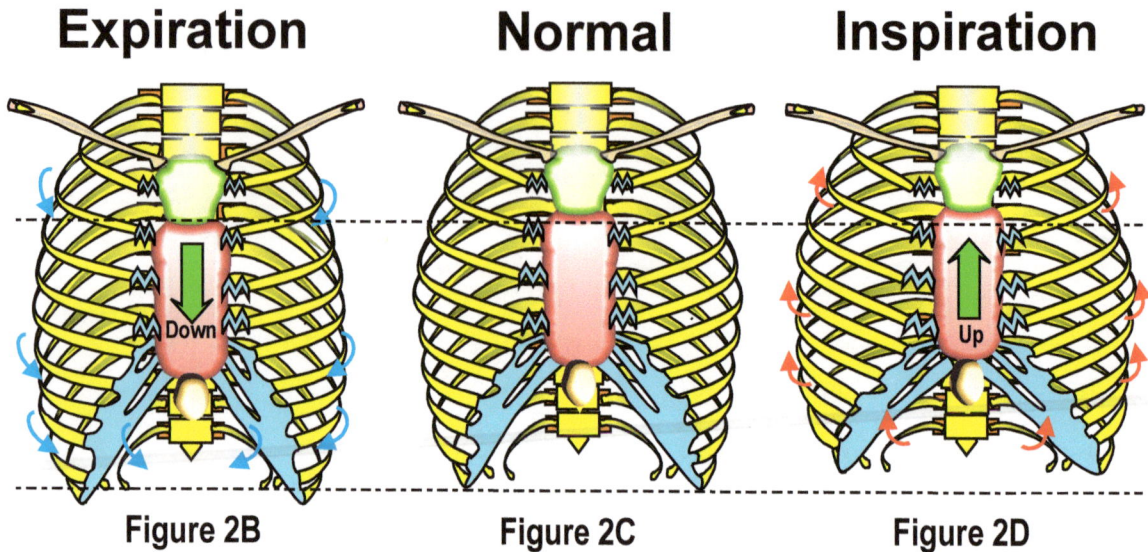

Expiration

Figure 2B

Normal

Figure 2C

Inspiration

Figure 2D

The process of breathing involves a method that has been likened to the trajectory of a bucket handle. This is shown in **figure 2E**. There are two distinct actions taking place 1) the anterior part of the rib is travelling up and down in an arc and 2) the rib itself is rotating horizontally as it completes this.

Internal muscles inspiration

External muscles expiration

Figure 2E
Rib bucket handle mechanism

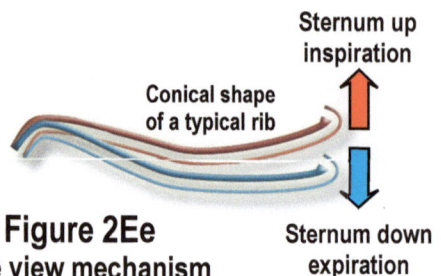

Inspiration

Figure 2D. The rib cage expands superiorly and laterally, when a person breaths in. This action is aided if the arms are raised above the head.

Expiration

Figure 2B. The rib cage contracts inferiorly and medially when a person breaths out. This action is aided if the arms are loose at the sides.

Figure 2Ee shows how the conical shape of the rib affects the rising and falling of the sternum.

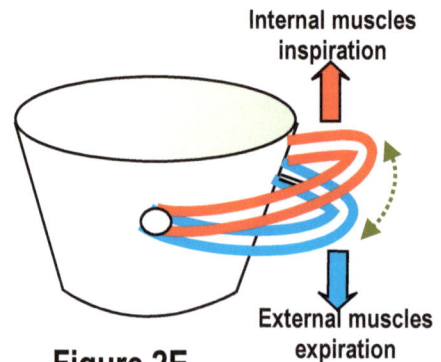

Sternum up inspiration

Conical shape of a typical rib

Sternum down expiration

Figure 2Ee
Side view mechanism

Articular Surface of a Typical T7 Rib

Working Rib Theory

For a rib theory to work, it must fulfil certain criteria. It has to make allowance for keeping the ribs level during the breathing mechanism in neutral, thoracic flexion, side-shift (side-bending) and rotation.

The detailed physiology shown in the following chapters explain how the above criteria can be satisfied.

The anterior end of a typical rib at its articulation with the costo-cartridge looks like it has been sawn through, as shown in **figures 2F** and **2G**. In contrast, the posterior end contains facets that give the surface a knobbly appearance.

There are three facets at the posterior end, shown in **figures 2G** and **2H**. Two of these facets are convex in shape and are located at the head of the rib. Their purpose is to articulate with the 'semi-dens' facets located on the bodies of the T7 and T8 vertebrae. The superior facet is angled vertically to articulate with T7 and the inferior facet is angled horizontally to articulate with T8 .

The third tubercle facet is located on the lateral posterior border of the rib. It is off-set inferio-anteriorly and convex horizontally and vertically. The facet articulates with the 'costo-transverse' facet located on the transverse process of the T7 vertebra.

The combination of these three rib joints provides the rib with the stability and the mobility it needs to perform the bucket handle breathing motion whilst in neutral, thoracic flexion, side-bending and rotation.

At the anterior end of the rib the bone fuses with fibro-cartilage which in turn fuses with the body of the sternum. This provides the 'true ribs' with large degrees of flexibility that allow superior, inferior, anterior and posterior planes of movement.

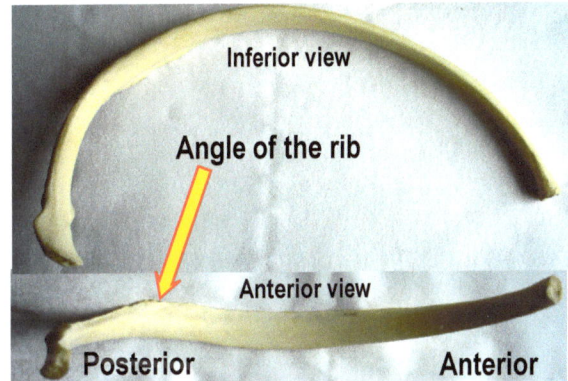

Figure 2F
Overview of a T7 rib

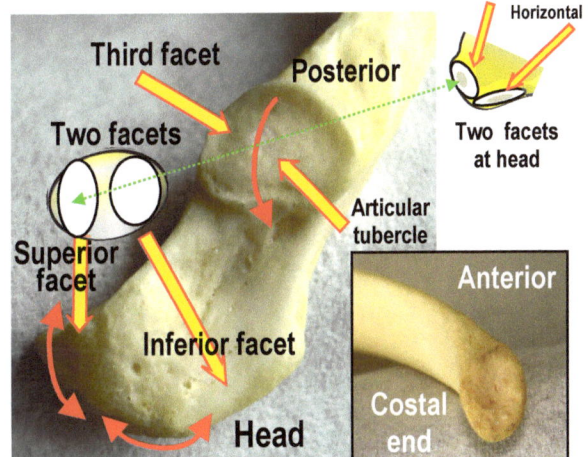

Figure 2G
Head and costal end of T7 rib

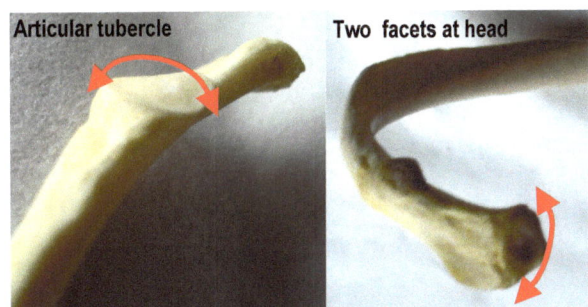

Figure 2H
Posterior facets

Articular Surface of a T1 Rib

The 1st ribs are small, wide and flat, as shown in **figures 2J and 2K**.

At the posterior end of the rib there are three facets. Two at the "head" and the third set back along the neck and off-set laterally. The latter is called the tubercle facet and is shown in **figure 2L**.

The facets at the head of the 1st rib articulate with the superior and inferior facets of the T1 and T2 vertebrae, as shown in **figure 2MA**. The 1st rib forms a canopy over the rib cage and acts as an anchor for some of the neck muscles. It would appear to play only a small role in the breathing mechanism.

Figure 2M shows the 1st rib in relation to its bony surroundings.

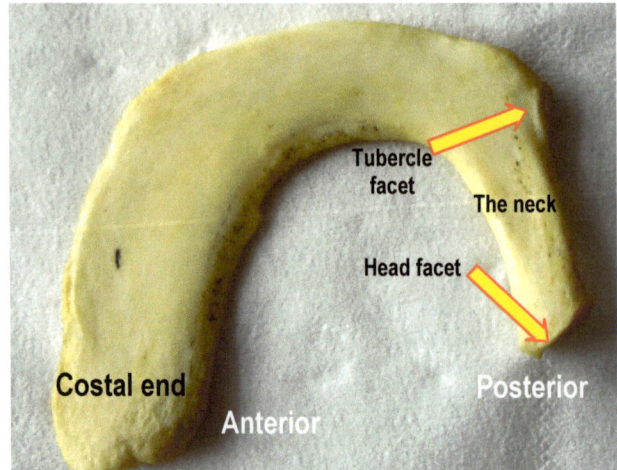

Figure 2J
Aerial view of a T1 rib

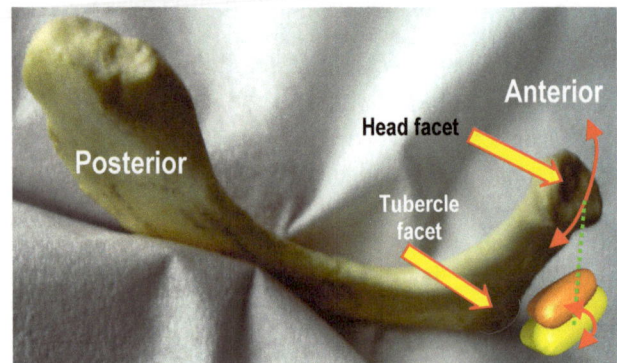

Figure 2K
Medial view of a T1 rib

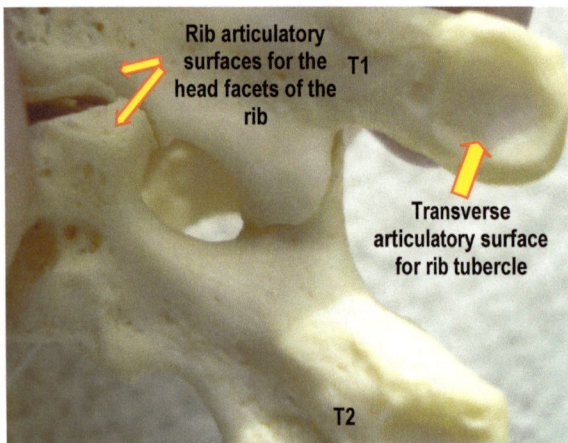

Figure 2MA
Side view of T1-T2 rib facets

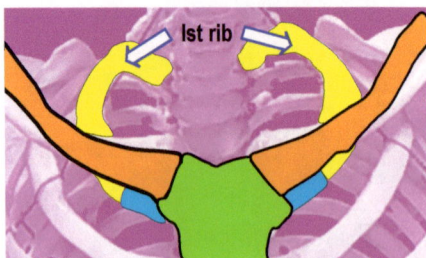

Figure 2M
Anterior view of a T1 rib

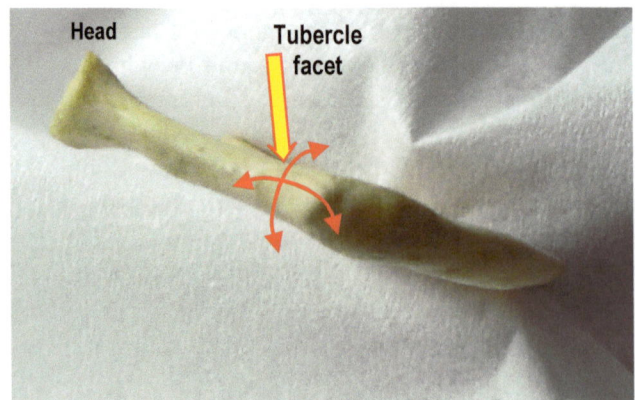

Figure 2L
Posterior view of a T1 rib

Rib Attachments to Body and Transverse Process

Figure 2N is a side-view of the demi-facets of the seventh and eighth vertebrae. Both facets are concave. The upper demi-facets of T7 are more vertical than the lower demi-facets of T8. The eighth demi-facets are predominantly horizontal. Note the proximity of the nerve.

To make it easier to visualize, the angles of the demi-facets are shown in illustration form, in **figure 2P**.

Figure 2Q is a photograph of the transverse facet. It is concave and off-set latero-medially.

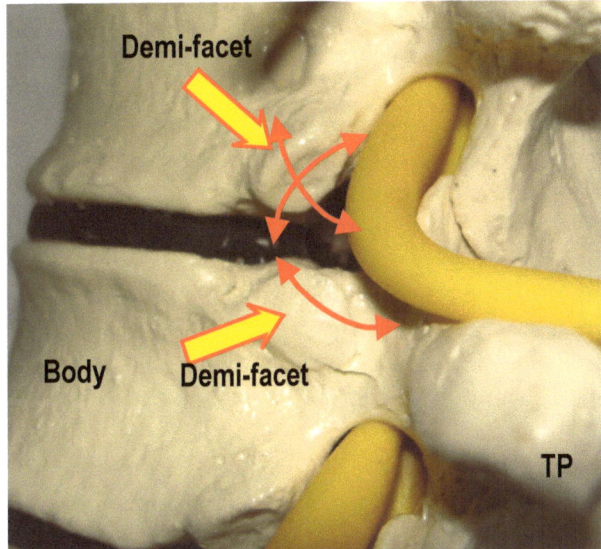

Figure 2N
Side-view of demi-facts

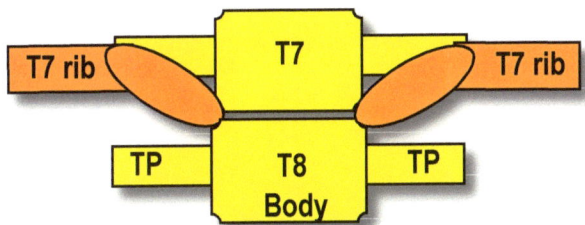

Figure 2P
Illustration of demi-facts

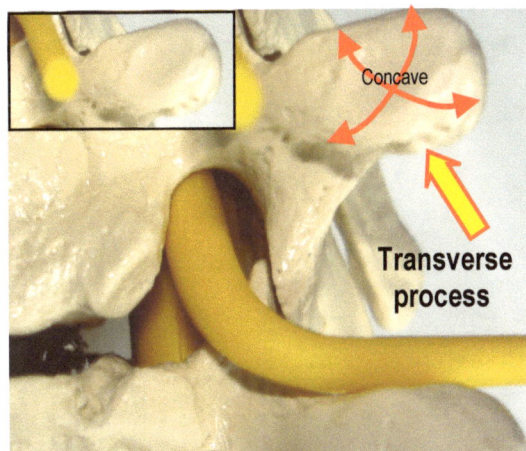

Figure 2R
Facet attachment
posterior View

The combined shape of these three facets allow the seventh rib to synchronously articulate with the seventh vertebra.

The facets are designed to accommodate the breathing action of the ribs in neutral, thoracic flexion together with rotation and side-bending (side-shift)

Figure 2R is a posterior view and illustration of how the seventh ribs attach to the seventh and eighth vertebrae.

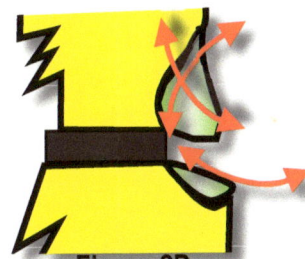

Figure 2Q
Anterior view of the T7
Transverse facet

The Rib Articulation During Breathing

Figure 2NA illustrates the articulator movements of the facets at the head and neck of a typical rib

During expiration the inferior facet at the head of the rib moves inferiorly against the demi-facet of the vertebra below, whilst swivelling superio-posteriorly over the host concave tubercle facet.

During inspiration the superior facet at the head of the rib moves superiorly against the inferior demi-facet of the host vertebra, whilst swivelling inferio-anteriorly over the tubercle facet.

Figure 2NB is a side-view and illustrates the lever effect that the change in facet position combined with muscle contraction has over the position of the ribs. Note, that the reason the rib in 'inspiration' goes up at the end is due to the conical shape of the rib, see **figure 2F**.

Figure 2ND is an aerial view of the rib cage illustrating the expansion and contraction that takes place during the breathing mechanism. This expansion and contraction is due to the conical shape of the ribs.

Figure 2NC is a horizontal cross section through three typical ribs and illustrates how the contraction of the internal and external muscles cause the ribs to behave in a similar manner to the blades of a Venetian blind.

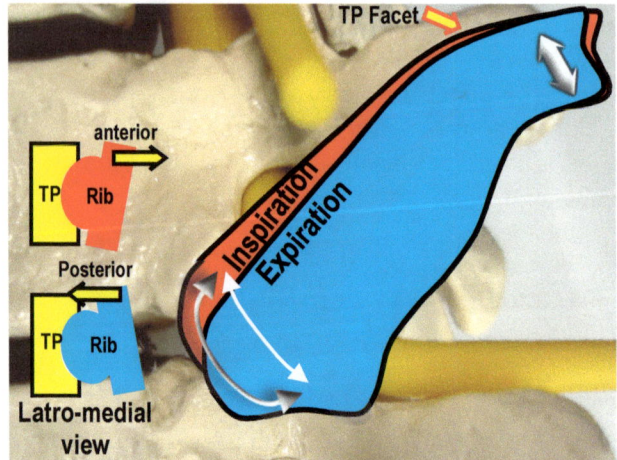

Figure 2NA
Anterior-view and cross section of the movement of a typical rib during the breathing articulation

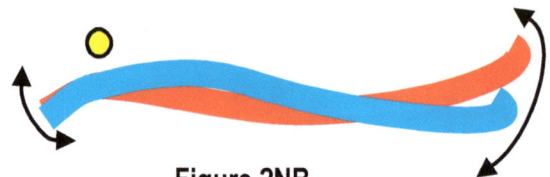

Figure 2NB
Side-view of rib trajectory during breathing

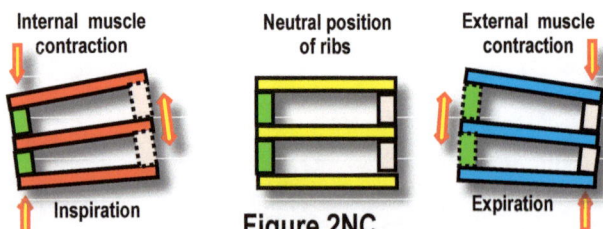

Figure 2NC
Transverse section through ribs during breathing

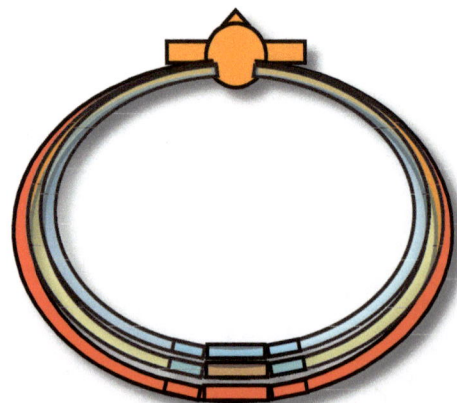

Figure 2ND
View from above of rib expansion and contraction during breathing

Rib Facet Surface Adaptation to Rotation

Figure 2S is a photograph of T7 rotating right in thoracic flexion. In order to complete this action and keep the ribs level and free for inspiration and expiration to take place, the seventh vertebra side-shifts to the right where the facets rotate right around the facets of T8. Note, breathing during thoracic rotation is not as deep as when the thoracic spine is in neutral or forward bending.

Figure 2T illustrates how the design of the demi-facets of T7 and T8 accommodate this sideways movement. In thoracic neutral or forward bending, observe that the head of the seventh rib on the right, swivels superiorly as it gets dragged along with the side-shift. Conversely the left rib swivels inferiorly against the demi-facet of T8 and counters the side-side shift. To make it easier to understand, **figure 2U** illustrates by exaggeration the shape of the demi-facets.

In reality this movement is a degree or so at the most thereby allowing the inferior and superior facets to be kept in contact with the vertebral demi-facets. One rib facet will play a more guiding role.

Figures 2V and **2W** illustrate the plane of movement the demi-facets offer to facilitate the rotational, vertical and side-ways movements of the ribs whilst they remain symmetrical and level.

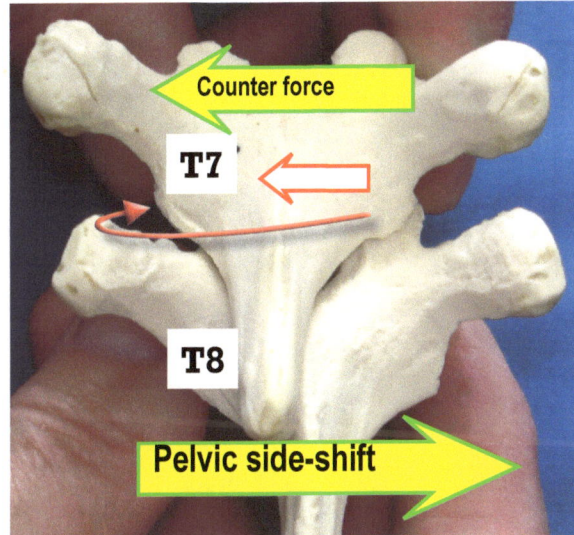

Figure 2S
Posterior view of
T7 vertebral rotation

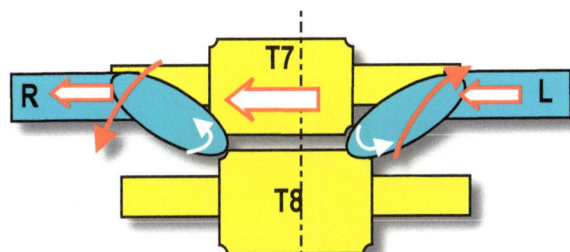

Figure 2T
Anterior view of rotation in
Neutral showing T7 rib accommodation

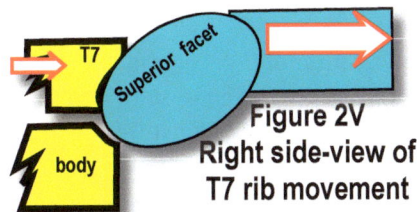

Figure 2V
Right side-view of
T7 rib movement

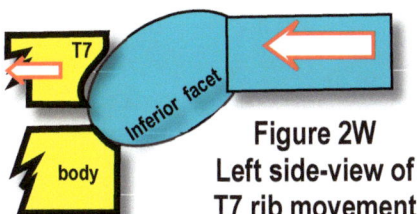

Figure 2W
Left side-view of
T7 rib movement

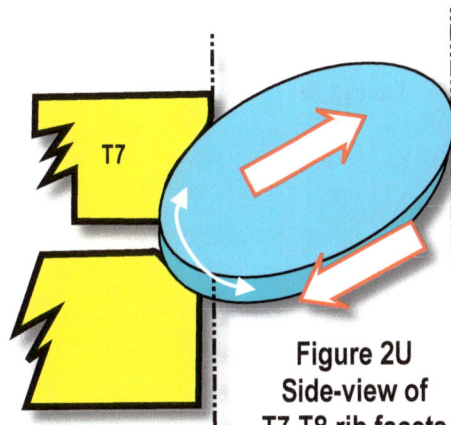

Figure 2U
Side-view of
T7-T8 rib facets

Rib Adaptations in Flexion Rotation

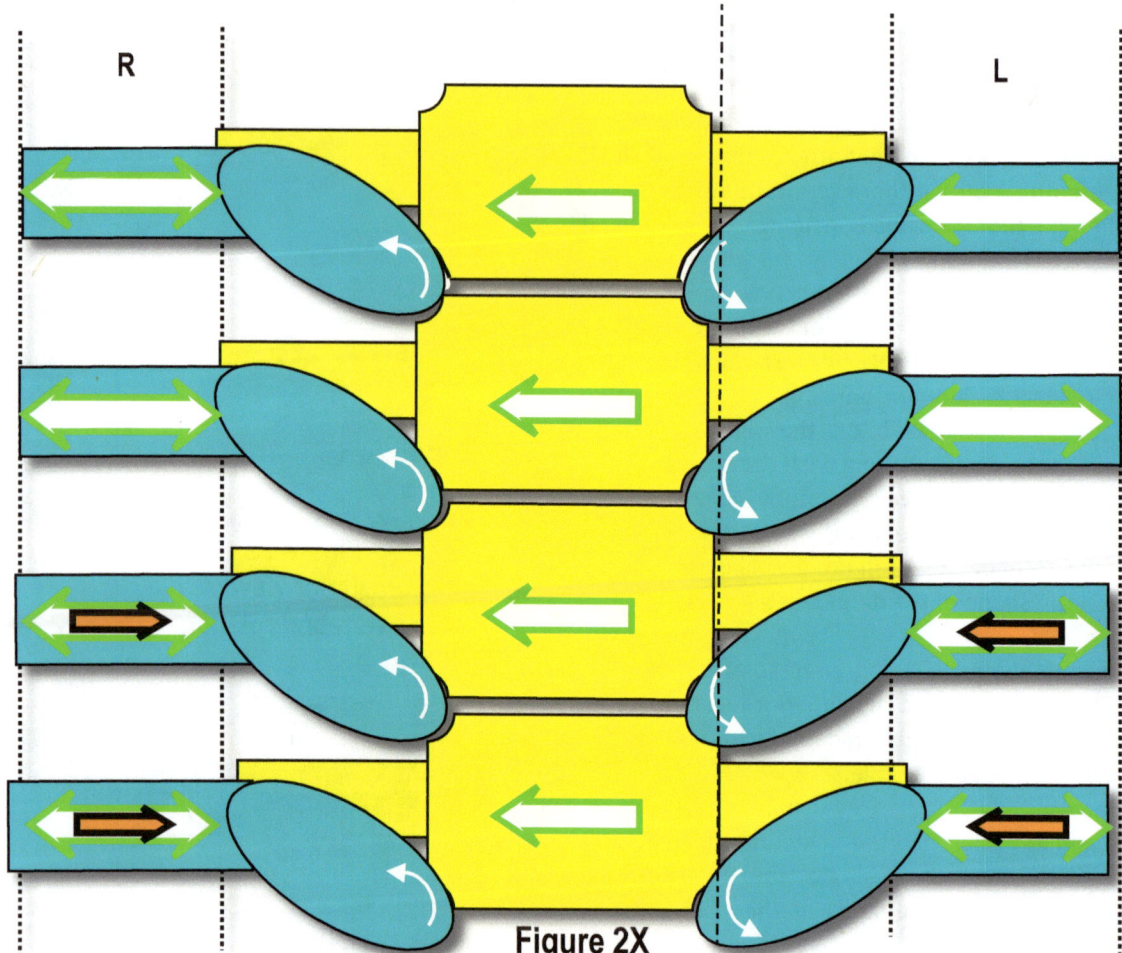

Figure 2X
Anterior view
Group flexion rotation
and rib accommodation

Figure 2X illustrates the overall positioning of the ribs and vertebrae during rotation right in thoracic flexion. Note that the ribs attempt to remain parallel and in position as the vertebrae side-bend (side-shift) and rotate. The arrows have been drawn in to represent the general counter-forces the ribs place against the vertebrae. The arrows on the previous page showed the forces the vertebrae placed on the ribs.

However, it is not possible to completely compensate for the lateral side-shift at the lower vertebrae. This is most probably one of the main reasons why false and floating ribs allow more flexibility than true ribs.

Where there is more flexibility there is more chance of problems arising and as the diaphragm attaches to the lower ribs and utilizes their increased flexibility, so the correct seating and articulation of the ribs becomes very important.

Chapter Fifteen

Physiology of the Manubrium and Clavicle

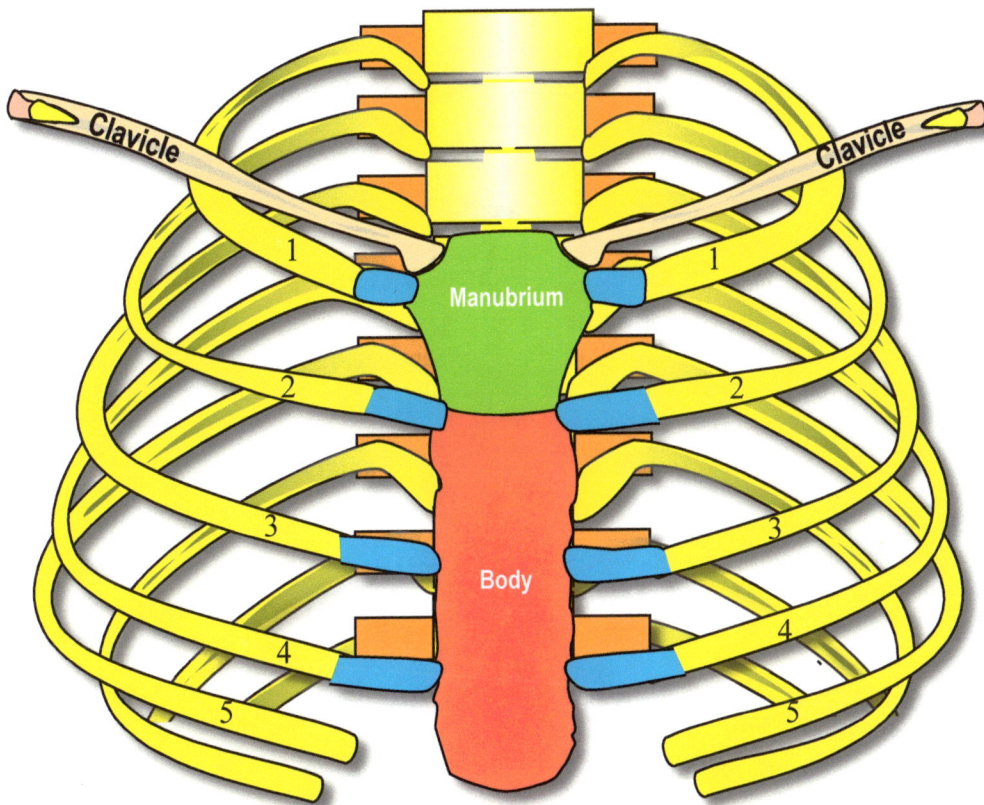

Figure 3A
Anterior view from slightly above
of the Manubrium and clavicle bones

The sternum comprises of three bones: The "Manubrium", the "Body" and the "Xiphoid process". This chapter is about the top bone, the Manubrium and its articulation with the clavicle bones, as illustrated in **figure 3A**.

The Manubrium

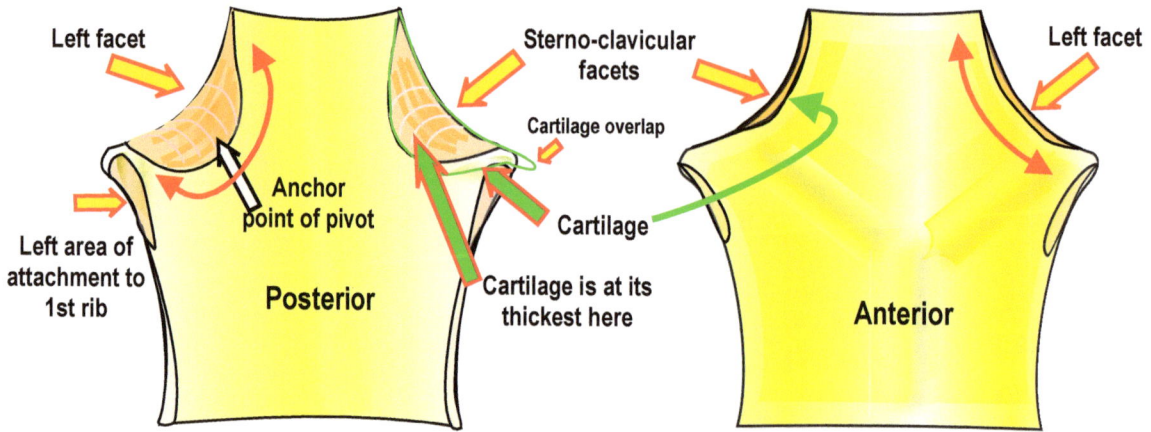

Figure 3B
Posterior and anterior views of the manubrium

Cut into the superior surface of the Manubrium there is a facet at either side, as illustrated in **figure 3B**. These facets are covered by cartilage and articulate with the sternal ends of the clavicle bones. The cartilage, shown in green, extends down the facets where it forms a slippery barrier between the clavicle and 1st rib.

The cartilage is thicker at the posterior part of the facet. Therefore, from an engineering point of view this is the most likely area for the point of pivot. See **figure 3D**.

Figure 3C shows photographs of the left side of the Manubrium and further illustrates the differences in the angles of the posterior and anterior facets. As can be seen, the posterior part of the sterno-clavicular facet slopes inferio-medially. Notice how close it is to the costal-cartilage of the 1st rib.

Figure 3D shows illustrations and a photograph of the sloping angle of the sterno-clavicular articular facets. The cross section is taken through the point of pivot shown in **figure 3B** and illustrates the convex shape of the facet.

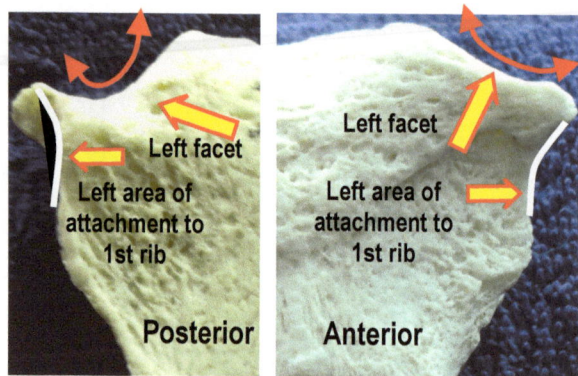

Figure 3C
Posterior and anterior views of the left side of the manubrium

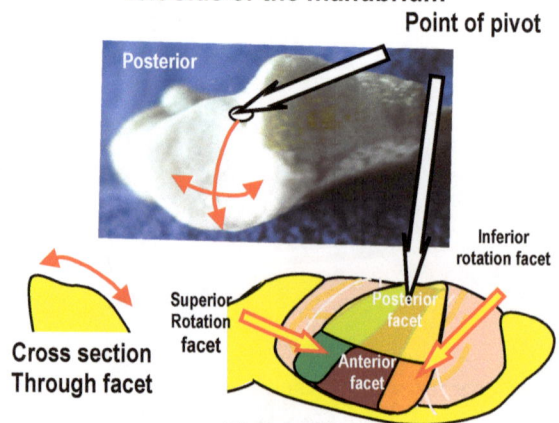

Figure 3D
Sterno-clavicular facets

The Clavicle

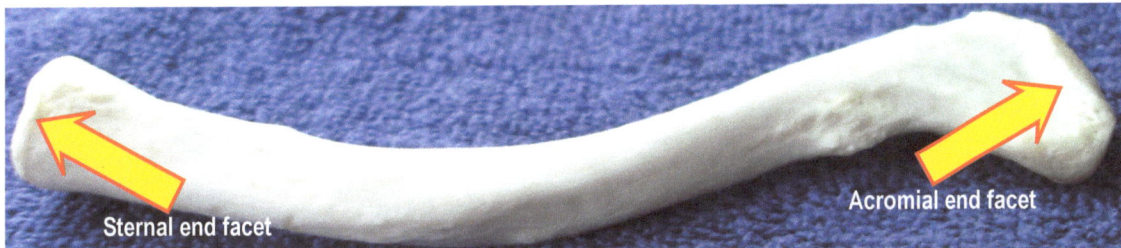

Figure 3E
Aerial view of a left clavicle

Figure 3E is an aerial view of a left clavicle bone. The clavicle has facets at either end.

The medial end articulates with the Manubrium and the lateral end with the acromial angle of the acromial process of the scapula.

Figure 3F illustrates the angles of the facet at the acromial end. Generally, the facet is inclined inferiorly and shaped like a rounded overhanging precipice, though this shape can vary. Across its anterio-posterior border it is generally convex. In some people there is a meniscus between this facet and the Acromion facet.

Figures 3G shows by illustration and photograph the complex surface contours of the clavicle facet at its sternal end.

The clavicle uses the thickened cartilage at the posterior part of the facet to anchor and pivot. This allows three basic planes of trajectory.

- The facet contours shown in illustration 'B' provide a shape that creates a sideways rocking action along the anterio-lateral and posterio-medial surface.

- The facet contours shown in photograph 'A' illustrate the swivel-like trajectory the facets follow when rotation takes place.

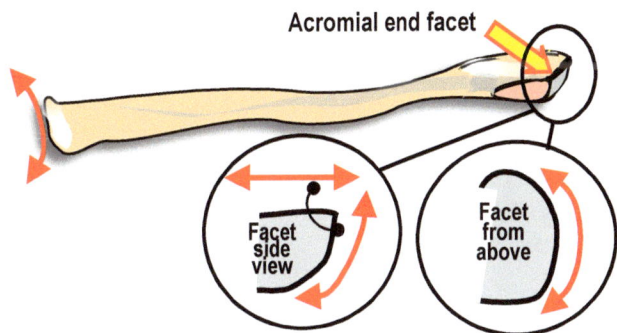

Figure 3F
Anterior view of a left clavicle

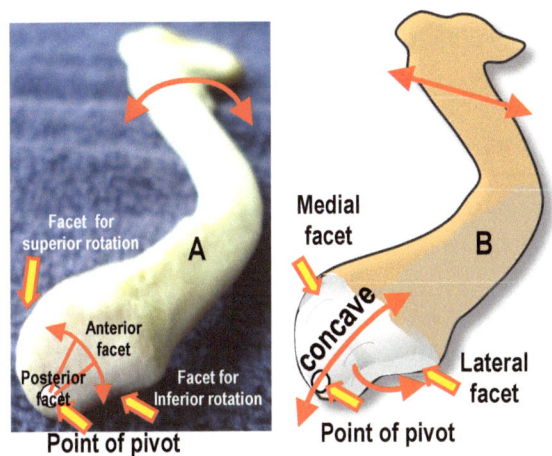

Figure 3G
View of sternal end of left clavicle

209

The Sterno-Clavicular Joint
Side-Bending and Rotation

Figure 3H shows three photographs of the sterno-clavicular joint during clavicular side-bending.

Figure 3HA shows the joint in neutral for comparison purposes.

Figure 3HB shows the plane of movement when the clavicle side-bends posterio-inferiorly. During this movement the facets of the clavicle engage at the posterior part (the pivot point) of the manubrial facet and rock in the line of the trajectory illustrated in **figure 3D**.

Figure 3HC shows the plane of movement when the clavicle side-bends anterio-superiorly. During this movement the facets of the clavicle engage at the anterior part of the manubrial facet and rock in the line of trajectory illustrated in **figure 3D**.

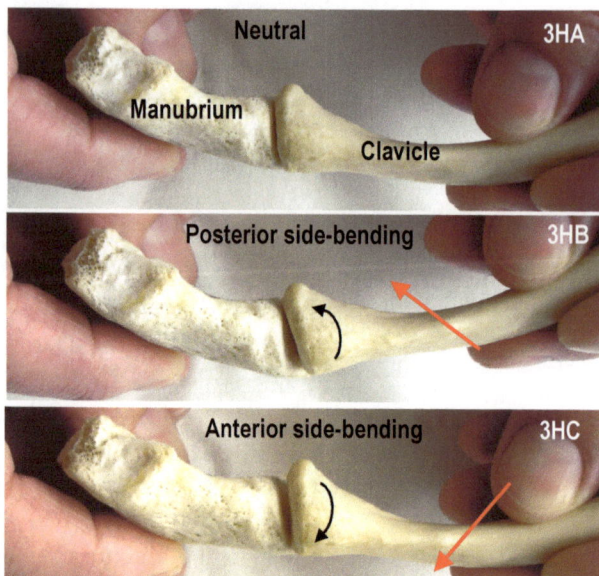

Figure 3H
View from above of the sterno-clavicular joint side-bending

Figure 3J shows three photographs of the sterno-clavicular joint during clavicular rotation. Again the same anchor point of pivot is used and works in a similar way to the axis of a singular central wind-screen wiper.

Figure 3JA shows the joint in neutral and is for comparison only.

Figure 3JB shows the plane of movement when the clavicle rotates superiorly. During this movement the facets of the clavicle rotate and slide medially over the anterior part of the manubrial facet, as shown in **figure 3D**.

Figure 3JC shows the plane of movement when the clavicle rotates inferiorly. During this movement the facets of the clavicle rotate and slide laterally over the anterior part of the manubrial facet, as shown in **figure 3D**.

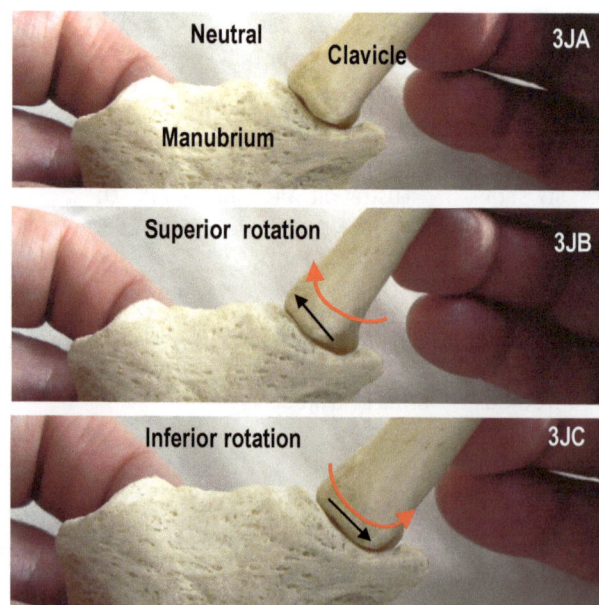

Figure 3J
Anterior view of the sterno-clavicular joint rotating

The Clavicle
Side-Bending and Rotation

This page should be read and compared with the previous page.

Figure 3K shows three photographs of the Acromion end of the clavicle during clavicular side-bending anteriorly and posteriorly.

Figure 3KA shows the joint in neutral for comparison purposes.

Figure 3KB shows the plane of movement when the posterior part of the manubrial facet is engaged. The distal end of the clavicle side-bends along an inferior-posterior plane.

Figure 3KC shows the plane of movement when the anterior part of the manubrial facet is engaged. The distal end of the clavicle side-bends along an superio-anterior plane.

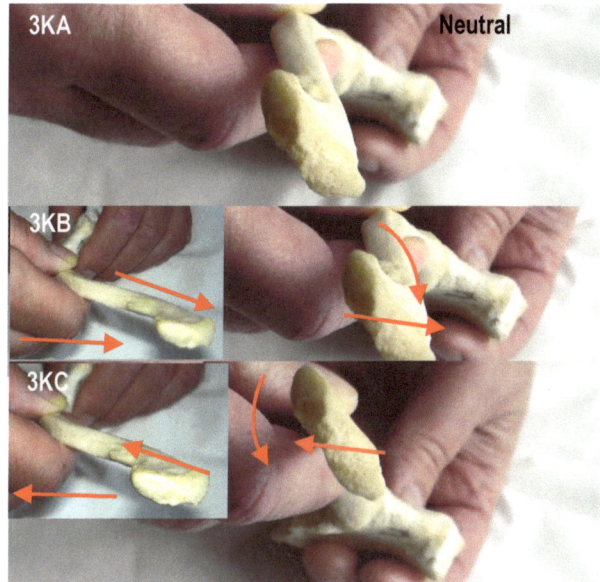

Figure 3K
Lateral view from above of the
sterno-clavicular joint side-bending

Figure 3L shows three photographs of the Acromion end of the clavicle during clavicular inferior and superior rotation.

Figure 3LA shows the joint in neutral and is for comparison only.

Figure 3LB shows the plane of movement at the distal end of the clavicle during superior rotation. During this movement the facets of the clavicle arc medially along the anterior manubrial facet. See **figure 3GA** .

Figure 3LC shows the plane of movement at the distal end of the clavicle during inferior rotation. During the movement the facets of the clavicle arc laterally along the anterior manubrial facet. See **figure 3GA**.

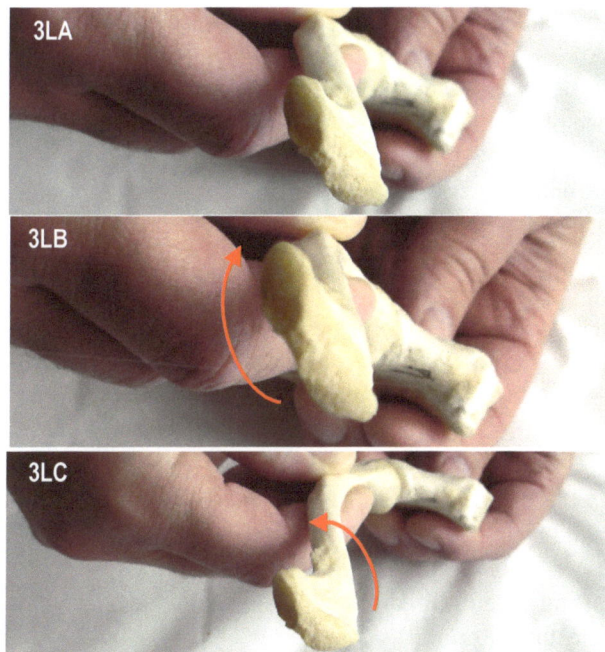

Figure 3L
Lateral view from above of the
sterno-clavicular joint rotating

Manubrium Facet in Summary

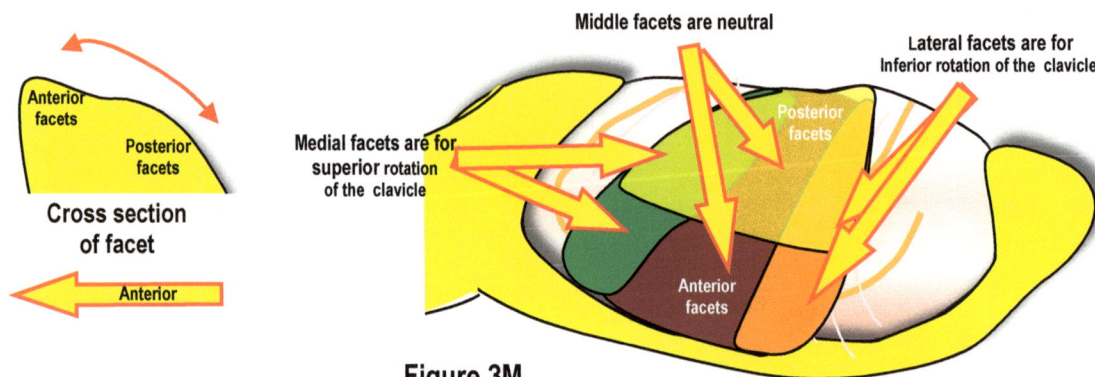

Figure 3M
The Manubrium facet surface areas

To summarize, the manubrial facets can be divided into six continuous segments:

When the clavicle engages with the middle posterior and anterior facets, the arm hangs in neutral. This means that the palmer surface of the hand will face the upper thigh.

When both the medial posterior and anterior facets are engaged the arm hangs in neutral and the palmer surface of the hand faces anteriorly.

When both the lateral posterior and anterior facets are engaged the arm hangs in neutral and the palmer surface of the hand faces posteriorly.

When the posterior middle facet is singularly engaged the arm moves in extension with the palmer surface of the hand in neutral.

When the posterior medial facet is singularly engaged the arm moves in extension with the palmer surface of the hand facing anteriorly.

When the posterior lateral facet is singularly engaged the arm moves in extension with the palmer surface of the hand facing posteriorly.

When the anterior medial facet is singularly engaged the arm moves in flexion with the palmer surface of the hand facing anteriorly.

When the anterior lateral facet is singularly engaged the arm moves in flexion with the palmer surface of the hand facing posteriorly.

Chapter Sixteen

Physiology of the Acromio-Clavicular Joint and Scapula

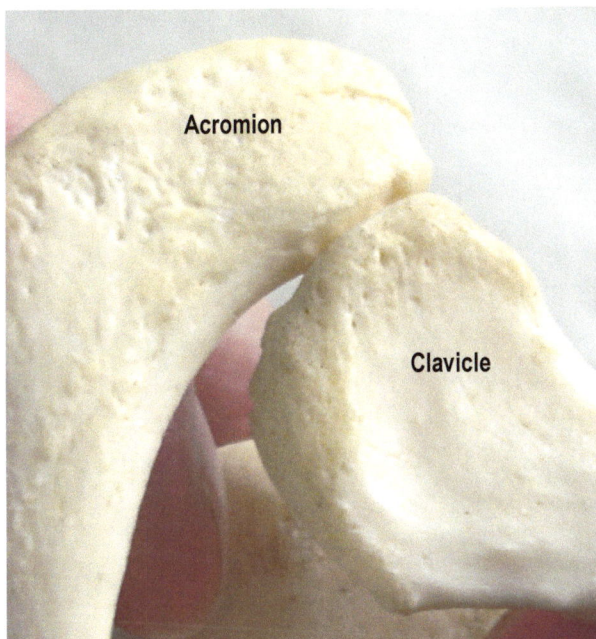

Figure 4A
Aerial view of
the sterno-clavicular joint

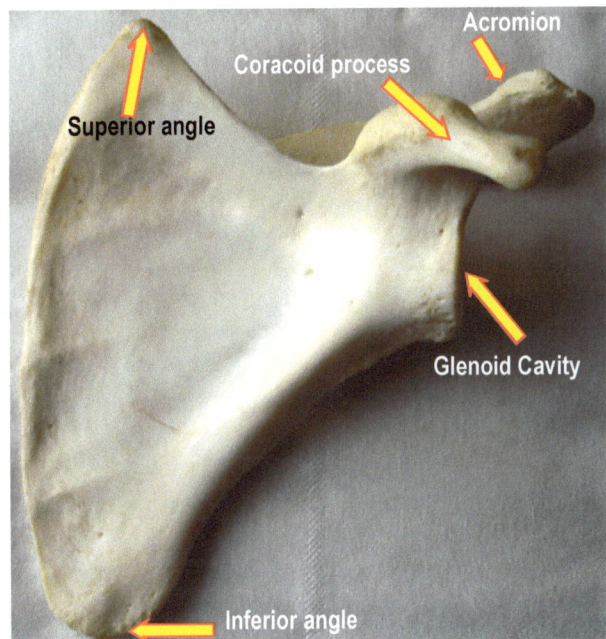

Figure 4B
Anterior view of
scapula

The acromio-clavicular joint, as shown in **figure 4A** is simple and multi-purpose. The articulation of the joint provides an anterio-posterior arc together with superio-inferior rotation of the scapula.

For reference purposes **Figure 4B** is an anterior photograph of a left scapula. The scapula is 'strapped' to the body by muscles which provide it with considerable mobility. It makes physical joint contact with the lateral end of the clavicle at the sterno-clavicular joint and with the head of the humorous at the gleno-humeral joint.

Overview of the
Acromio-Clavicular Ligament

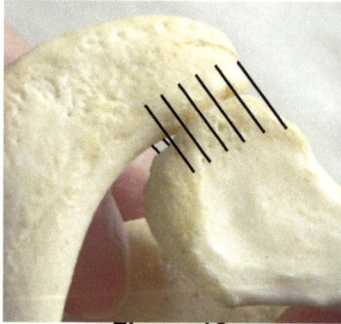

Figure 4C
Aerial view of
The sterno-clavicular
ligaments

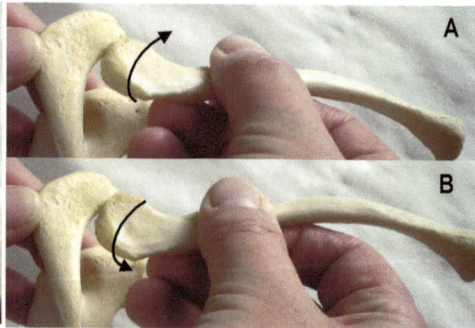

Figure 4D
Aerial view of
The sterno-clavicular joint
incorrect rotation

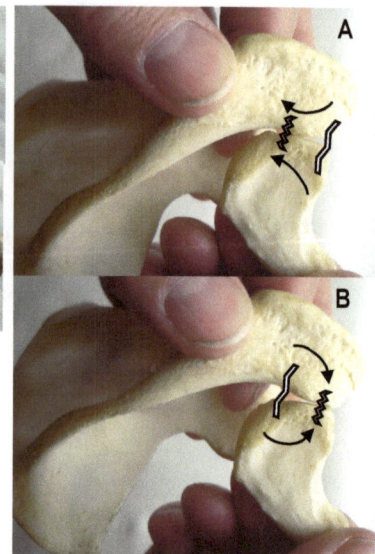

Figure 4E
Aerial view of
The sterno-clavicular joint
horizontal side-bending

Although the acromio-clavicular articular facets and ligaments look simple they are very cleverly designed and provide a dual function. The fibres of the coraco-clavicular ligaments run in a medial to lateral direction, above and below the joint, as shown in **figure 4C**. With such a ligament configuration, obvious rotation as that shown in **figures 4D A** and **B** would have the ligaments at a disadvantage and lead to a buckling of the joint. Nature would be unlikely to have allowed this type of vulnerability to have evolved. Therefore, it can be deduced that this is not the way the acromio-clavicular accommodates arm rotation.

Figure 4E, **A** and **B** illustrate how the ligaments make allowance for a horizontal side-bending swivel type action. This action is required when the arm moves along an anterio-superior (flexion) or inferio-posterior (extension) plane of direction. As can be seen, this movement fits in perfectly with the line of the ligaments.

Figure 4F, **A** and **B** illustrate how the line of the ligament fibres make allowance for vertical side-bending. It will be explained later in this chapter why vertical side-bending is integral to arm rotation.

In summary, the position of the ligament and the line of its fibres accommodate both side-bending horizontally and vertically, either independently, or at the same time.

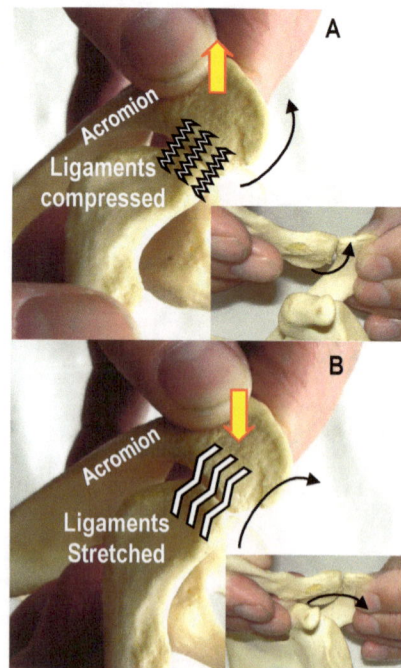

Figure 4F
Aerial view of
The sterno-clavicular joint
vertical side-bending

Acromio-clavicular Joint Movements

Figures 4GA, B and **C** illustrate the action that takes place at the acromio-clavicular joint during arm movements.

Figure 4GA shows the joint in neutral. When the arm is in neutral the arm and hand hang at the side of the body with the palmer surface of the hand facing the thigh.

Figure 4GB shows the joint in extension. The arm and hand with the palmer surface facing medially moves posteriorly and medially. The scapula moves inferiorly and posteriorly drawing the lateral end of clavicle along with it in the same plane. At the apex of this movement the anterior section of the acromio-clavicular joint side-bends open.

Figure 4GC shows the joint in flexion. The arm and hand with the palmer surface facing medially moves anteriorly, laterally and superiorly. The scapula moves superiorly and anteriorly drawing the lateral end of the clavicle along with it in the same plane. At the apex of this movement the posterior section of the acromio-clavicular joint side-bends open.

Figure 4HA illustrates the acromio-clavicular joint in neutral.

Figure 4HB illustrates the Acromion side-bending in a vertical plane inferiorly when the arm is extended.

Figure 4HC illustrates the Acromion side-bending in a vertical plane superiorly when the arm is flexed.

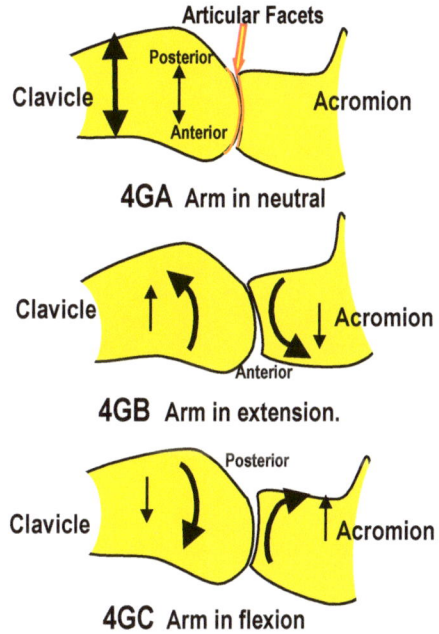

4GA Arm in neutral

4GB Arm in extension.

4GC Arm in flexion

Figure 4G
Aerial view of the right sterno-clavicular joint showing horizontal side-bending

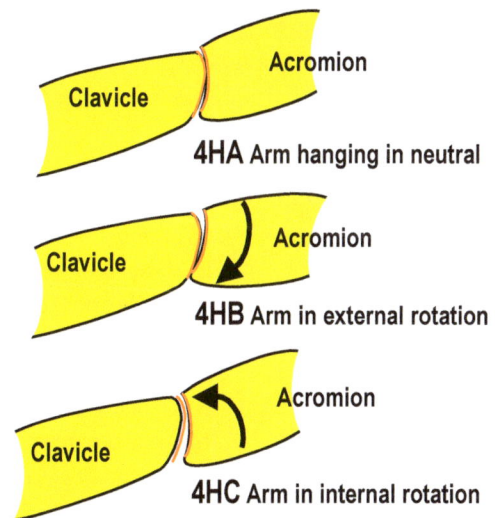

4HA Arm hanging in neutral

4HB Arm in external rotation

4HC Arm in internal rotation

Figure 4H
Anterior view of the right sterno-clavicular joint showing vertical side-bending

Arm Rotation and the Scapula

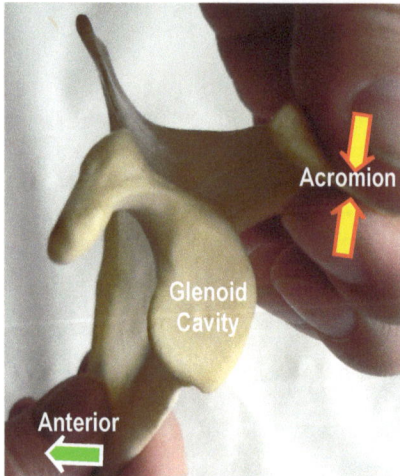

Figure 4J
Side-view of
the scapula in neutral

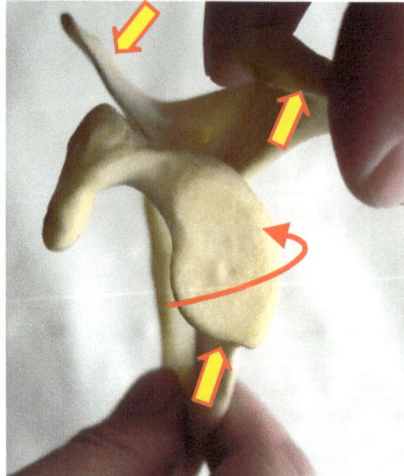

Figure 4K
Side-view of
the scapula in external rotation

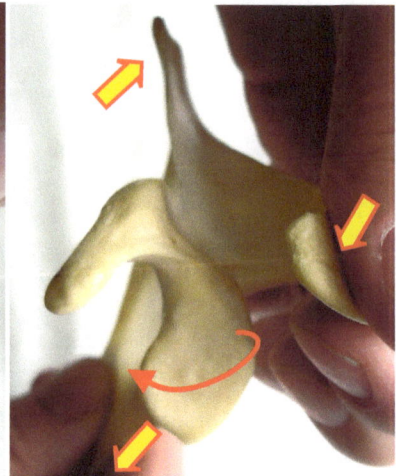

Figure 4L
Side-view of
the scapula in internal rotation

Try this experiment: Let your arm hang loose at your side, in neutral. Be aware of the height of your shoulder and make finger tip contact with your thigh. If you internally rotate your hand your finger tips and shoulder will move inferiorly. If you externally rotate your arm your shoulder and fingers will move superiorly. Most arm rotation comes from the gleno-humeral joint. However, the scapula also has an important role to play in these movements.

Figure 4 M is a side-view of the glenoid cavity and the Acromion. Note that the angle of the Acromion is off-set. Therefore, superio-lateral and inferio-medial rotational movements at the acromio-clavicular joint will produce superior and inferior rotational movements at the glenoid cavity.

These rotational movements are illustrated in **figures 4J**, **4K** and **4L**. When gleno-humeral and acromio-clavicular rotation has taken place; further rotation takes place at the sterno-clavicular joint.

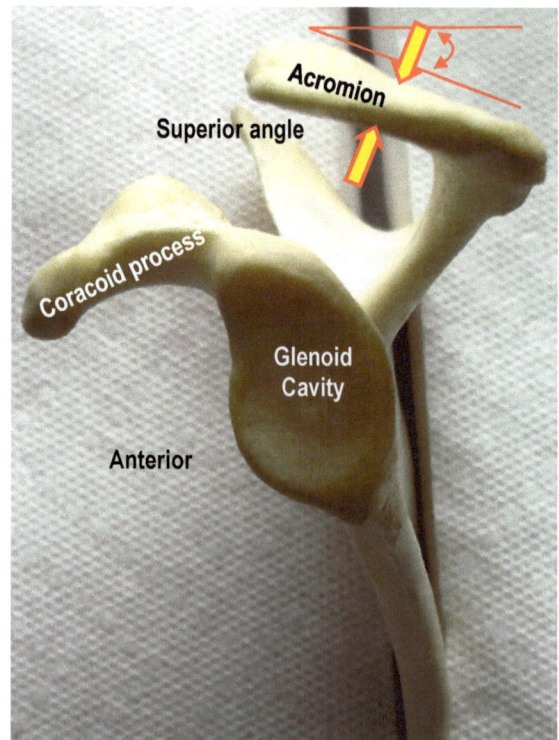

Figure 4M
Side-view of
the scapula

216

Chapter Seventeen

Rib Cage and Clavicle Lesions

Ribs can become subluxated in either inspiration or expiration, as illustrated in **figures TSHa,b** and **c,** and **TSEa, b** and **c.**

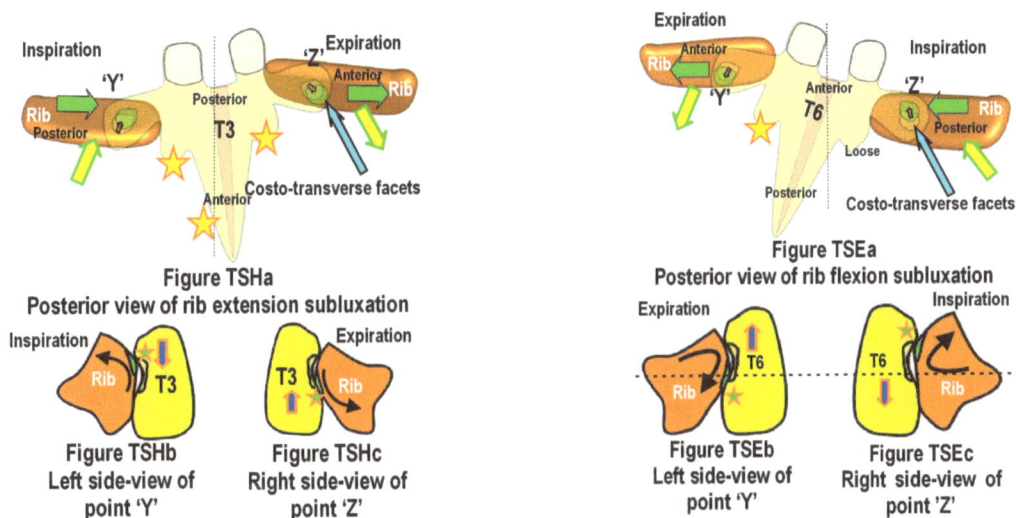

Figure TSHa
Posterior view of rib extension subluxation

Figure TSHb
Left side-view of point 'Y'

Figure TSHc
Right side-view of point 'Z'

Figure TSEa
Posterior view of rib flexion subluxation

Figure TSEb
Left side-view of point 'Y'

Figure TSEc
Right side-view of point 'Z'

Because ribs move in a similar way to the blades of a Venetian blind it only takes one blade to lock and go out of alignment, as shown in **figure 5A**, to cause the surrounding blades to become entangled and displaced. If more than one blade locks and goes out of alignment, the disarray as will be shown later in this chapter, will cause the rib cage and sternum to distort.

This could theoretically effect the efficiency of the breathing mechanism and would definitely distort the symmetry and therefore, the efficiency of the shoulder girdle.

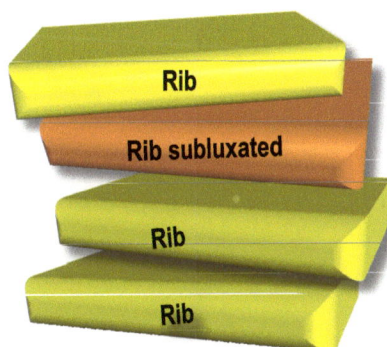

Figure 5A
Illustration of rib misalignment

Rib Displacements in Flexion and Extension

Figures 5AA and **5AAA** illustrate the facet positioning within a flexion lesion. The right 7th rib, shown in red, is pulled superiorly and away from the demi-facets with a consequent loss of stability. The reason it is pulled laterally is due to the pull of the ligaments at the transverse facet of T7. If it were not for these ligaments the rib would dislocate. The left rib, shown in blue is pushed inferiorly and becomes lodged against the superior demi-facet of T8. This entrapment locks the rib and causes a band of rib rigidity around that side of the torso.

Figures 5AB and **ABA** illustrate the positions of the 7th ribs lesioned in extension. Extension subluxations are more serious than flexion lesions because two violations of the thoracic laws of movement take place.

1) The vertebra rotates in the opposite direction to that intended while at the same time compressing the lesioned vertebra against its neighbour below.

2) The compression placed on the ribs leaves no room to manoeuvre. Therefore, when side-shift takes place the ribs on either side of T7 are pushed into the side of the demi-facets where they lock. This locking results in a band of rigidity around the trunk far more rigid than that found in ribs lesioned in thoracic flexion.

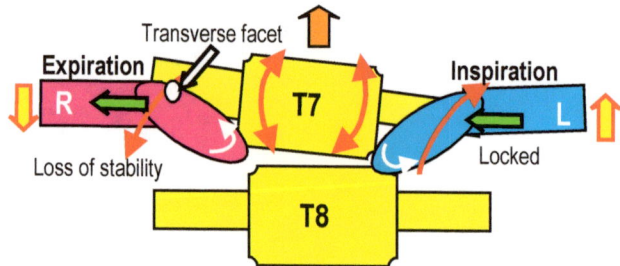

Figure 5AA
Anterior view of rotation left within flexion subluxation showing T7 rib displacement

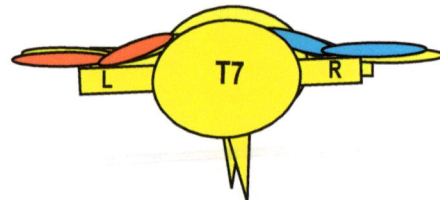

Figure 5AAA
Aerial view of rotation left in flexion subluxation showing T7 rib displacement

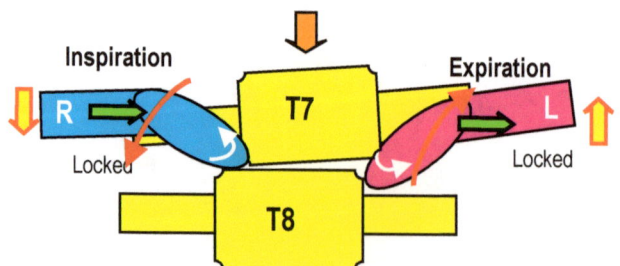

Figure 5AB
Anterior view of rotation right within extension subluxation showing T7 rib displacement

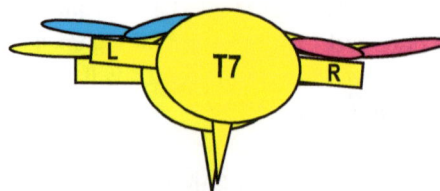

Figure 5ABA
Aerial view of rotation right with in extension subluxation showing T7 rib displacement

Rib Displacements in Flexion and Extension

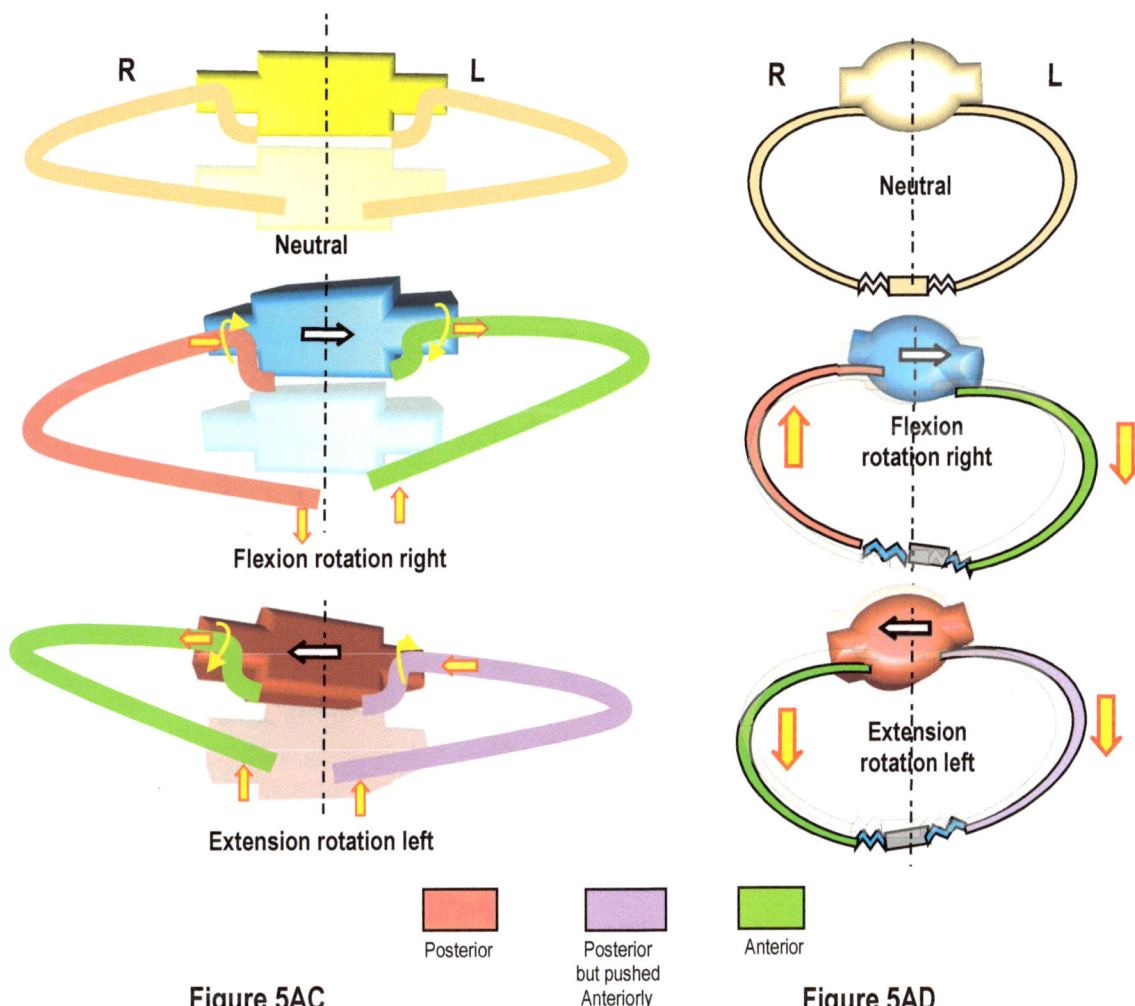

Neutral

Flexion rotation right

Extension rotation left

Neutral

Flexion rotation right

Extension rotation left

| Posterior | Posterior but pushed Anteriorly | Anterior |

Figure 5AC
Anterior view of rib distortions in
flexion and extension

Figure 5AD
Aerial view of rib distortions in
flexion and extension

Figures 5AC and **5 AD**, which are self-explanatory, show the extent to which the ribs become distorted when certain vertebrae become subluxated. The distortions have been exaggerated for clarity, nevertheless they are not as far from reality as it may at first seem.

Above; these distortions will affect the alignment of the sternum and therefore the general symmetry of the rib cage and have implications for the correct seating and alignment of the clavicle.

Below; these distortions have serious consequences regarding the efficiency of the diaphragm.

Rib Cage Distortions in the L3-Right-Right Lesion Pattern

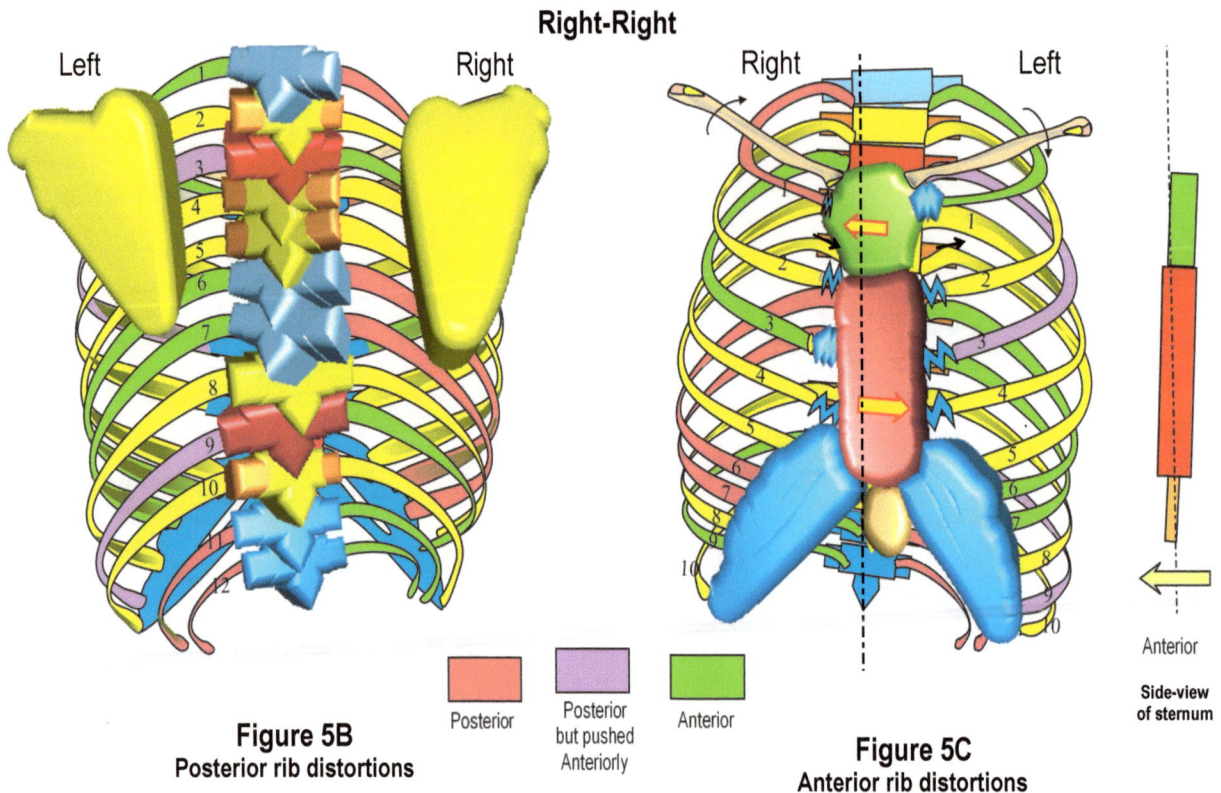

Figure 5B
Posterior rib distortions

Figure 5C
Anterior rib distortions

The illustrations above are based upon the concluded lesion pattern. The red ribs are those that lesioned and became levered posteriorly. The purple ribs are those that should be posterior but due to the angle of the corresponding vertebral transverse process become levered anteriorly. The green ribs are those that became levered anteriorly.

Figure 5B shows the lesion pattern and the effect this pattern inflicts on the rib cage. It looks grossly distorted with obvious general rotation to the left and oblique side-bending that splits the rib cage at T8. When I first drew this I thought that it must be a mistake but when I compared it to the L3-right-right model it fitted exactly.

Figure 5C shows the lesion pattern and the effect the ribs lesion have on the sternum. Note that the sternum has become side-sifted to the right around the inferior ribs and to the left at the Manubrium. It has also incurred an element of rotation to the right.

This displacement has a direct effect on the seating of the clavicle bones and therefore has implications for the alignment and efficiency of the shoulder joints.

Rib Cage Distortions in the L3-Right-Right Lesion Pattern

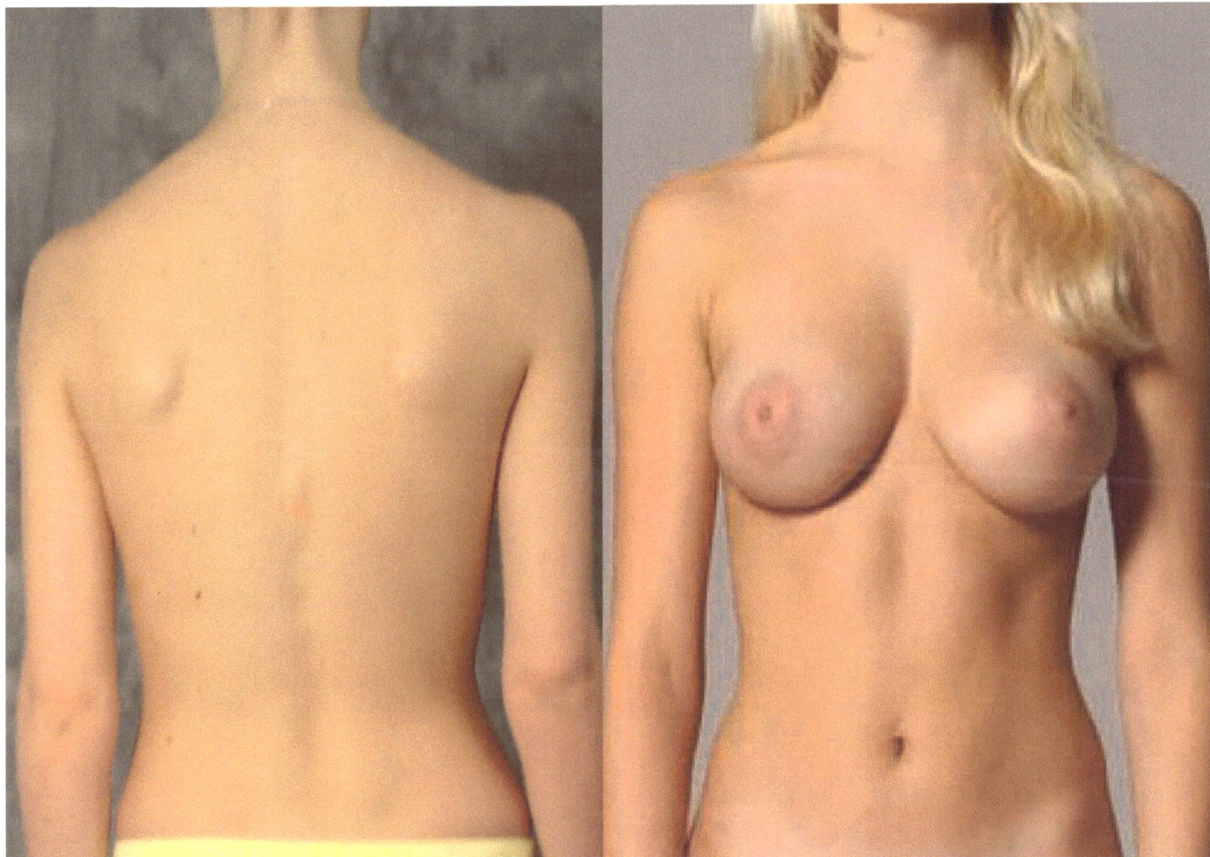

Figure 5D
Posterior rib distortions

Figure 5E
Anterior rib distortions

Compare the above photographs with the illustrations on the previous page and a marked similarity can be seen.

Look particularly at the waist lines of both women. Remember, the diaphragm attaches to this area and so it is of particular importance.

Observe the protruding clavicle on the right in **figure 5E** and how it squares and tightens the shoulder posteriorly. This posterior pull causes the right arm to be drawn backwards and the elbow to flex.

Rib Cage Distortions in the L3-Left-Right Lesion Pattern

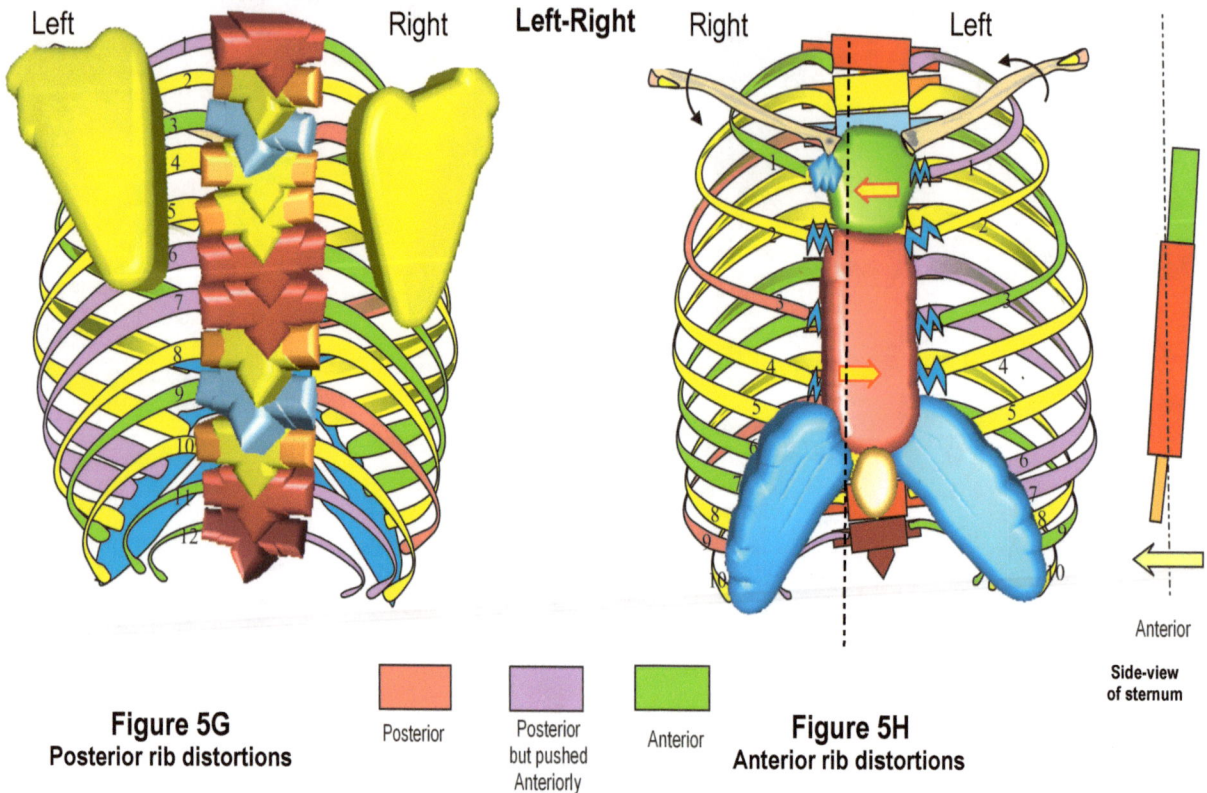

Figure 5G
Posterior rib distortions

Posterior | Posterior but pushed Anteriorly | Anterior

Figure 5H
Anterior rib distortions

Side-view of sternum

The illustrations above are based upon the concluded lesion pattern. The red ribs are those that sub-lesioned and became levered posteriorly. The purple ribs should be posterior but due to the angle of the corresponding vertebral transverse process became levered anteriorly. The green ribs are those that became levered anteriorly.

Figure 5G shows the lesion pattern and the effect this pattern inflicts on the rib cage. It looks distorted with obvious general rotation to the left and oblique side-bending that splits the rib cage at T8. This illustration fits exactly with the L3-left-right model.

Figure 5B shows the lesion pattern and the effect the rib lesions have on the sternum. Note that the sternum has side-sifted and side-bent to the left. It has also incurred an element of rotation to the left.

This displacement has a direct effect on the seating of the clavicle bones and therefore has implications for the alignment and efficiency of the shoulder joints.

Rib Cage Distortions in the L3-Left-Right Lesion Pattern

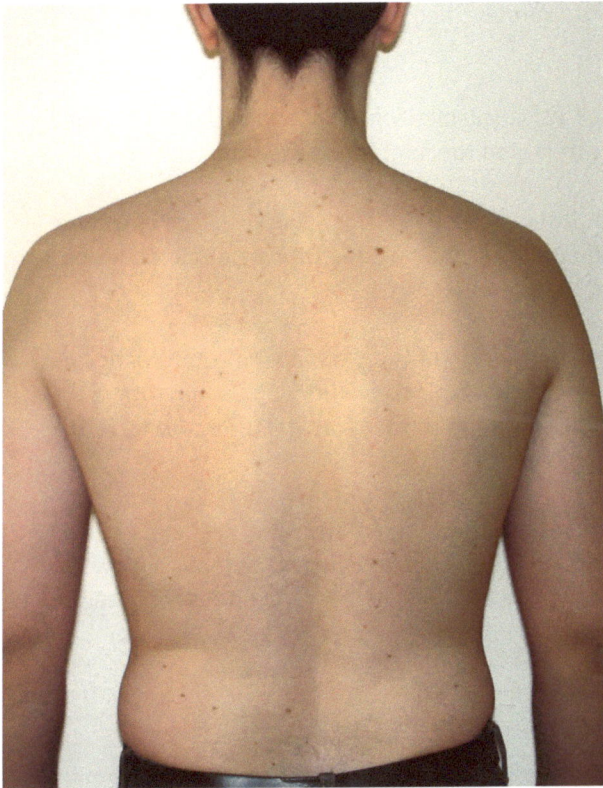

Figure 5J
Posterior rib distortions

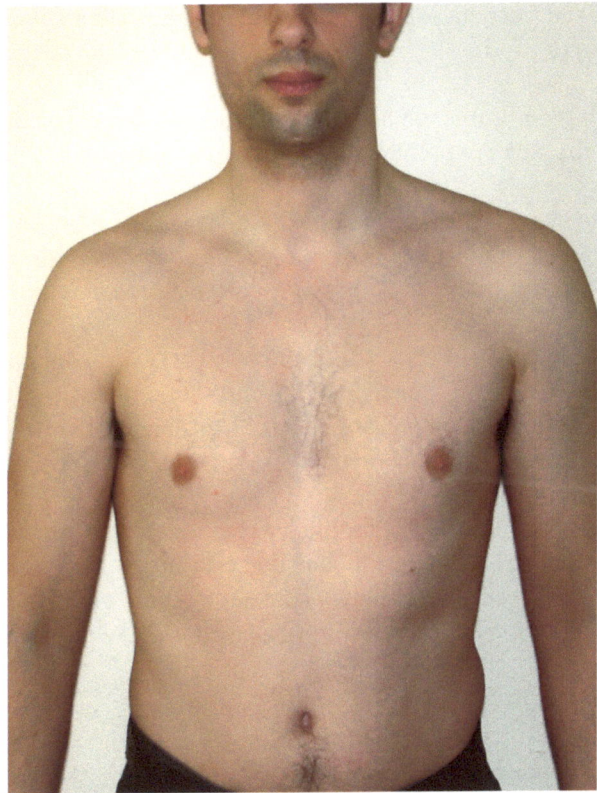

Figure 5K
Anterior rib distortions

Compare the photographs above with the illustrations on the previous page and a marked similarly can be seen.

Look particularly at Dan's waist line. The diaphragm attaches to this area and so this distortion is of particular importance.

Compare **figure 5k** with **figure 5E** on page 217 and notice how the mid-line of the rib cage side-bends and rotates to the left in the L3-left-right pattern and how it side-bends and rotates to the right in the L3-right-right pattern.

In the photographs of all the models they are standing on both legs with their feet in alignment.

Direct Trauma to Ribs

Ribs can become subluxated by other causes than spinal misalignment and for completeness this has been included.

From the chapters on how the thoracic vertebrae articulate, it was explained why thoracic backward bending and rotation are prohibited in normal physiology and why if attempted the joint/s and rib/s subluxate.

Some everyday tasks can put extreme levering forces on the ribs and cause them to severely lesion. This type of trauma can result in extreme sharp pain and breathing difficulties for the person. Direct trauma rib lesions can occur in both inhalation, which is the more common, and exhalation.

To recap on the mechanics, in thoracic backward bending if the intension of the person is to rotate right, the thoracic vertebrae depending on their integrity at the time will either block this movement or rotate the vertebrae to the opposite side, left.   This means that any forced rotation to the right will lever and force the ribs in a non-physiological manner that risks their severe lesion.

As the arms are usually the guiding rotational force, rib trauma subluxations tend to be found higher up the rib cage, between T7 and T1. They do occur below this at around T9-T10 but are much less common. Below are some photographs of Lindsey completing some of the everyday tasks that people regularly do that can lead to direct trauma rib lesions.   They all involve backward leaning and rotation.

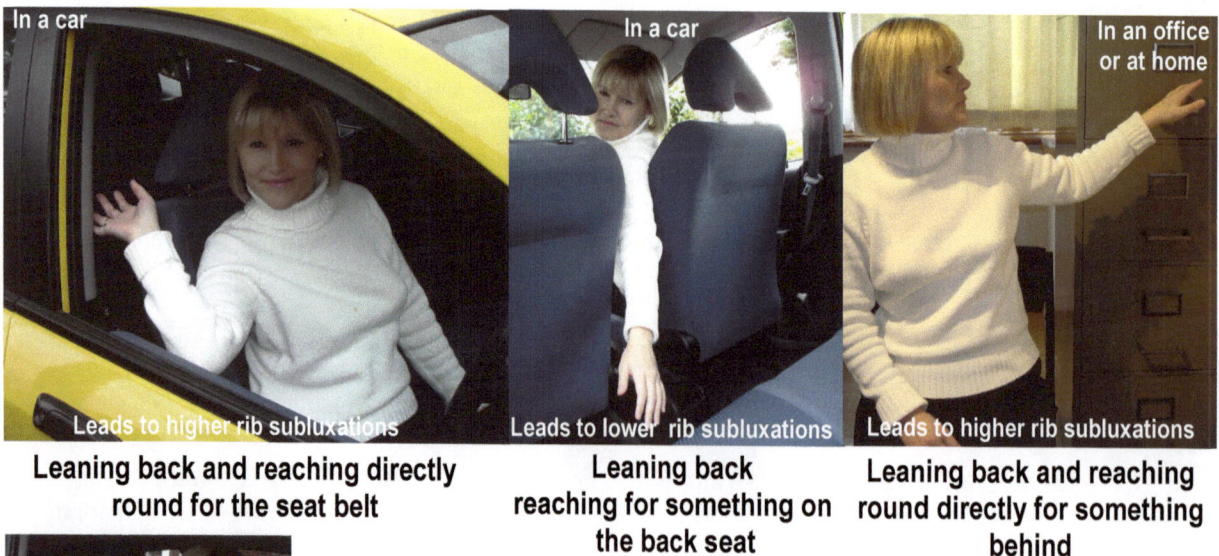

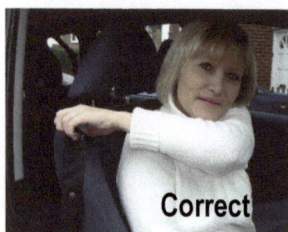

Leaning back and reaching directly round for the seat belt

Leaning back reaching for something on the back seat

Leaning back and reaching round directly for something behind

Showing how to put a seat belt on. Lean forward and bring the furthest arm round.

Clavicle Misalignments

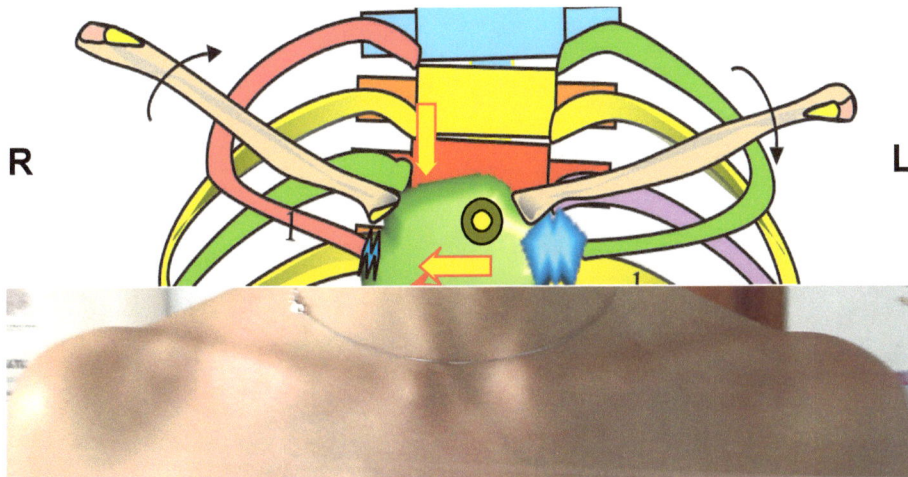

Figure 5L
Clavicle misalignments in the L3-right-right
Subluxation pattern distortions

Key:
◎=Anterior

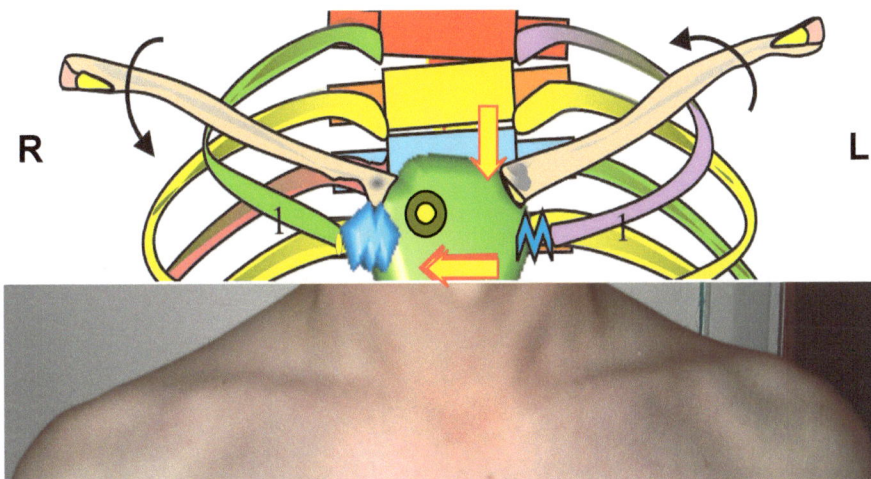

Key:
◎=Anterior

Figure 5M
Clavicle misalignments in the L3-left-right
Subluxation pattern distortions

In **figure 5L**, **L3-R-R**, observe the distorted position of the Manubrium. It has side-shifted, side-bent and rotated to the right and altered the seating of the clavicle bones. The right clavicle is angled higher than the left. Note that the right shoulder is anterior.

In **figure 5M**, **L3-L-R**, observe the distorted position of the Manubrium. It has side-shifted right, side-bent and rotated to the left and altered the seating of the clavicle bones. The left clavicle is angled higher than the right. Note that the right shoulder is anterior.

Clavicle Rotated Superiorly and Laterally

Figure 5N is anterior view of the left side of the sterno-clavicular joint for reference purposes.

The illustrations apply to the sterno-clavicular subluxations that can present on the left side in the L3-left-right lesion pattern and on the right in the L3-right-right pattern.

Figure 5P shows the Manubrium rotated posteriorly on the affected side caused by the leverage exerted on the body of the sternum by the myriad of rib lesions below.

This rotation causes the posterior part of the manubrial facet to part away from the posterior part of the clavicle facet. This parting destabilizes the joint.

Figure 5Q shows the secondary force of side-bending placed on the sterno-clavicular joint by the distortion of the sternal body.

The Manubrium on the affected side is forced to side-bend inferiorly. This causes the already destabilized anterior facets of the clavicle to swivel medially along the anterior margin of the manubrial facet towards point A. At the same time the posterior part of clavicle facet is forced to swivel towards point B. At this point the joint locks in subluxation.

This lesion places the medial facet of the clavicle medially and therefore superiorly against the manubrial facet..

This is a sterno-clavicular lesion, in other words the Manubrium becomes displaced against the clavicle, not the other way round.

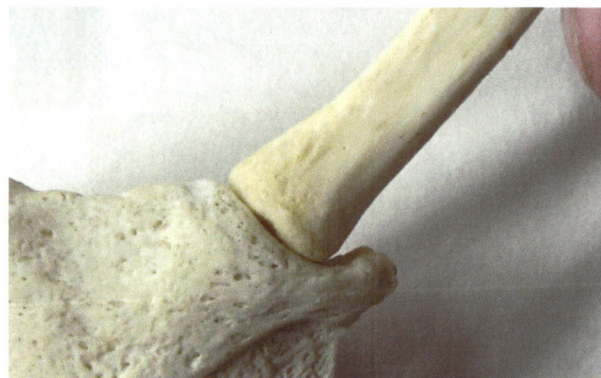

Figure 5N
Clavicle in Neutral

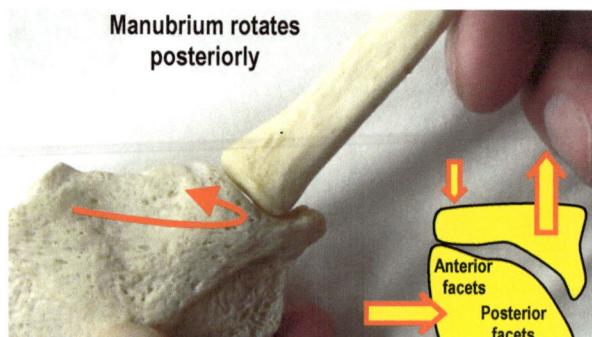

Manubrium rotates posteriorly

Anterior facets

Posterior facets

Figure 5P
Anterior view of manubrium when forced to rotate posteriorly

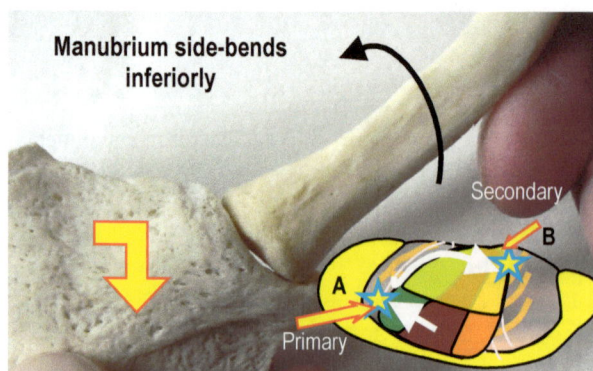

Manubrium side-bends inferiorly

Secondary

B

A

Primary

Figure 5Q
Anterior view of manubrium when forced to side-bend

Clavicle Rotated Inferiorly and Medially

Figure 5R is an anterior view of the left side of the sterno-clavicular joint for reference purposes.

The illustrations apply to the sterno-clavicular subluxations that can present on the right side in the L3-left-right lesion pattern and on the left in the L3-right-right pattern.

Figure 5S shows the Manubrium rotated anteriorly on the affected side. This rotation was caused by the leverage exerted on the body of the sternum by the myriad of rib lesions. As the Manubrium moves anteriorly on the effected side, the anterior areas of the facets of both the Manubrium and the clavicle become parted. This parting destabilizes the joint.

Figure 5T shows the secondary superior force of side-bending that is also inflicted on the sterno-clavicular joint by the unruly forces placed on the body of the sternum by the myriad rib lesions.

This causes the already destabilized posterior facet of the clavicle to side-shift medially up the posterior manubrial facet towards point A. At the same time the anterior part of the clavicle facet swivels laterally along the anterior margin towards point B where the joint locks in lesion.

This lesion causes the medial facet of the clavicle to rotate inferiorly and therefore inferiorly against the manubrial facet.

This is a sterno-clavicular lesion; in other words the Manubrium becomes displaced against the clavicle, not the other way round.

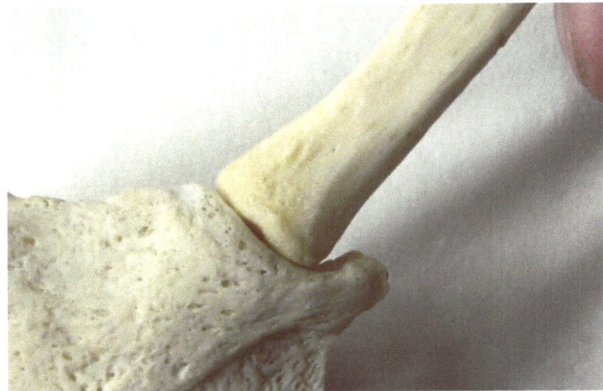

Figure 5R
Clavicle in Neutral

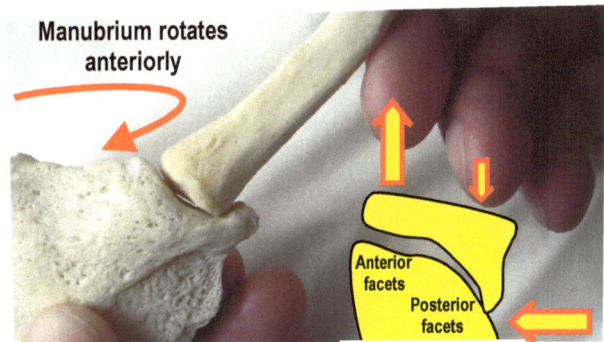

Manubrium rotates anteriorly

Anterior facets

Posterior facets

Figure 5S
Anterior view of manubrium when forced to rotate posteriorly

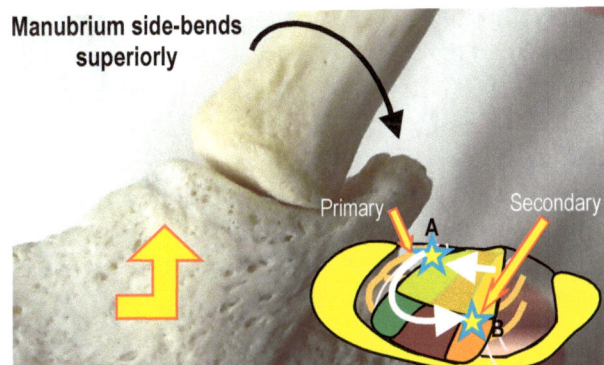

Manubrium side-bends superiorly

Primary   Secondary

A

B

Figure 5T
Anterior view of manubrium when forced to side-bend

Displacement of the Acromion in L3-Right-Right Pattern

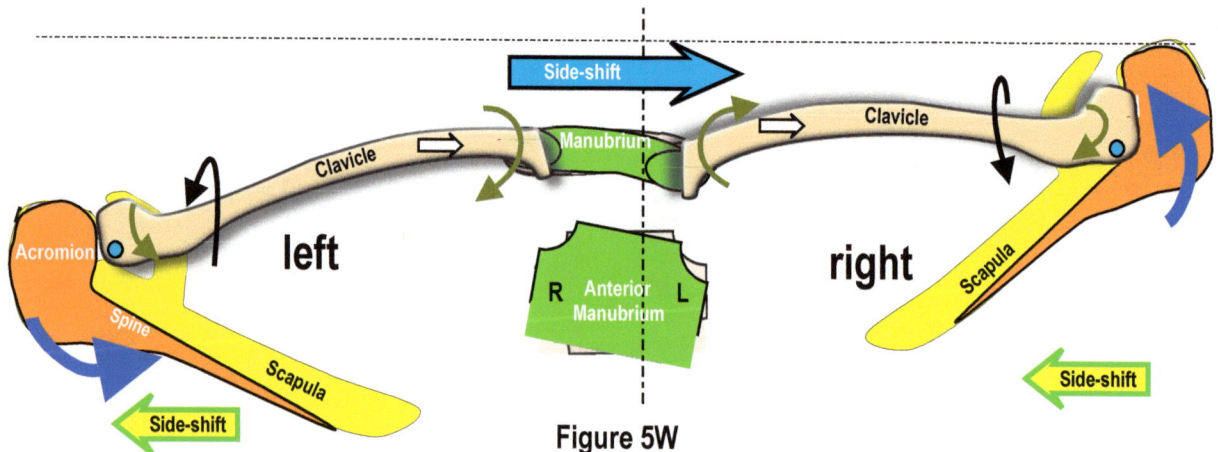

Figure 5W
Aerial view of shoulder girdle
in the L3-right-right pattern

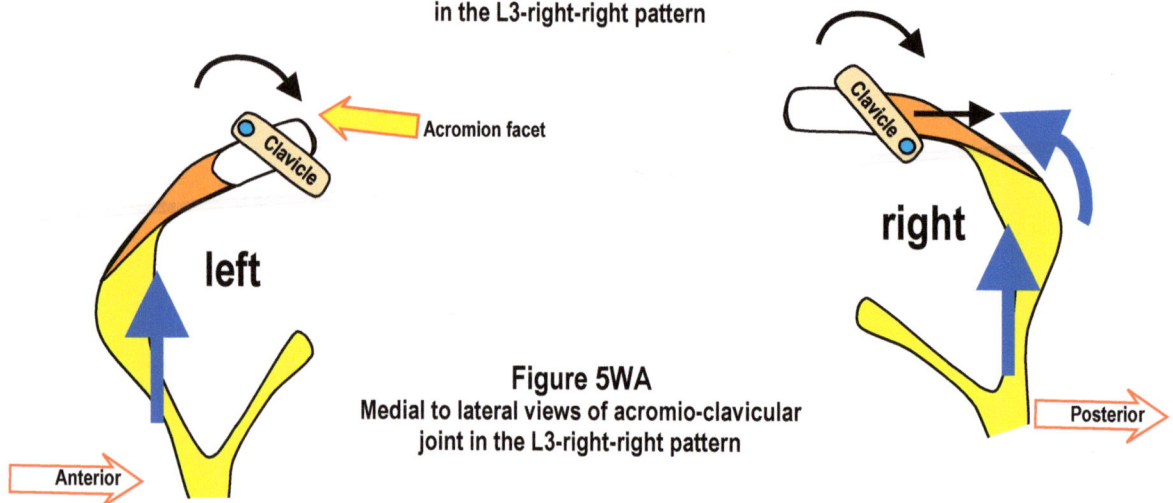

Figure 5WA
Medial to lateral views of acromio-clavicular
joint in the L3-right-right pattern

It was demonstrated earlier in this book how the scapula becomes misaligned. This has serious implications on the alignment of the acromio-clavicular joint.

L3-right-right

The above illustrations have been drawn to show the positions of the facets at the acromio- clavicular joint.

Both the left and right scapulae are raised with a general side-shift to the left. This side-shift exerts side-shift forces to the right at the Manubrium. See **figure 5L**

Both scapula bones are rotated to the left. See **figure 5W.** Because the side-shift forces exerted on the scapula are to the left, see **figure 17A** on page 131, the right scapula and therefore the right acromio-clavicular joint becomes the focus of most of the force.

Displacement of the Acromion
in L3-Left-Right Pattern

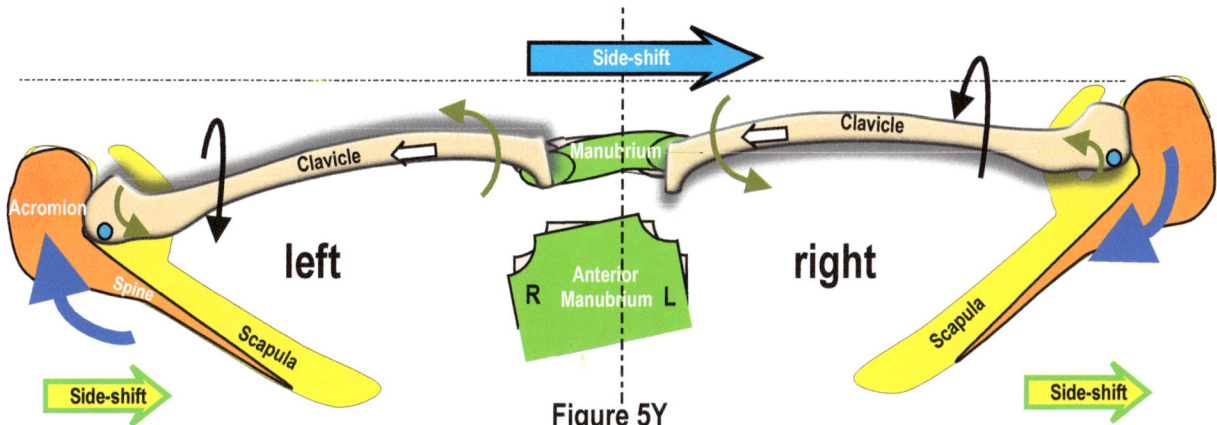

Side-shift

Clavicle

Manubrium

Clavicle

Acromion

left

right

Spine

Scapula

Scapula

Anterior
Manubrium

R   L

Side-shift

Side-shift

Figure 5Y
Aerial view of shoulder girdle
in L3-left-right pattern

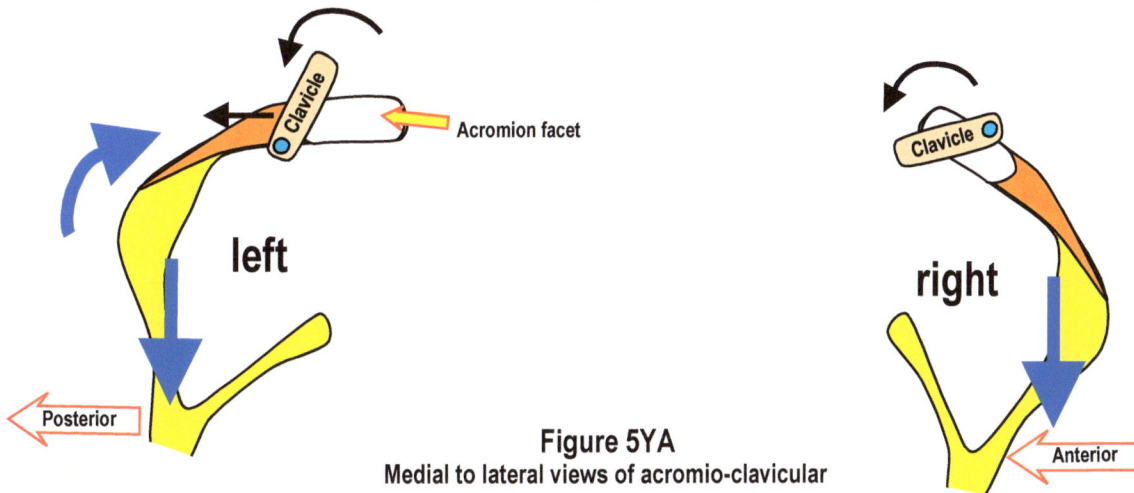

Clavicle

Acromion facet

Clavicle

left

right

Posterior

Anterior

Figure 5YA
Medial to lateral views of acromio-clavicular
joint in the L3-left-right pattern

L3-left-right

The above illustrations have been drawn to show the positions of the facets at the acromio- clavicular joint.

Both the left and right scapulae are lowered with a general side-shift to the right. This side-shift moves round the torso and exerts side-shift forces to the left at the Manubrium. See **figure 5M**.

Both scapula bones are rotated right, see **figure 5Y**. Because the side-shift forces exerted on the scapula are to the right, see **figure 17C** on page 137, the left scapula and therefore the left acromio-clavicular joint becomes the focus of most of the force.

Aids to Rib Diagnosis

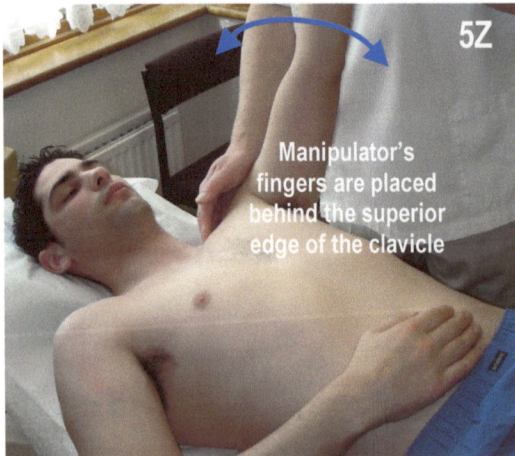

5Z

Manipulator's fingers are placed behind the superior edge of the clavicle

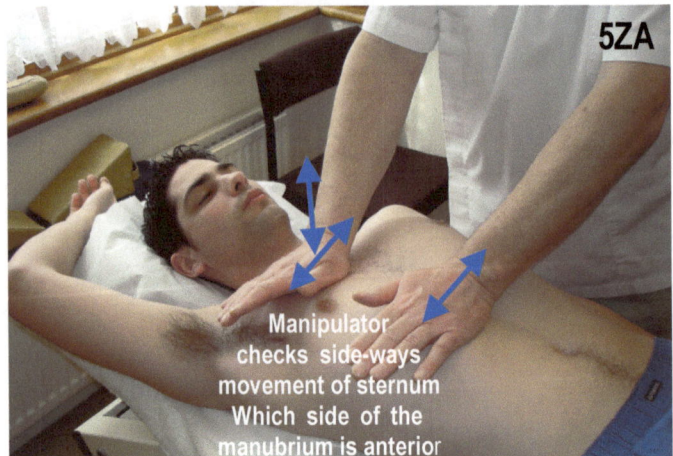

5ZA

Manipulator checks side-ways movement of sternum Which side of the manubrium is anterior

Due to complications of trauma etc, rib cage and shoulder diagnosis may need verification. **Figure 5Z** shows how the angle of the clavicle can be checked. Both sides are compared. With an inferior clavicle, resistance is felt when the arm is raised. To check the distortion of the sternum, **figure 5ZA** shows how the direction can be diagnosed. Check for side-ways movement. The side that feels easiest to move is the side the rib cage is veering. By putting the results of these two tests together, the angles of the manipulation can be confirmed.

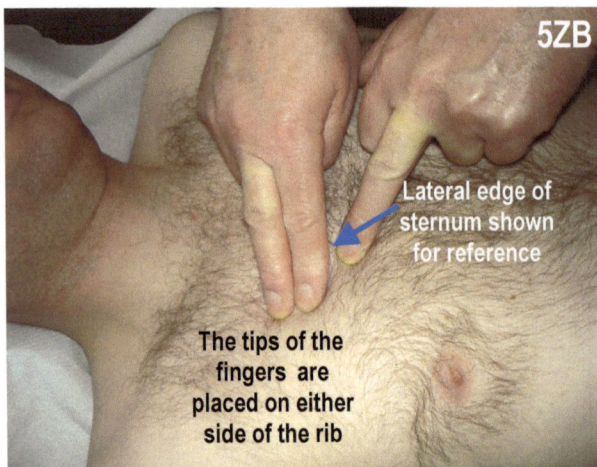

5ZB

Lateral edge of sternum shown for reference

The tips of the fingers are placed on either side of the rib

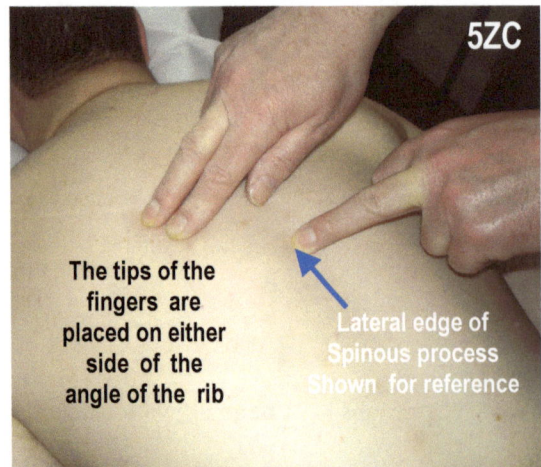

5ZC

The tips of the fingers are placed on either side of the angle of the rib

Lateral edge of Spinous process Shown for reference

Again due to complications of trauma etc. the diagnosis of whether a rib is locked in inhalation or exhalation may need verification. **Figure 5ZB** and **5ZC** show the position the manipulators fingers should be placed. The patient is then asked to breath in or out. If the patient breaths in and the rib does not move the rib is locked in exhalation. If the patient breathes out and the rib does not move the rib is locked in inspiration.

The displaced angle of the subluxated rib feels like the head of a pea. It can be difficult to locate with up to a ¼ of an inch of soft tissue above. Palpation requires considerable skill, but it can be done.

Chapter Eighteen

Rib Cage Manipulation

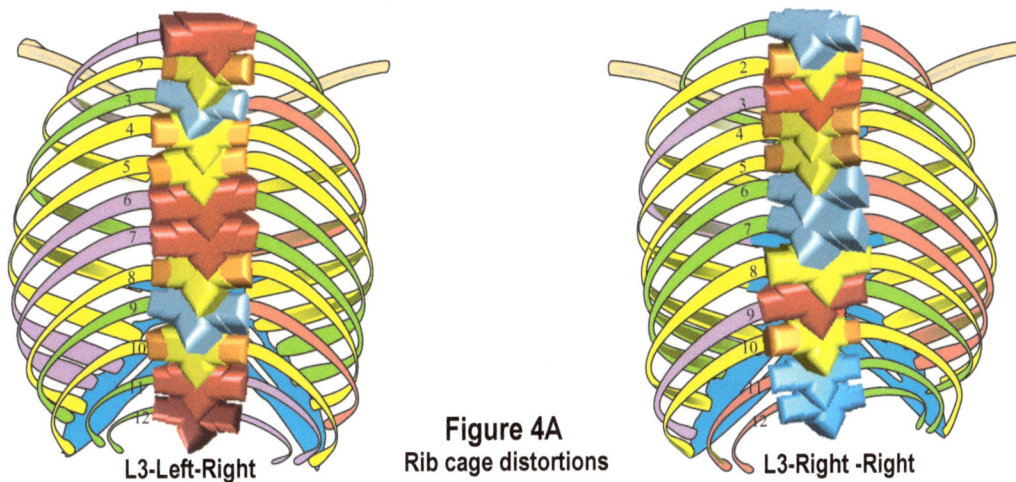

Figure 4A
Rib cage distortions

L3-Left-Right   L3-Right-Right

Secondary rib cage and shoulder joint misalignments follow on when the sacroiliac joints become lesioned. These misalignments have the potential to affect the efficient function of the breathing mechanism.

Unfortunately, rib cage and shoulder joint distortions by their very nature double back and compound the locking of the already lesioned spine. Each area locks-in the previous area. With this catch 22 situation taking place it makes it very difficult to know where to start. But a start has to be made. This is where the science behind this type of manipulation becomes exciting.

A lot of manipulation takes place during a single treatment session if 'true alignment' is your goal. When PPT's are correctly applied, only a minimal trauma footprint is left behind so that in a single treatment session every joint in the spine and torso can be manipulated several times, when necessary, with minimal after-affect.

The chest is a very sensitive and painful area to palpate and often patients can feel uncomfortable during palpation and in particular during stretching articulation techniques. However, because PPT's are so quick and gentle, discomfort is minimal.

Manipulation
Rib Expiration Technique

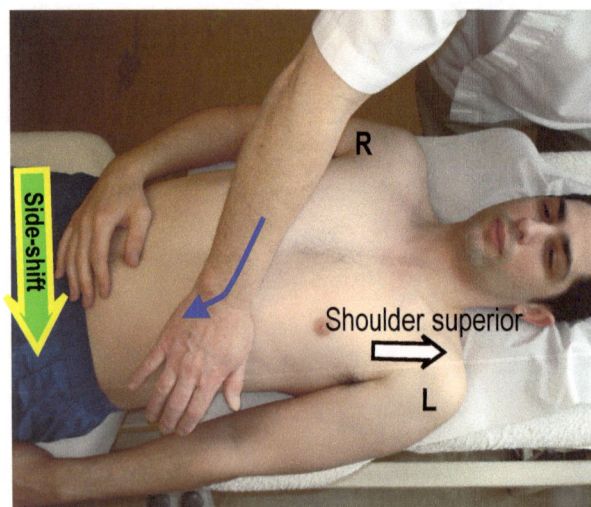

Figure 6A
Anterior view of patient
receiving CST rib manipulation

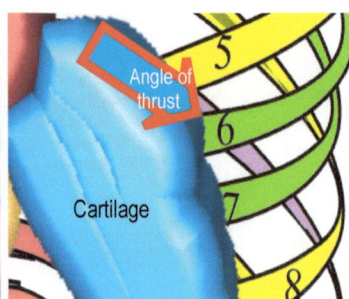

Side-shift

R

Shoulder superior

L

Angle of thrust

Cartilage

Figure 6B
Anterior views T6 and T7

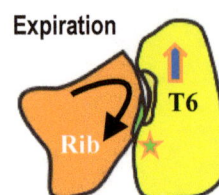

5

6

7

8

Expiration

T6

Rib

Figure TSEb
Left side-view of
point 'Y'

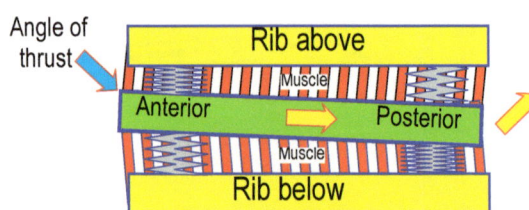

Angle of thrust

Rib above

Muscle

Anterior

Posterior

Muscle

Rib below

Figure 6C
Side-view of subluxated rib

This rib expiration correction technique uses the subluxated rib as a long lever. For this reason very little force is needed. The technique can be used for correcting ribs locked in both flexion and extension. The patient has no control over when the manipulation will be made therefore, they are less likely to tense prior to the gentle push.

Technique
The patient is placed in a supine position on a flat couch with their left shoulder raised. Their knees are supported and flexed by a pillow and their pelvis side-shifted to the left, as shown in **figure 6A**. The manipulator asks the patient to breathe-in, 'inspiration'. A gentle push in then made in a posterior inferio-lateral direction, using the hypo-thenar eminence, against the superior surface of the rib. This is shown in **figures 6A, B** and **C**.

How does it work
The ribs are made malleable by the pelvic side-shift left which causes all of the individual vertebrae up the spine to attempt to shift towards the right. This is away from the lesioned rib and therefore this lessens the tension within the vertebral/rib lesion.

The raised left shoulder opens and lifts the rib cage on the left. When the patient breathes-in the anterior part of the ribs move superiorly. A push is then made in a posterior inferior lateral direction, as shown in **figure 6C**, (the mechanics of this are explained in **figure 6D**) and this pushes the posterior end of the rib medially and superiorly to mate correctly with the corresponding vertebrae.

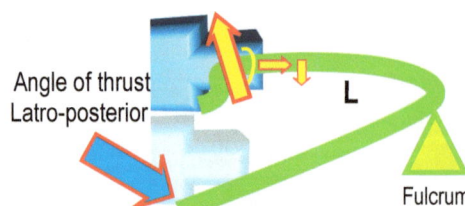

Angle of thrust
Latro-posterior

L

Fulcrum

Figure 6D
Anterior views of T6
Showing angle of thrust

Rib Manipulation
Inspiration Technique

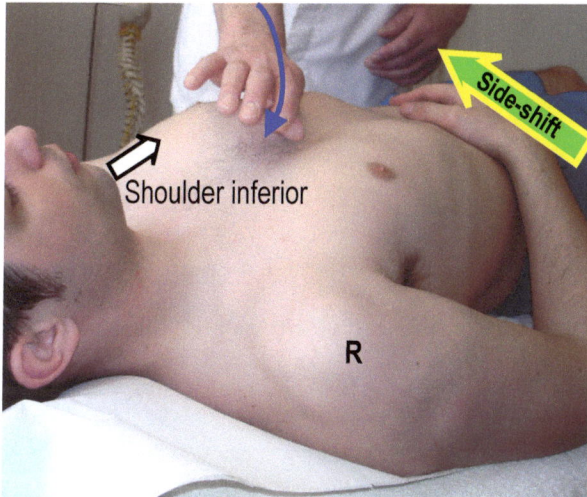
Figure 6F
Anterior view of patient
receiving CST rib manipulation

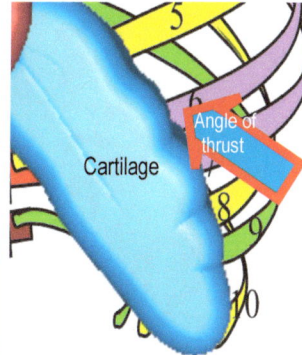
Figure 6G
Anterior views T6 and T7

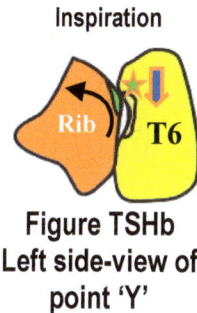
Inspiration
Figure TSHb
Left side-view of
point 'Y'

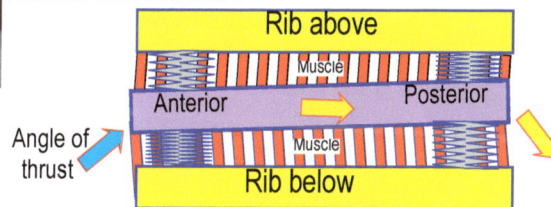
Figure 6H
Side-view of subluxated rib

This rib inspiration correction technique is only suitable for ribs subluxated in extension. The rib is used as a long lever and for this reason very little force is needed.

Technique
The patient is placed in a supine position on a flat couch with their left shoulder lowered. Their knees are supported and flexed by a pillow and their pelvis side-shifted to the left with their left arm at their side. The manipulator stands to the left side of the table parallel to the patient's abdomen. The patient is then asked to breathe-out, 'expiration'. A superio-medial a push is then made against the anterior surface of the rib. Only a light push is needed and is shown in **figures 6F, G** and **H.** Note that the palmer surface of the hand is steeply angled to avoid any accidental contact with breast tissue.

How does it work
The rib is made malleable by the pelvic side-shift to the left which causes all the individual vertebrae up the spine to attempt to shift towards the right. This is away from the rib, and therefore removes the tension from the joint.

The lowered left shoulder closes the rib cage on the left. When the patient breathes-out the anterior part of the ribs move inferiorly. A gentle push is then made in a superio-medial direction, as shown in **figure 6H,** (the mechanics of this are explained in **figure 6J),** and this pushes the posterior end of the rib laterally and inferiorly to mate correctly with the corresponding vertebra.

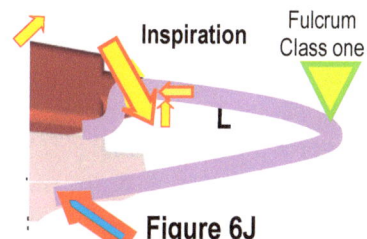
Figure 6J
Anterior view of T6
Showing angle of thrust

Rib Trauma Manipulation Technique in Inspiration

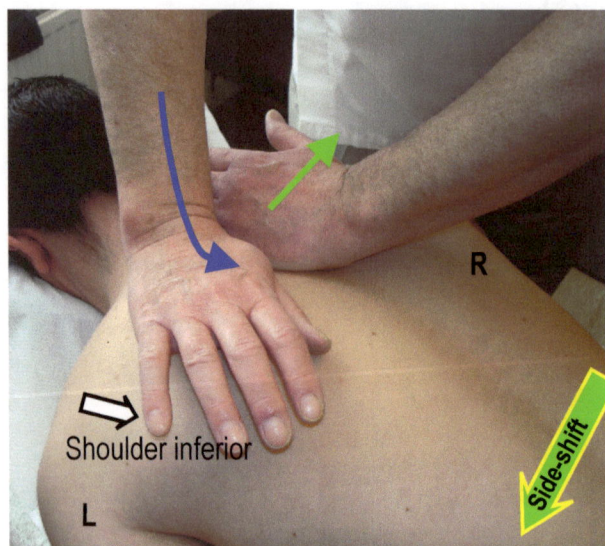

Figure 6K
Posterior view of patient
receiving CPT rib manipulation

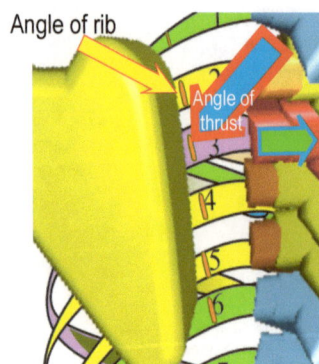

Labels on 6K: Shoulder inferior, Side-shift, R, L

Figure 6L
Posterior view of T3

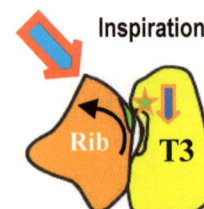

Labels on 6L: Angle of rib, Angle of thrust

Figure TSHb
Left side-view of point 'Y'

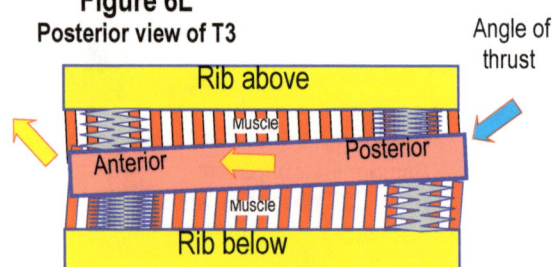

Labels on TSHb: Inspiration, Rib, T3

Figure 6M
Side-view of subluxated rib

Labels on 6M: Angle of thrust, Rib above, Muscle, Anterior, Posterior, Muscle, Rib below

This correction technique is suitable for ribs lesioned in inspiration caused by inappropriate lever or trauma. The rib is used as a short lever and for this reason a little force is needed. The patient has no control over when the manipulation will be made, therefore they are less likely to tense before the push. This is a fairly standard technique; the only difference is that the pelvis is side-shifted to the left, which reduces the trauma of the manipulation.

Technique

The patient is placed in a prone position on a flat couch with their shins supported by a pillow to flex their knees. Their pelvis is side-shifted to the left, as shown in **figure 6K** and the left shoulder is lowered. The manipulator stands to the right side of the table parallel with patient's shoulder. The patient is then asked to breathe-out, 'expiration'. The heel of the manipulator's left hand stabilizes the spinous process of the vertebra at the same time as the thenar eminence of the right hand makes a gentle push against the superior angle of the rib in an anterior latero-inferior direction, as shown in **figures 6K, L** and **M.**

How does it work

The Pelvic side-shift to the left causes the T3 vertebra to side-shift to the right and therefore away from the subluxated rib. The combination of the lowered arm and the patient breathing out causes the ribs to move generally inferiorly. This therefore highlights the angle of the rib locked in inspiration. A gentle push is made in a latero-inferior direction to lever the rib away from the vertebra in a direction that allows the rib to reseat against the vertebra. There can be an audible click.

Rib Trauma Manipulation Technique in Expiration

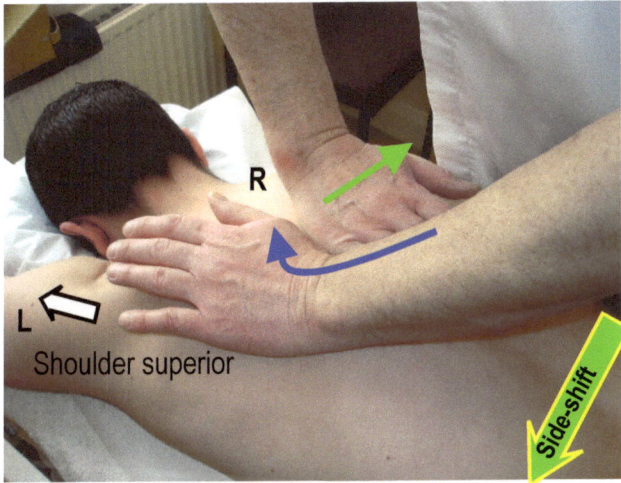

Figure 6KA
Posterior view of patient receiving CPT rib manipulation

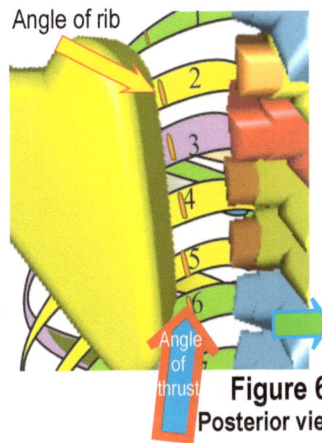

Angle of rib

Figure 6KB
Posterior view of T6

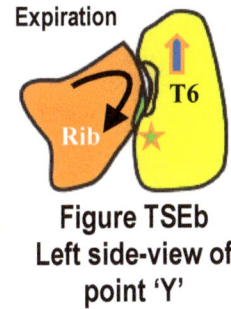

Expiration

Figure TSEb
Left side-view of point 'Y'

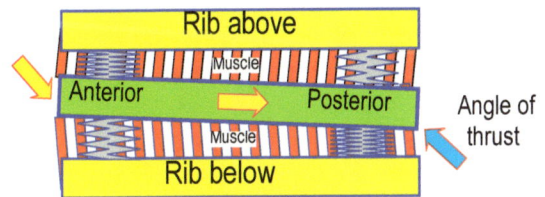

Figure 6KC
Side-view of subluxated rib

This correction technique is suitable for ribs lesioned in expiration caused by inappropriate lever or trauma. The rib is used as a short lever and for this reason a little force is needed. The patient while co-operating has no control over when the manipulation will be made, therefore they are less likely to tense before the thrust. This is a fairly standard technique, with added knee flexion and pelvic side-shift to make the manipulation less traumatic.

Technique

The patient is placed in a prone position on a flat couch with their shins supported by a pillow to flex their knees. Their pelvis is side-shifted to the left, as shown in **figure 6KA** and the left shoulder and arm are raised. The manipulator stands to the right side of the table parallel with patient's torso. The patient is then asked to breathe-in, 'Inspiration'. The heel of the manipulator's left hand stabilizes the spinous process of the vertebra, while at the same time the thenar eminence of their right hand makes a gentle push against the inferior angle of the rib in a medio-superior direction, as shown in **figures 6KA** and **6KB.**

How does it work

The Pelvic side-shift to the left causes the T6 vertebra to side-shift to the right and therefore away from the subluxated rib. The combination of the raised arm and the patient breathing in causes the ribs generally to move in a superior direction. This therefore highlights the angle of the rib locked in expiration. The gentle push is made in a medio-superior direction to lever the rib away from the vertebra in the direction that allows the rib to reseat against the vertebrae. There can be an audible click. In this type of lesion the angle of the rib is hidden, therefore it can be difficult to locate a rib lesioned in expiration.

Rib Manipulation
Elevated First Rib

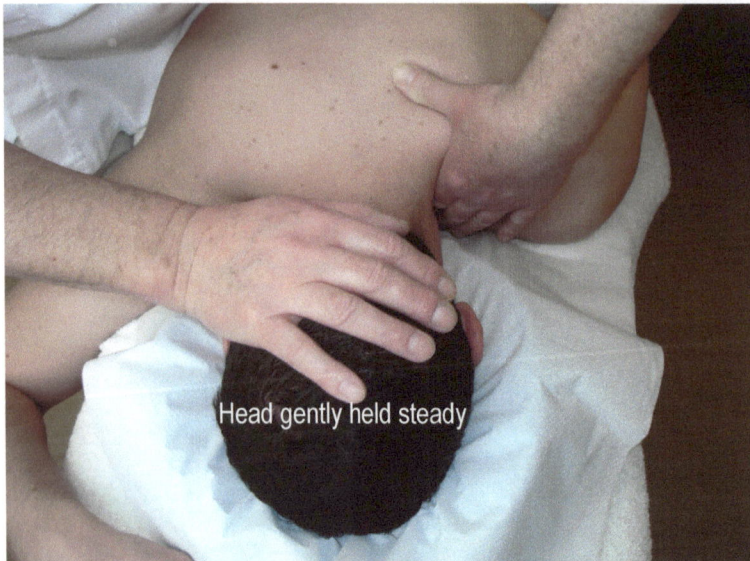

Figure 6MA
Posterior view of patient
receiving CPT rib manipulation

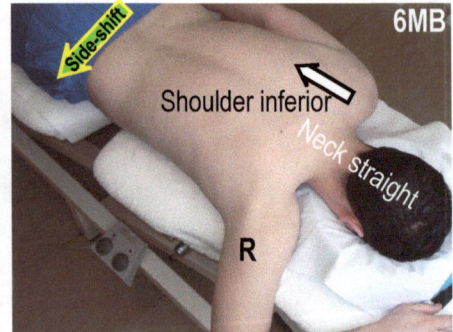

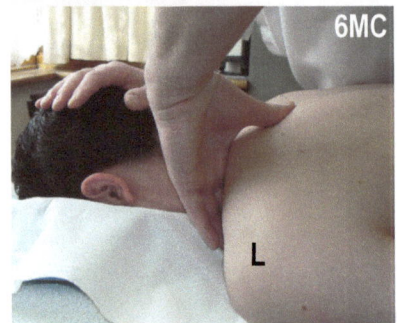

This rib technique is suitable for correcting a subluxated 1st rib locked in elevation. Unlike most 1st rib correction techniques the neck and head are kept in the mid-line and only a gentle push is needed. This keeps the neck safe.

Note. T1 must be aligned before attempting this manipulation.

Technique

The patient is placed in a prone position on a flat couch with their shins supported by a pillow to flex their knees. Their pelvis is side-shifted to the right, as shown in **figure 6MB** and the left shoulder is lowered. The patient's right arm should be at a minimum of 90 degrees.

The manipulator stands to the left side of the table parallel with patient's lower torso. The patient is then asked to breathe-out, 'expiration'. The manipulators' right hand stabilizes the head and neck ensuring that they are kept in the mid-line while the thenar eminence of the left hand makes contact with the superio-medial part of the 1st rib. The thrust is made in an inferior medial direction. See **figures 6MA** and **6MB.**

How does it work

The Pelvic side-shift to the right destabilizes the lesioned 1st rib. The combination of the lowered arm and the patient breathing out causes the ribs on the left to generally move inferiorly. This highlights any ribs locked in inspiration. The gentle push is made in an inferior medial direction, as shown in **figure 6MD** and allows the 1st rib to effortlessly reseat.

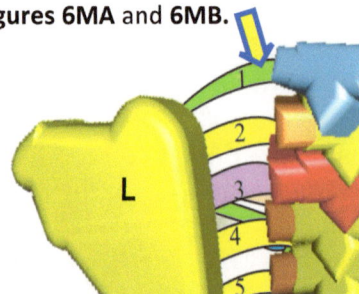

Figure 6MD
Posterior view showing angle of thrust

Inferiorly Rotated Clavicle
Acromio-Clavicular Manipulation

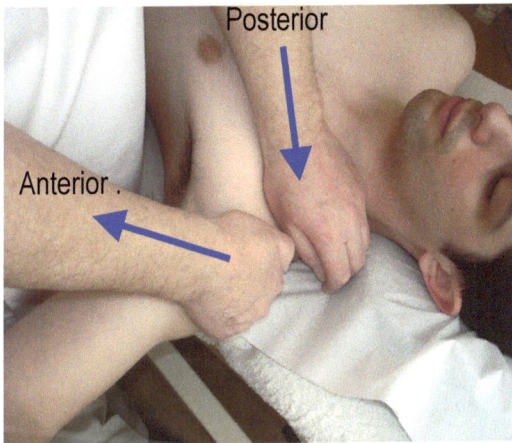

Figure 6N
Acromio-clavicular manipulation

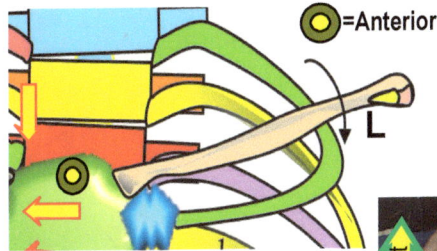

Figure 6P
Anterior view showing the
inferior rotation of the left clavicle

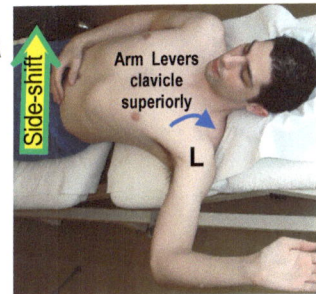

Figure 6Q
Position prior to manipulation

This technique is used to correct a left acromio-clavicular joint subluxated in the L3-right-right lesion pattern.

This manipulation is used to correct an inferiorly rotated clavicle on the left. In the L3-left-right lesion pattern the exact same procedure is carried out on the right shoulder.

Technique

The patient adopts a supine position on a flat couch. A pillow is placed under their knees to induce mild knee flexion and the pelvis side-shifted to the right. The left elbow is bent and the forearm raised parallel with the head with the palmer surface of the hand upward, as shown in **figure 6Q**. The manipulator stands to the side of the left shoulder and places the heel of their left hand over the anterior surface of the left clavicle while the right hand is placed under the humeral head. The joint is then gently aligned by pushing down (posteriorly) on the clavicle while the right hand pulls the humeral head in the opposite direction (anteriorly).

How does it work

The pelvic side-shift to the right destabilizes the left acromio-clavicular joint, making the joint malleable. The raised left arm rotates the clavicle superiorly and correctly aligns it with Acromion process.

As can be seen from **figure 6R** the lateral end of the clavicle is anterior in relation to the Acromion. By gently pushing down on the clavicle and upwards on the humeral head the joint is sliced and eased back into place.

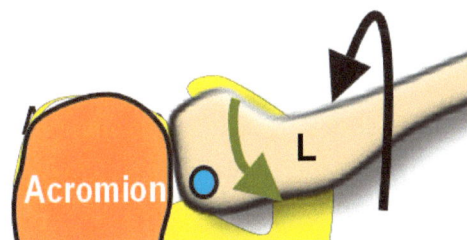

Figure 6R
View from above of the left
acromio-clavicular joint

Superiorly Rotated Clavicle
Acromio-Clavicular Manipulation

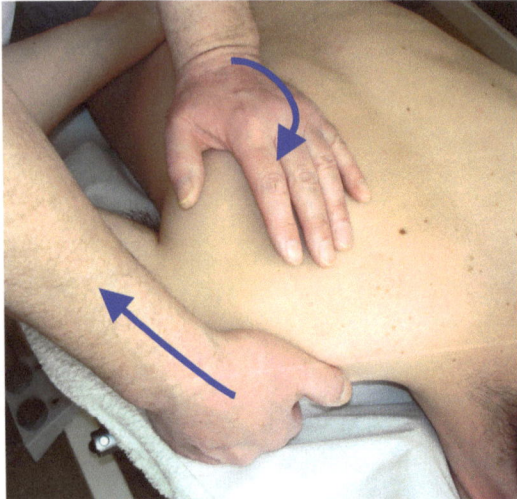

=Anterior

Figure 6T
Anterior view showing the superior rotation of the right clavicle

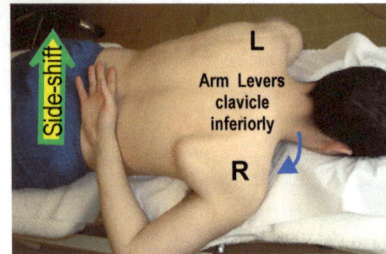

Side-shift

L

Arm Levers clavicle inferiorly

R

Figure 6S
Acromio-clavicular manipulation

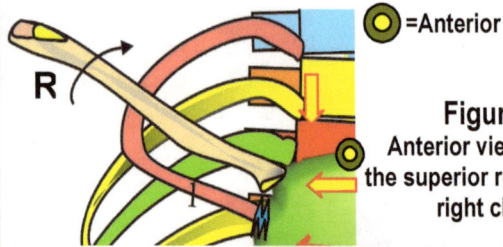

Figure 6U
Position prior to manipulation

This technique is used to correct a right acromio-clavicular joint lesioned in the L3-right-right subluxation pattern. This manipulation is used to correct a superiorly rotated clavicle on the right.

In the L3-left-right lesion pattern the exact same procedure is carried out on the left shoulder. The left scapula can be guided inferiorly to refine the technique.

Technique

The patient adopts a prone position on a flat couch. A pillow is placed under their shins to induce mild knee flexion and the pelvis side-shifted to the left. The right arm is either placed along side the torso or behind the back, as shown in **figure 6U**. The manipulator stands to the side of the right shoulder and places their right hand under the humeral head and their left hand over at medial border of the right scapula. The joint is then gently aligned by pulling the humeral head up (posteriorly) while the right hand pushes the scapula laterally and anteriorly in such a way as to toggle the scapula posteriorly at its lateral border.

How does it work

The pelvic side-shift to the left destabilizes the right acromio-clavicular joint, making the joint malleable. The neutral position of the arm rotates the clavicle inferiorly and correctly aligns it with Acromion process.

As can be seen from **figure 6V** the lateral end of the clavicle is posterior in relation to the Acromion. By toggling and laterally side-shifting the scapula whilst gently pulling up on the humeral head the joint is sliced and eased back into place.

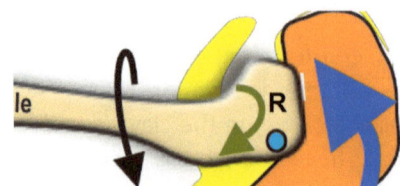

Figure 6V
View from above of the right acromio-clavicular joint

Sterno-Clavicular-Rib Cage Manipulation

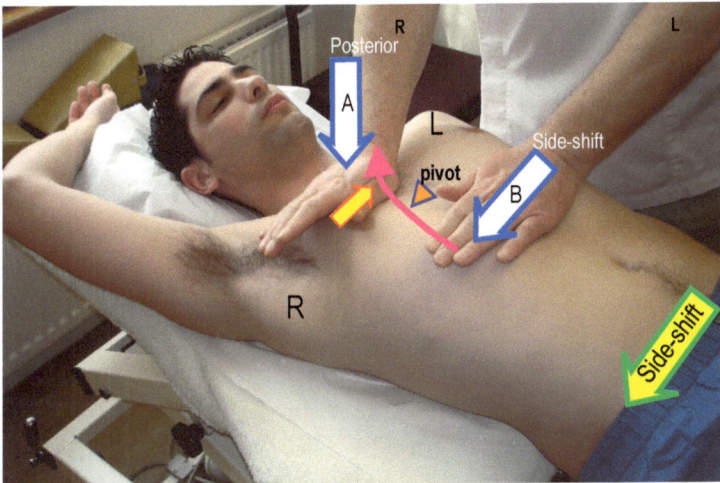

Figure 6W
Sterno-clavicular manipulation

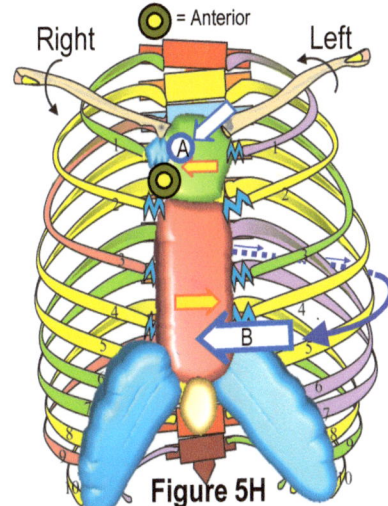

Figure 5H
Anterior rib distortions in
the L3-left-right pattern

This is a sterno-clavicular technique and as the name suggests the emphasise of the correction should be placed on correcting the position of the sternum relative to the clavicle, not the other way round. The L3-left-right rib cage lesion pattern is being used as an example. In the L3-right-right lesion pattern the left arm would be raised.

Technique

The patient adopts a supine position on a flat couch and raises their right arm parallel to their head, as shown in **figure 6W**. The left arm is positioned in neutral to the side of the torso. A pillow is placed under the patient's knees to induce mild knee flexion and the pelvis side-shifted to the right. The manipulator stands to the left of the patient's torso and places the heel of their left hand against the left side of the body of the sternum, just above the Xiphoid process, shown as 'B' in **figure 5H**. At the same time they place the heel of their right hand over the right anterior part of the Manubrium, at point 'A' shown in **figure 5H**. In one movement the body of the sternum is gently pushed to the right and the Manubrium posteriorly. A slight feeling of give is experienced as the sternum and sterno-clavicular joints re-align.

How does it work

The upper left side of the sternum is made malleable by the side-shift of the pelvis to the right. The raised right arm attempts to de-rotate the right clavicle that is subluxated inferiorly. The left arm is held in neutral at the side and de-rotates the left lesioned clavicle superiorly. The pelvic side-shift to the right, causes the lower thoracic vertebrae and ribs to side-shift to the left. This force is carried round the rib cage so that at the front the ribs tend to side-shift towards the right. Note, if the pelvic side-shift were to the left the upper ribs would move towards the left.

The side-ways push to the right on the sternum is aided by the lower rib side-shift to the right. This combined force causes the sternum to act as a long lever and swivel the Manubrium, which is being eased posteriorly by the manipulators right hand, to the left. In doing this all the forces are aligned and therefore the sternum, rib cage and the sterno-clavicular joints unlock and reseat in their correct and mobile position.

Skeleton
L3-Right-Right Subluxation Pattern

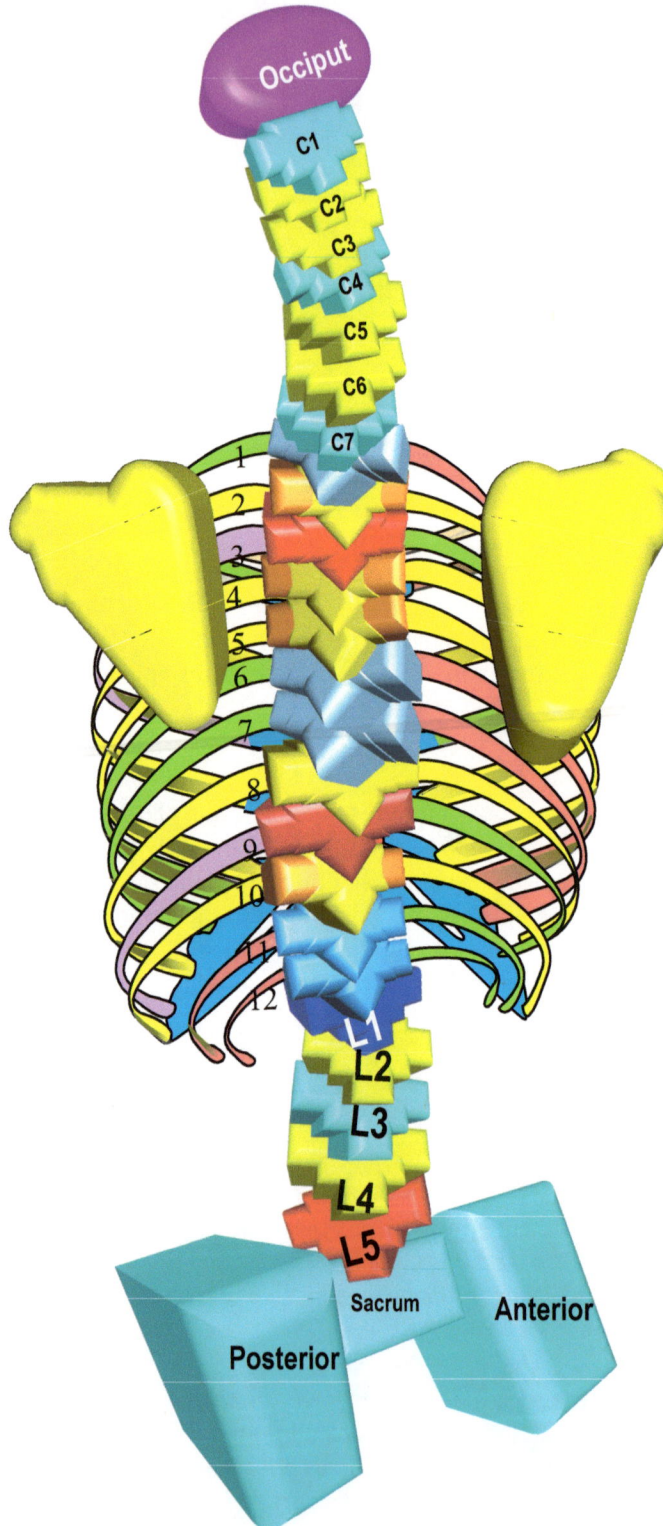

Skeleton
L3-Left-Right Subluxation Pattern

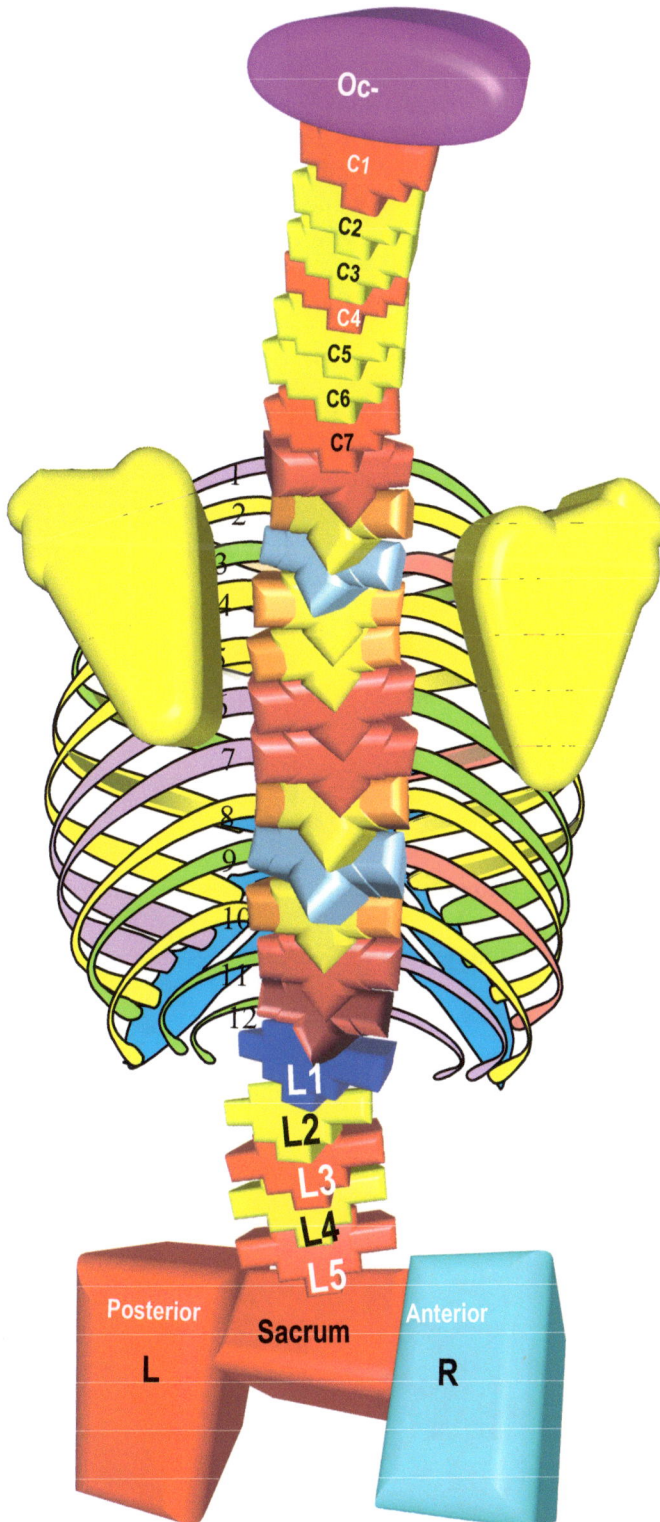

Where do we go from here?

A new door has opened in the history of bio-mechanics and manipulation

With this new understanding of the how spine, sacroiliac, ribs and shoulder joints articulate and how these same joints lesion, a new era in the science of spinal bio-mechanics has begun.

The monopoly of muscle based treatments so favoured by the medical profession is ebbing to give way to a more structured and scientific approach to the treatment of joint and nerve pain.

Some critics claim manipulation is dangerous and should never be practiced. In future they will not be able to accuse professional manipulators who use PPT's of this because these techniques leave such a small trauma footprint behind.

In an Osteopathic patient research survey, when asked 50% of the research group did not realise that they had been manipulated, and those that did felt the manipulation was less traumatic than conventional techniques. 100% felt PPT's were effective and caused them no anxiety and pain. 89% said that would be more likely to recommend a friend to a therapist using these techniques. 94% felt PPT's relieved their pain effectively. 72% felt PPT's relieved their pain faster than conventional manipulation.

So where do the professions who use PPT manipulation at the heart of their treatments go from here? *Forwards, with pride.*

Research survey by J.R.Bayliss completed by patients in summer 2006. A small group of 27 patients were chosen at random by the order they attended the clinic were asked to take part in the PPT survey. Of these eighteen filled in the questionnaire and returned it anonymously that is 67%. The research survey was only meant as a toe in the water test.

Another title by the author of this book to help you to expand your knowledge of spinal mechanics is:

PAL DVD: Spinal Mechanics and Bony Locking *For Heath Professionals*

If a picture is worth a thousand words, a moving picture is worth many more. To see the close up movement of joints, from many angles, helps the viewer to more clearly understand and appreciate how the sacroiliac and spinal joints articulate and subluxate.

The DVD is 1 hour and 38 minutes long and presented from the point of view of posture dysfunction. The two models are again sited for reference. There is also a PPT technique DVD available.

The DVD is available through: www.spinalmechanics.com

T3Z2-JRB

References

Gray's Anatomy Edition 36 by Williams & Warwick published by Churchill Livingstone

Weisl H. Movements of the sacroiliac joint. *Acta anat* 1955:23:80-91

The Anatomy Coloring Book by Wynn Kapit/Lawrence M. Elson published by Churchill Livingstone

Strruresson B. Movements of the sacroiliac joint: A fresh look. In: Vleeming A, Mooney V, Snijders C, Dorman T, Stoeckart R, editor. Movement, stability and low back pain. The essential Role of the pelvis. First edition New York: Churchill Livingstone 1997:171-185

The Physiology of the Joints Volume 3 The Trunk and the Vertebral Column By I. A. Kapandji published by Churchill Livingstone

Lavignolle B, Vital JM, Senegas J, Destandau J, Toson B, Bouyx P, *et al* An approach to functional anatomy of the sacroiliac joints in vivo. Anatimica Clinica 1983:5: 169-176

Journal of Osteopathic Medicine volume 7 Number 1 Clinical Considerations of Sacroiliac Anatomy by M.C.McGrath April 2004 published by Research media Pty Ltd/ Journal of Osteopathic medicine

Mooney V. Sacroiliac Joint Dysfunction. In: Vleeming A, Mooney V, Snijders C, Dorman T, Stoeckart R, editors Movement stability and low back pain. The essential role of the pelvis. First edition New York: Churchill Livingstone; 1997:37-52

Joint Motion: Method of Measuring and Recording published by American Academy of Orthopaedic Surgeons

Principles of Osteopathic Technic By H Fryette.

Bernard TN, Cassidy JD, The SIJ syndrome. Pathophysilogy, diagnosis and management. New York:Raven Press:1991.

Osteopathy: Notes on the Technique and Practice by John Wernham published by The Maidstone Osteopathic Clinic

An Illustrated Manual of Osteopathic Technique by John Wernham and Mervyn Waldman: published by The Maidstone Osteopathic Clinic

Yullberg T, Bloomberg S, Branth B, Johnson R. Manipulation does not alter the position of the sacroiliac joint. Roentgen stereophotogrammetric analysis: 1998:23:1124-9

Interactive Spine: Chiropractic Edition. CD ROM published by Primal

www.ingramcontent.com/pod-product-compliance
Lightning Source LLC
Chambersburg PA
CBHW050825220326
41598CB00006B/312